MANUAL OF PULMONARY
FUNCTION TESTING

SIXTH EDITION

Manual of Pulmonary Function Testing

Gregg E. Ruppel, M.Ed., R.R.T.

Director
Pulmonary Function Laboratory
St. Louis University Hospital
St. Louis, Missouri

With 89 illustrations

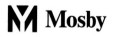 Mosby

St. Louis Baltimore Boston Chicago London Madrid
Philadelphia Sydney Toronto

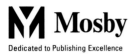
Dedicated to Publishing Excellence

Publisher: George Stamathis
Editor: James F. Shanahan
Developmental Editor: Jennifer Roche
Assistant Director/Production, Editing, Design: Frances M. Perveiler
Project Manager: Nancy C. Baker
Proofroom Manager: Barbara M. Kelly
Designer: Nancy C. Baker
Manufacturing Supervisor: Kathy Grone

Printed in the United States of America
Composition by Graphic World, Inc.
Printing/binding by R.R. Donnelly

Mosby–Year Book, Inc.
11830 Westline Industrial Drive
St. Louis, Missouri 63146

Library of Congress Cataloging in Publication Data
Ruppel, Gregg, 1948–
    Manual of pulmonary function testing / Gregg Ruppel. — 6th ed.
      p.   cm.
    Includes bibliographical references and index.
    ISBN 0-8016-7789-0
    1. Pulmonary function tests — Handbooks, manuals, etc.   I. Title.
    [DNLM: 1. Respiratory Function Tests.   WB 284 R946m 1993]
  RC734.P84R86 1993
  616.2'4075 — dc20
  DNLM/DLC
  for Library of Congress   93-27962
                                                    CIP

1 2 3 4 5 6 7 8 9 0 98 97 96 95 94

to Carol
for her continued patience and encouragement

The primary function of the lung can be stated as twofold: first, the oxygenation of mixed venous blood, and second, the removal of carbon dioxide from that same blood. These two functions depend on the integrity of the airways, pulmonary vascular system, alveolar septa, respiratory muscles, and respiratory control mechanisms. Tests that could assess each part of the pulmonary system separately would be most appropriate. Most lung function tests, however, measure the status of the lungs' components in an overlapping way.

The beginning of modern pulmonary function testing can be traced to the studies of John Hutchinson in the period from 1840 to 1850. Hutchinson developed the prototype of the modern water-sealed spirometer. He performed measurements of "vital capacity" on thousands of subjects and developed tables to predict lung volume divisions. These studies of the various lung compartments form the basis for modern spirometric and lung volume tests. In 1951 Gaensler and others began recording timed vital capacity maneuvers. These studies were the basis for parameters such as the FEV_1. Leuallen and Fowler described the measurement of the maximal midexpiratory flow (MMEF) in 1955. Measurement of flows during forced expiration quickly became standard in the evaluation of obstructive lung disorders.

The first measurements of residual volume are attributed to Davy in the early 1800s. He used hydrogen to perform a closed circuit dilution measurement of the gas remaining in the lung at the end of a maximal expiration. The hydrogen dilution technique was used sporadically by various investigators until 1940. Modern techniques for measuring lung volumes depended on the development of gas analyzers. In 1939, McMichael used a katharometer to make hydrogen dilution measurements of functional residual capacity. The development of a katharometer to measure helium concentration allowed Meneely and Kaltreider to measure functional residual capacity using a dilution technique similar to that of McMichael. At about the same time Darling and co-workers developed an open-circuit method of measuring functional residual capacity using oxygen breathing.

In 1956, Dubois and Comroe resurrected a concept that had been introduced as early as the 1880s, that of the body plethysmograph. The introduction of sensitive pressure transducers and a cathode ray oscilloscope capable of reproducing rapidly changing signals permitted them to measure lung volumes and airway resistance. The techniques used for plethysmography today differ very little from those introduced almost 40 years ago.

Many of the tests used in clinical practice today were developed in the investigation of pulmonary physiology. In 1910 Marie and August Krogh set out to demonstrate that the lung did not actively excrete oxygen into the pulmonary capillaries. They used carbon monoxide (CO) to show that gas moved from the lung into the pulmonary blood by diffusion. In the 1950s, Forster and his co-workers resurrected this technique as the basis for the modern diffusing capacity test using a simple ten-second breathhold maneuver. At about the same time Filley was developing a steady-state methodology that also used carbon monoxide to assess diffusion, both at rest and during exercise.

Although many of the principles used in blood gas analysis had been described previously, it was not until the decade of the 1950s that blood gases became part of pulmonary function testing. In 1957 Sanz introduced a glass electrode system to measure the pH in blood. In 1958 Severinghaus developed a combination Ph electrode that responded specifically to the partial pressure of CO_2 in a specimen. In 1956, Clark modified a platinum electrode that reduced oxygen at its tip by covering it with a membrane. This membrane covered electrode allowed the partial pressure of oxygen in blood to be determined by preventing immediate contamination of the platinum wire. The combination of these three electrodes produced blood gas analysis in the form used today.

In the mid-1960s, Hyatt and his co-workers began using computers to display analyses of flow, volume, and pressure as three dimensional graphs. They applied these techniques to the analysis of forced expiratory maneuvers. Within ten years, the flow-volume curve became a standard part of spirometry. The widespread application of microprocessors beginning in the late 1970s paved the way for sophisticated pulmonary function testing applications. The wide variety of flow-sensing spirometers, metabolic measurement systems, and pulse oximeters are just a few of the applications that have been made possible by microprocessor control.

The evaluation of pulmonary function in the laboratory or at the bedside may be indicated for the following reasons:

1. To determine the *presence* of lung disease or abnormality of lung function
2. To determine the *extent* of abnormalities
3. To determine the *extent of impairment* caused by abnormal lung function
4. To determine the *progression* of the disease
5. To determine the *nature of the physiologic disturbance*
6. To determine a *course of therapy* for treatment of a particular lesion

Pulmonary function tests are commonly used to evaluate obstructive lung diseases such as asthma, chronic bronchitis, emphysema, and cystic fibrosis. Lung function tests are often used to determine the presence and extent of abnormalities classified as restrictive disorders. These include diseases that interfere with the bellows action of the lungs or chest wall. Chief among these are lesions produced by inhalation of toxic dusts or chemicals, diseases related to cardiovascular dysfunction, neuromuscular disorders, and defects caused by lung resection or chemotherapy. Specialized applications of pulmonary function tests are often directed at determining the physiologic causes for the patient's symptoms. A prime example of this is cardiopulmonary exercise testing, in which various components of the lung and cardiovascular system are evaluated to determine the cause(s) of dyspnea on exertion. Many types of pulmonary function tests are directed at answering clinical questions regarding how to best treat lung disorders. Before and after-bronchodilator studies, inhalation challenge studies, and nutritional assessment using exhaled gas analysis are all examples of pulmonary measurements that help determine which therapies might be most effective.

This text presents explanations of many commonly used pulmonary function tests, the techniques used, and the pathophysiology that may be evaluated by each test. Included are sections on pulmonary exercise evaluation, metabolic testing, pediatric pulmonary function testing, and test regimens for specific purposes, such as disability or preoperative evaluation. Pulmonary function testing equipment, computers, and quality assurance are addressed.

This sixth edition elaborates on material presented in the first five editions, and reflects the suggestions of users of those editions. The chapters on pulmonary function equipment and computers have been expanded to cover the newer technologies commonly available. Chapter 11, dealing with quality assurance issues, has been expanded to include recommendations of the American Thoracic Society and the Centers for Disease Control regarding testing protocols and safety. Chapter 12 has been extended to include case studies involving quality assurance issues, serial pulmonary function studies, and metabolic measurements.

As in previous editions, Chapters 1 through 11 are followed by self assessment questions. The self assessment questions are new to this edition, and answers may be found in the Appendix. Entries in the selected bibliographies at the end of each chapter are arranged according to specific topics within the chapter. As with previous editions, prediction regressions and nomograms for reference values are contained in the Appendix, along with information on the use of reference values. Sample calculations for lung volumes, plethysmography, diffusion, and exercise tests are also included in the Appendix.

This manual is intended to serve as a text for students of pulmonary function testing and as a reference for technologists and physicians. Because of the diversity of testing methods and equipment currently in use, some aspects of certain tests are treated in a general way. For this reason, readers are encouraged to make use of the bibliographies provided. The presentation of the pathophysiology and significance of various tests presumes a basic knowledge of the pulmonary anatomy and physiology. Again, readers are urged to refer to the General References included in the selected bibliography to refresh or support their background in lung function. The terminology used is that of the American College of Chest Physicians-American Thoracic Society Joint Committee on Pulmonary Nomenclature. In some instances test names reflect very common usage that does not follow the ACCP-ATS recommendations.

Gregg Ruppel, M.Ed., R.R.T.

ACKNOWLEDGMENTS

My thanks to Drs. William Kistner, John Winter, and James Wiant for their encouragement in the development of the original text. My special thanks to Drs. Roger Secker-Walker, Susan Marshall, and Gerald Dolan for comments and constructive criticism in the preparation of the revised editions. Special thanks also go to Ronald Gilmore and Jack Tandy for their contributions to the illustrations in previous editions. A note of thanks also to Thomas Anderson, MEd, RRT, David Shelledy, MA, RRT, Patricia Dent, BS, MS, RPT, and Barbara Disborough, MA, RRT for their reviews of and suggestions for the 4th edition. Louis Metzger, RPFT, Donald Barker, BS, PA, RPFT, David Hoover, RRT, RPFT, Randall Krohn, James Kemp, MD, Alan Hibbett, RPFT, and Michael Snow, RPFT all provided guidance and suggestions for the 5th edition. Cesar Keller, MD, and Deborah Stanger, RD, provided insight for case studies for the 6th edition.

My appreciation for materials and illustrations provided goes to Warren E. Collins Inc., Radiometer America, Jones Medical Instrument Co., Vitalograph Medical Instrumentation, Instrumentation Laboratories, Medical Graphics Inc., Hewlett Packard, Hans Rudolph Inc., Biochem International, Ohmeda, Abbott Critical Care Systems, Clement-Clarke, HealthScan Products, Inc., Pulmonary Data Services, and SensorMedics Corp.

Gregg Ruppel, M.Ed., R.R.T.

CONTENTS

11 QUALITY ASSURANCE IN THE PULMONARY FUNCTION LABORATORY   *343*

12 CASE STUDIES   *393*

1

Lung Volume Tests

VITAL CAPACITY (VC), INSPIRATORY CAPACITY (IC), AND EXPIRATORY RESERVE VOLUME (ERV)

Description

The vital capacity (VC) is the volume of gas measured on a slow, complete expiration after a maximal inspiration, without forced or rapid effort (Fig. 1–1). The VC is normally recorded in either liters or milliliters and reported at body temperature, pressure, and saturation (BTPS). The VC sometimes is referred to as the slow vital capacity (SVC), distinguishing it from the forced vital capacity (FVC) as discussed in Chapter 3. The inspiratory capacity (IC) and expiratory reserve volume (ERV) are subdivisions of the VC. The IC is the largest volume of gas that can be inspired from the resting expiratory level (see Fig. 1–1). The IC sometimes is divided further into the tidal volume (V_T) and the inspiratory reserve volume (IRV). The ERV is the largest volume of gas that can be expired from the resting end-expiratory level (see Fig. 1–1). Both the IC and ERV are recorded in liters or milliliters and corrected to BTPS.

Technique

The VC is measured by having the subject inspire maximally and then exhale completely into a spirometer capable of recording change in lung volume, with no time limit imposed on the maneuver. The spirometer need not be able to produce a tracing of the maneuver if only the VC is to be measured. If the subdivisions of the VC are to be determined (see Fig. 1–1), some means of recording the tracing is required. The recording can be done with a mechanical device (see Chapter 9) or a computer (see Chapter 10). The VC can also be measured from maximal expiration to maximal inspiration. This latter method

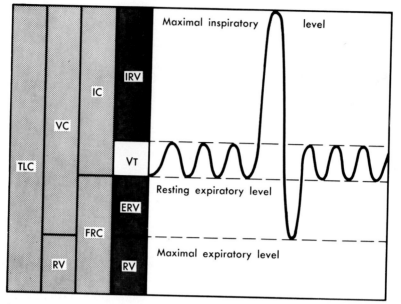

FIG 1–1.
Lung volumes and capacities. Diagrammatic representation of various lung compartments based on a typical spirogram. *TLC,* total lung capacity; *VC,* vital capacity; *RV,* residual volume; *FRC,* functional residual capacity; *IC,* inspiratory capacity; *VT,* tidal volume; *IRV,* inspiratory reserve volume; *ERV,* expiratory reserve volume. *Shaded areas* indicate relationships between the subdivisions and relative sizes as compared with the TLC. The resting expiratory level should be noted, since it remains more stable than other identifiable points during repeated spirograms, and hence is used as a starting point for FRC determinations, etc. (Modified from Comroe JH Jr, Forster RE, Dubois AB, et al: *The lung: clinical physiology and pulmonary function tests,* ed 2. Chicago, 1962, Year Book Medical Publishers, Inc.)

is sometimes termed the *inspiratory vital capacity* (IVC or SIVC), while the former is simply the VC or SVC.

The IC may be measured by having the subject breathe normally for several breaths and then inhale maximally (from the resting expiratory level). The volume inspired is measured from an appropriate spirogram, usually as part of an SVC maneuver. The IC also may be estimated by subtracting the ERV from the VC.

The ERV may be measured by having the subject breathe normally for several breaths and then exhale maximally from the level of resting exhalation, while recording the changes on a spirogram. The ERV also may be estimated by subtracting the IC from the VC. The accuracy of the measurement of both the IC and ERV depends on the determination of the passive end-expiratory level and patient effort. This is best accomplished by recording at least three tidal breaths that vary by less than 100 mL before the SVC maneuver.

Significance and Pathophysiology

Normal values for VC as well as for many other lung function parameters are computed using the following equation:

$$VC = XH - YA - Z$$

where:

H = height (cm or inches)

A = age (years)

X, Y, Z = constants

Nomograms and equations for men, women, and children appear in the Appendix. The VC may vary as much as 20% from predicted normal values in healthy individuals and may vary from time to time in the same individual depending on the position of the body or time of day. The VC in adults varies directly with height and inversely with age and is generally smaller in females than in males. Recent evidence indicates that lung volumes may differ significantly according to race or ethnic origin; thus, the interpretation of the measured volumes in regard to predicted normal values should consider these factors in addition to age, height, weight, and sex (see Using Predicted Values in the Appendix).

Decreases in VC can be caused by a loss of distensible lung tissue, as in bronchogenic carcinoma, bronchiolar obstruction, pulmonary edema, pneumonia, atelectasis, pulmonary restriction, pulmonary congestion, or surgical excisions. Restriction results from tissue destruction, space-occupying lesions, or changes in the composition of the parenchyma itself. Tissue loss may be illustrated by resection (as in a lobectomy), where the decrease in VC is roughly proportional to the tissue removed. A good example of a space-occupying lesion is a tumor, which directly displaces lung tissue. Fibrotic diseases such as silicosis may cause changes in the elastic properties of the parenchyma. The VC is often reduced in obstructive lung disease, while other lung compartments show increased volumes (see section on Residual Volume, below). There are some causes for decreases in VC not related to lung lesions, such as depression of the respiratory centers or neuromuscular diseases; reduction of available thoracic space possibly caused by pleural effusion, pneumothorax, hiatal hernia, or cardiac enlargement; limitation of movement of the diaphragm possibly resulting from pregnancy, ascites, or a tumor; and limitation of thoracic movement possibly occurring because of scleroderma, kyphoscoliosis, or pain.

When the VC is reduced, other pulmonary function measurements may be indicated. Forced expiratory maneuvers will typically reveal whether an obstructive process is the cause of the reduced VC. A reduction in VC without evidence of expiratory slowing is a nonspecific finding and measurement of other lung volumes (FRC, RV, and total lung capacity [TLC]) may be indicated to ascertain if a restrictive defect is present.

When the VC is reduced to less than 80% of predicted or less than the 95% confidence limit (see Appendix), the interpretation of the measured VC value should be correlated with the patient's history and physical findings. The terms *mild, moderate,* and *severe* may be used to qualify the extent of reduction of the VC, and should be based on a comparison of the measured VC vs. the predicted VC. Artificially low estimates of the VC may result from poor subject effort or inadequate instruction in the performance of the test maneuver. Reproducible values for at least three maneuvers should produce acceptable results (see Chapter 11).

The IC and ERV normally are approximately 75% and 25% of the VC, respectively. Changes in the absolute volumes of the IC or ERV usually parallel increases or decreases in the VC. Increased tidal volumes, in response to exertion or acid-base disorders, may encroach on both the inspiratory reserve volume (IRV) and ERV, as both the end-inspiratory and end-expiratory levels are altered. This pattern also may be seen when subjects are asked to breathe into a spirometer through a mouthpiece with noseclips in place. Changes in the IC or ERV are of minimal diagnostic significance when considered alone. Reduction of either the IC or ERV is consistent with restrictive defects. Erroneous estimates of ERV may confound the measurement of residual volume (RV) as described below, because the ERV is usually subtracted from the functional residual capacity (FRC) to calculate the RV. An underestimated ERV causes the computed RV to appear larger than the actual RV.

FUNCTIONAL RESIDUAL CAPACITY (FRC) AND RESIDUAL VOLUME (RV)

Description

The FRC is the volume of gas remaining in the lungs at the end of resting expiration. The RV is the volume of gas remaining in the lungs at the end of a maximal expiration (see Fig. 1–1). Both are recorded in liters or milliliters, corrected to BTPS.

Technique

There are two gas dilution methods of measuring the FRC that employ a foreign gas (i.e., a gas not normally present in the lungs). The FRC and its subdivision, the RV, must be measured indirectly because the gas filling these compartments cannot be exhaled from the lungs.

Open-circuit method. The concentration of nitrogen (N_2) in the lungs is presumed to be in equilibrium with the atmosphere, or approximately 80%. By having the subject breathe 100% oxygen (O_2) for several minutes, the nitrogen in the lungs can be washed out gradually. Because all of the N_2 cannot be washed out, the test is usually continued until the concentration of alveolar N_2 is less than 1%; then an alveolar sample is taken. The exhaled gas may be collected in a spirometer or bag that has been flushed previously with pure O_2. First the concentration of N_2 is measured; then the original volume of gas in the lungs at the end-expiratory level can be computed using this formula:

$$FRC = \frac{F_EN_{2_{final}} \times \text{expired volume} - N_{2_{tiss}}}{F_AN_{2_{alveolar\,1}} - F_AN_{2_{alveolar\,2}}}$$

where:

$F_EN_{2_{final}}$ = fraction of N_2 in volume expired

$F_AN_{2_{alveolar\,1}}$ = fraction of N_2 in alveolar gas initially

$F_AN_{2_{alveolar\,2}}$ = fraction of N_2 in alveolar gas at end
(determined from an alveolar sample)

$N_{2_{tiss}}$ = volume of N_2 washed out of blood/tissues

Corrections for the amount of N_2 washed out of the blood and tissue and for small amounts of nitrogen in pure O_2 must be made when computing the FRC. For each minute of oxygen breathing, approximately 30 to 40 mL of N_2 are removed from blood and tissue, so $0.04 \times T$ (where T is the time of the test) is subtracted from the volume of N_2 in the spirometer. Because not all of the N_2 in the lungs may be washed out, even after 7 minutes of O_2 breathing, the $F_AN_{2_{alveolar2}}$ may be measured by taking an alveolar sample near the end of the test, and subtracting this value from the alveolar N_2 present at the beginning. The FRC must be corrected to BTPS, (see Appendix).

To obtain the RV, a previously determined expiratory reserve volume is subtracted from the FRC as just measured:

$$RV = FRC - ERV$$

A newer method for performing the open-circuit procedure uses a rapid N_2 analyzer in combination with a spirometer to provide a ''breath-by-breath'' analysis of expired N_2 (Fig. 1–2). The exhaled concentration and volume for each breath are measured and values are accumulated for the duration of the test. The values for all breaths are summed to provide the total volume of N_2 washed out. The test is continued for 7 minutes or until the N_2 in alveolar gas has been reduced to less than 1%. The FRC is calculated by dividing the total volume of N_2 washed out by the fractional concentration of alveolar N_2 at the beginning of the test and making the necessary corrections (i.e., blood/tissue washout, temperature). In addition, a breath-by-breath plot of the %N_2 (or log %N_2) vs.

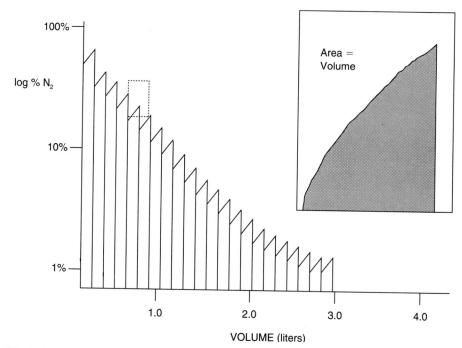

FIG 1–2.
Nitrogen (N_2) washout (open-circuit) determination of functional residual capacity (FRC). The concentration (or the log concentration) of N_2 is plotted against time or against the volume expired as the subject breathes through a circuit such as that in Figure 1–4, B. The volume of N_2 expired with each breath is determined by integrating flow and N_2 concentration to determine the area under each curve (see *inset*). The volume of N_2 expired with individual breaths is summed and the test continued until most of the N_2 in the lung has been washed out (usually 1% or less). The FRC is then determined by dividing the volume of N_2 expired by the change in alveolar N_2 from the beginning to the end of the test, with corrections, as described in the text.

volume or number of breaths can be obtained to derive indexes of the distribution of ventilation (see Chapter 4).

In systems employing a pneumotachometer, a device sensitive to the composition of gas (see Chapter 9), corrections must be made for changes in the viscosity of the gas as oxygen replaces nitrogen in the expired gas. This is usually easily accomplished by software or electronic correction of the analyzer output.

Closed-circuit method. The FRC can also be calculated indirectly by diluting the gas in the lungs with a gas of known concentration. A suitable spirometer is filled with a known volume of gas to which helium (He) has been added. The amount (usually about 600 mL) and concentration of He (usually about 10%) are measured and recorded before the test is begun. Then the subject breathes the gas in the spirometer, with a carbon dioxide (CO_2) absorber in place, until the concentration of He falls to a stable level. This usually requires less than 7 minutes. Oxygen is added to the spirometer system in order to maintain the fractional concentration at a level near or above that of room air and to keep the system volume relatively constant, as O_2 is absorbed by tissue and blood.

An older method added a large bolus of oxygen at the beginning of the procedure and allowed the subject to gradually consume the O_2. Because of the possibility of equilibrium not being attained before the added oxygen was depleted, this method is no longer commonly employed.

If the 10% He mixture is prepared in an appropriate system volume (usually 6 to 8 L), equilibration between the normal lungs and the rebreathing system takes place quickly, typically in about 3 minutes. The final concentration of He is then recorded. The system volume (the volume that was in the spirometer before the test was begun) can then be calculated using this formula:

$$\text{system volume} = \frac{\text{He}_{\text{added}}(\text{mL})}{F_{\text{He}_{\text{initial}}}}$$

where:

$F_{\text{He}_{\text{initial}}}$ is the %He converted to a fraction (%He/100)

Once the system volume is known, the FRC (and RV) can be computed:

$$\text{FRC} = \frac{(\%\text{He}_{\text{initial}} - \%\text{He}_{\text{final}})}{\%\text{He}_{\text{final}}} \times \text{system volume}$$

Either percent or fractional concentration of He may be used since the term is a ratio.

Some automated systems employ the same method to calculate the system volume; a small amount of He is added to the closed system, followed by a known volume of air. The change in He concentration after the addition of the air is used to determine the system volume as described previously. As in the open-circuit technique, RV = FRC − ERV.

Rebreathing is normally continued until the He concentration changes by no more than 0.02% over 30 seconds (see Chapter 11 for criteria for acceptability of lung volumes).

Several corrections are frequently made to the FRC value obtained by the above equation. Because a small volume of He dissolves in the blood during the test, the final helium reading is lower than it would have been had the decrease in He resulted solely from dilution by the subject's FRC. The loss of He to the blood results in a slight increase in the apparent FRC. A volume of 100 mL is usually subtracted from the FRC to correct for this effect. The dead space volume of the breathing valve likewise should be subtracted from the measured FRC.

Most manufacturers recommend a "switch-in" error correction to be applied when the subject is turned into the system at a point either above or below the actual end-expiratory level (FRC). Depending on the subject's breathing pattern, a volume difference of several hundred milliliters may result. However, the effect of the switch-in error may be insignificant because equilibrium does not occur instantaneously at switch-in, and because the total volume of the spirometer and lungs is constantly changing with tidal breathing, removal of CO_2, and addition of O_2. If the switch-in error is large, or if the subject's end-expiratory level appears to be changing or irregular during the maneuver, the test should be restarted after allowing several minutes of air breathing to clear any residual He from the lungs. The FRC must be converted to BTPS (Fig. 1–3). Sample calculations of both the open- and closed-circuit techniques can be found in the Appendix.

Significance and Pathophysiology

In both the open- and closed-circuit techniques, the RV is measured indirectly as a subdivision of the FRC. This is the preferred method because the resting end-expiratory level is more reproducible than the points of complete inspiration or complete expiration. The end-expiratory level (and the ERV) must be accurately measured; if the tidal breathing pattern is irregular, the ERV may be overestimated or underestimated, thus affecting the calculation of the RV.

The validity of both techniques depends on the assumption that all parts of the lung are reasonably well ventilated. In subjects who have obstructive disease, a 7-minute test period may not be long enough to wash out N_2 or mix He to a stable level in the poorly ventilated parts of the lungs. Thus, the FRC, RV, and TLC will appear less than the true values. Prolongation of the test improves results somewhat, but will not account for *completely* trapped gas, as found in bullous emphysema.

In either of the foreign gas techniques, leaks in the valving or circuitry, or at the subject connection, will affect gas concentrations and cause erroneous estimates of FRC. Leaks most commonly result in overestimates of lung volumes. Likewise, malfunction of the gas analyzer in either method will produce spurious values. Integrity of the breathing circuit or analyzer (Fig. 1–4, A and B) should be questioned whenever FRC values appear inconsistent with the subject's clinical history or with other lung function parameters such as spirometry results or carbon monoxide diffusing capacity ($D_{L_{CO}}$)(discussed in Chapter 5).

An increase in the FRC is considered pathologic. An FRC value of greater than approximately 120% of that predicted represents hyperinflation, which may result from emphysematous changes, asthmatic or bronchiolar obstruction, compensation for surgical removal of lung tissue, or in some instances from thoracic deformity. An increase in FRC usually results in muscular and mechanical inefficiency, causing an increase in the effort required to breathe.

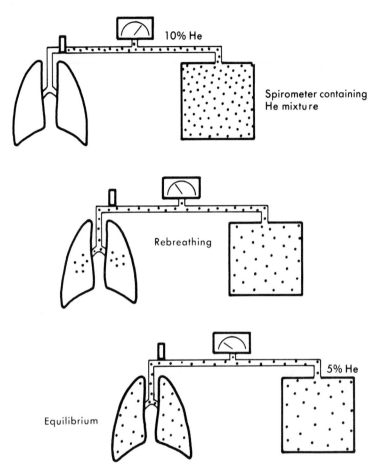

FIG 1–3.
Helium *(He)* dilution (closed-circuit) determination of functional residual capacity (FRC). At the beginning of the test, the subject's lungs contains no He. The subject then rebreathes a mixture of He and air or O_2 from a system such as that shown in Figure 1–4, A. Helium is diluted until an equilibrium is reached. The volume of He present initially and its concentration is known, and the volume of the rebreathing system can be calculated. At the end of the test, the same volume of He has been diluted in a larger volume (rebreathing system + lungs), and the total volume is computed from the initial He volume ($V_{He_{final}}$) and the final He concentration ($F_{He_{final}}$) values, as follows:

$$\frac{V_{He_{initial}}}{F_{He_{final}}} = \text{total volume of system (after rebreathing)}$$

The FRC is derived by subtracting the rebreathing system volume (see text). The switch from air to the He mixture must be made at the end-expiratory level for accurate measurement of FRC. The residual volume is derived by subtracting the expiratory reserve volume. (Modified from Comroe JH Jr, Forster RE, Dubois AB, et al: *The lung: clinical physiology and pulmonary function tests,* ed 2. Chicago, 1962, Year Book Medical Publishers, Inc.)

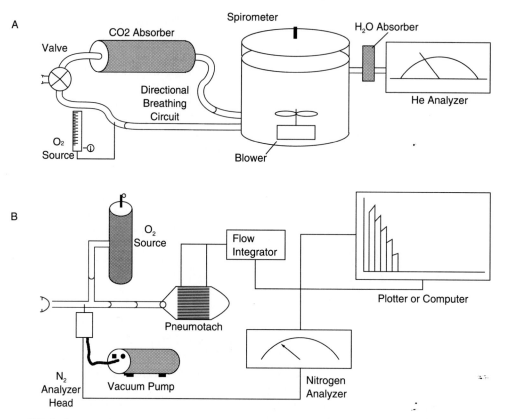

FIG 1–4.

Typical circuits for functional residual capacity (FRC) determination. **A,** closed-circuit components used for helium *(He)* dilution FRC determination include a volume-based spirometer with an He analyzer, CO_2 absorber, and directional breathing circuit and blower fan to promote mixing between the spirometer system and the subject's lungs. A breathing valve near the mouth allows the subject to be "switched in" to the system after He has been added and the system volume determined. An oxygen (O_2) source allows the addition of O_2 during the test to replenish that taken up by the subject and to maintain a relatively constant system volume. **B,** open-circuit components used for the nitrogen (N_2) washout determination of FRC. The subject inspires O_2 from a regulated source and expires past a rapid responding N_2 analyzer into a pneumotachometer. Flow and gas concentration signals are integrated and displayed on a plotter or computer screen. The FRC is calculated from the total volume of N_2 expired and the change in alveolar N_2 from the beginning to the end of the test (see Fig. 1–2 and text).

An increase in RV indicates that despite the subject's maximal expiratory effort, the lungs still contain an abnormally large amount of gas. This type of change appearing in young asthmatic patients is usually reversible. Increases of RV are also characteristic of emphysema and bronchial obstruction, both of which may cause chronic air trapping. The RV and FRC usually increase together. As RV becomes larger, more ventilation may be required to adequately exchange O_2 and CO_2 in the lung. This usually requires an increase in tidal volume, rate, or both. At the same time, the work of breathing is increased. Subjects with increased RV often display gas exchange abnormalities such as hypoxemia or CO_2 retention.

The FRC and RV, and the total lung capacity derived from them, are typically decreased in restrictive diseases that interfere with the bellows action of the chest or the lungs. Such decreased values are seen in those diseases associated with extensive fibrosis, such as sarcoidosis, asbestosis, and complicated silicosis. Restrictive disorders affecting the chest wall include kyphoscoliosis, pectus excavatum, neuromuscular weakness, and obesity. The FRC and RV may also be decreased in diseases that occlude many alveoli, such as pneumonia.

Table 1–1 lists typical values for lung volumes for a normal adult male, a subject with hyperinflation (as in emphysema), and a subject with restriction (as in sarcoidosis). It should be noted that generalized restrictive processes cause the lung volumes to be reduced approximately equally. Thus, the proportional relationship between different lung volume compartments, such as the RV/TLC ratio, may be relatively normal.

In obstructive patterns, one of two changes in the proportions of the various compartments is usually observed. The RV may be increased; this increase may be at the expense of a reduction in VC (see Fig. 1–7), with the TLC remaining close to the expected value. In other cases, the RV may increase while the VC remains fairly well preserved; thus, the TLC value is actually greater than predicted. The term *air trapping* is sometimes used to describe the increase in FRC and RV, while the term *hyperinflation* is often used to describe the absolute increase in TLC.

THORACIC GAS VOLUME (V$_{TG}$)

Description

The V$_{TG}$ is the volume of gas contained in the thorax, whether in communication with patent airways or trapped in any compartment of the thorax. The V$_{TG}$ is usually measured at the end-expiratory level, and is then equal

TABLE 1–1.

Comparative Lung Volumes for a Normal Adult Male, a Subject With Hyperinflation, and a Subject with Restriction

Value	Normal	Hyperinflation	Restriction
VC (mL)	4800	3000	3000
FRC (mL)	2400	3600	1500
RV (mL)	1200	3000	750
TLC (mL)	6000	6000	3750
RV/TLC (%)	20	50	20

to FRC. It may also be measured at other lung volumes and then corrected to relate to FRC. The V$_{TG}$ is recorded in liters or milliliters.

Technique

The V$_{TG}$ is measured using the body plethysmograph (Fig. 1–5). The technique is based on Boyle's law, which states that the volume of gas varies in inverse proportion to the pressure to which it is subjected, if the temperature remains constant. At the start of the test, the subject has an unknown volume of gas in the thorax (i.e., the FRC). By occluding the airway and allowing the subject to decompress the gas in the chest by making an inspiratory effort, a new volume and a new pressure are generated. The change in pulmonary gas pressure is easily measured at the airway, as mouth pressure theoretically equals alveolar pressure when there is no airflow. The change in pulmonary gas volume is measured by monitoring the change in pressure in a constant volume plethysmograph, or by measuring the flow of gas into and out of a flow box (see Plethysmographs in Chapter 9). In a constant volume plethysmograph, the transducer measuring box pressure is calibrated directly in terms of volume

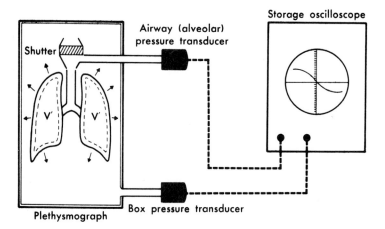

FIG 1–5.
Thoracic gas volume (V$_{TG}$). The body plethysmograph is used to measure V$_{TG}$. Boyle's law states that the volume varies inversely with the pressure if the temperature is held constant. A pressure-type plethysmograph, with pressure transducers for measurements of box pressure and airway (alveolar) pressure, is shown. An electronic shutter momentarily occludes the airway so that airway pressure is approximately equal to alveolar pressure. Simultaneously, the alveolar gas is decompressed because of enlargement of the thorax, without gas flow. This change in alveolar volume is reflected by an increase in box pressure, and an estimation of the volume change can be derived by calibration. When the original pressure *(P)*, the new pressure (P'), and the new volume (V' or V + ΔV) are known, the original volume (V or V$_{TG}$) can be computed from Boyle's law (see text and Appendix).

change by introducing a small, known volume of gas into the sealed chamber and expressing the pressure change as an index of volume.

In a constant volume (or pressure-type) plethysmograph, the subject breathes against a closed airway that has been occluded by means of an electrical shutter. The air within the chest is alternately compressed and decompressed by the action of the ventilatory muscles. The signal measuring mouth pressure (which equals alveolar pressure) is plotted on the vertical axis of an oscilloscope or computer screen, while the signal measuring box pressure (calibrated as volume change) is plotted on the horizontal axis (see Fig. 1–5). Changes in each parameter are graphed continuously and appear as a sloping line, which is equal to $\Delta P / \Delta V$, where ΔP is the change in alveolar pressure and ΔV is the change in alveolar volume. (The change in alveolar volume is measured indirectly by noting the reciprocal change in plethysmograph volume.)

The original volume contained in the thorax at the time the shutter was closed then can be obtained from the slope of the tracing by applying a derivation of Boyle's law:

$$V_{TG} = \frac{P_B}{\lambda V_{TG}} \times \frac{P_{box}cal}{P_{mouth}cal} \times K$$

where:

V_{TG} = thoracic gas volume

P_B = barometric pressure minus water vapor pressure

λV_{TG} = slope of the oscilloscope trace equal to $\Delta P / \Delta V$

$P_{box}cal$ = box pressure transducer calibration factor

$P_{mouth}cal$ = mouth pressure transducer calibration factor

K = correction factor for volume displaced by the subject

For the complete derivation of the equation and sample calculations, see the Appendix.

The measurements are usually made with the subject panting shallowly at a rate of 1 to 2 breaths/sec with an open glottis. This type of breathing allows small pressure changes to be recorded at or near FRC, eliminates some artifacts related to temperature fluctuations, and improves the signal-noise ratio. Some plethysmograph systems allow V_{TG} measurements by occluding the airway during normal breathing without panting. If the mouth shutter is closed precisely at end-expiration, V_{TG} equals FRC. Several determinations can be made quickly to obtain an average for the slope of $\Delta P / \Delta V$; the averaged slope is then used in the equation above to derive the V_{TG}.

Computerized plethysmograph systems permit the measurement of the VC as well as its subdivisions (ERV, IC, etc.) in conjunction with the V_{TG} maneuver.

By continuously integrating the flow through the plethysmograph's pneumo-tachometer, instantaneous changes in lung volume can be monitored and the resting ventilatory level recorded. The subject then begins to pant with the shutter open, and the computer records the change in lung volume above or below the resting level (i.e., FRC). When asked to pant, most subjects do so slightly above FRC. The mouth shutter is then automatically closed while the subject continues panting, and the V_{TG} is measured as described above. The computer then adds or subtracts the difference in volume from the resting breathing level (before the subject began panting) in reference to the actual volume in the thorax when the shutter was closed to calculate the true FRC. This computerized technique allows the subject to pant at the correct frequency and depth before the shutter is closed, and eliminates the necessity of closing the shutter precisely at end-expiration. In addition to the VC and its subdivisions, the airway resistance (Raw) can be measured simultaneously by recording the ratio of flow to box pressure during the open-shutter panting (see Chapter 3).

Significance and Pathophysiology

The V_{TG} offers a quick and precise means of measuring FRC and may be used in combination with simple spirometry to derive other lung volume compart-ments. The plethysmograph's principle advantage is that it measures the volume of gas in the thoracic cavity whether it is in ventilatory communication with the atmosphere or not. The V_{TG} measurement of FRC is often larger than the FRC as measured by He dilution or N_2 washout, especially in emphysema, other diseases characterized by air trapping, and in the presence of uneven distribution of ventilation. When dilution tests are extended beyond 7 minutes, the results for FRC determinations approach the V_{TG} figure.

Recent evidence suggests that in severe obstructive patterns, the FRC actually may be overestimated when the V_{TG} technique is used, primarily due to inaccuracies in measuring alveolar pressure at the mouth during airway occlusion. Normal lungs, however, show similar results by either method.

When two or more methods of determining lung volumes are employed, it is often instructive to compare the FRC determined by each method, particularly in subjects with suspected obstructive disease. The ratio of FRC_{box}/FRC_{gas} may be used as an index of gas trapping. The ratio is usually near unity (i.e., 1) in persons with normal lungs or in subjects with mild restriction. Values greater than 1 indicate gas volumes detectable by the plethysmograph but "hidden" from the gas techniques. Care must be taken to determine that the lung volumes ascertained by the two separate methods are reliable before the values can be expressed as a ratio.

By appropriate integration of the pneumotachometer flow signal, spiromet-ric indexes (FVC, FEV, SVC, etc.) may be obtained with the same equipment normally used in plethysmography, allowing measurements of both lung volumes and flows in a single sitting. The V$_{TG}$ maneuver requires that the technician carefully instruct and monitor the subject in order to obtain acceptable data (see Chapter 11). Thoracic gas volume cannot be measured in subjects who have claustrophobia or physical limitations that preclude entry into the box, or in those unable to perform the panting maneuver acceptably.

RADIOLOGIC ESTIMATION OF TOTAL LUNG CAPACITY (TLC)

Description

Total lung capacity can be determined according to several methods using standard posterior-anterior (P-A) and lateral radiographs of the chest. A commonly used procedure involves dividing the films into ellipsoidal segments and estimating the volumes of each segment. A planimeter can also be used to estimate the thoracic volume.

Technique (Ellipsoidal segment method)

Posterior-anterior and lateral chest radiographs are taken at a standard distance of 72 inches. The borders of the lungs, heart, and diaphragms are outlined using a china marker or similar pencil. Figure 1–6 illustrates the necessary outlines for the measurements. If the lung apex is not visible on the lateral film, it can be determined after some preliminary measurements are made. The P-A film is first subdivided (see Fig. 1–6) as follows:

1. A horizontal line is drawn 2.75 cm from the apices (#1).
2. A second line is drawn 2.75 cm below the first line (#2).
3. A horizontal line is drawn through the upper diaphragm dome (#4).
4. A horizontal line is drawn midway between lines #2 and #4 (#3); these lines determine segments I through IV.

The lateral film is then subdivided (see Fig. 1–6) as follows:

1. A horizontal line is drawn through the upper diaphragm dome (#4).
2. The apex of the lung on the lateral view then can be determined by measuring the distance from the apex to line #4 on the P-A film and transposing to the lateral.
3. Line #1 is drawn 2.75 cm below the apex.
4. Line #2 is drawn 2.75 cm below line #1.
5. Line #3 is drawn midway between lines #2 and #4, just as on the P-A film.
6. A fifth horizontal line is drawn through the posterior sulcus forward to the anterior limit of the diaphragm. The distance from line #4 to

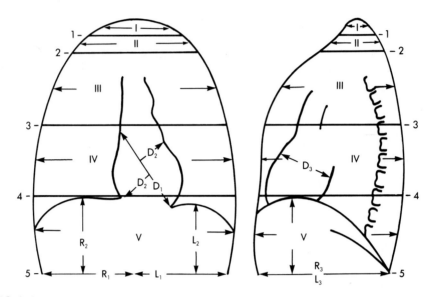

FIG 1–6.
Radiologic estimation of total lung capacity *(TLC)*. Standard posterior-anterior *(P-A)* and lateral x-ray films are outlined as indicated with wax pencil or marker. *Lines 1, 2, 3, 4,* and *5* divide each film into five segments (*I* to *V*). R_1, R_2, and R_3 define the volume under the diaphragms. (L_1, L_2, and L_3 are taken from the left diaphragm; $R_1 = L_1$, $R_3 = L_3$, and L_2 is the height of the left hemidiaphragm, while R_2 is the height of the right side.) D_1, D_2, and D_3 allow the calculation of the volume occupied by the heart. All measurements are made in centimeters, and each respective segment is measured at the points indicated by the *arrows* (see text).

> line #5 is then transposed to the P-A film to determine segment V; perpendicular lines are added from the margins of the diaphragms to line #5 on the P-A film.

The heart is outlined as indicated in Figure 1–6; line D_1 is drawn through the long axis from the right atrium to the apex. Perpendiculars D_2 to D_1 are drawn to the farthest borders of the heart outline. Line D_3 is drawn noting the longest distance across the heart shadow on the lateral film.

Measurements such as the following are then made from each segment and recorded on a data sheet (Fig. 1–7):

1. The width and depth of each segment is recorded in centimeters, measuring from the midpoint of the segment; the height is also recorded.
2. The measurements are then multiplied (width × depth × height) and added together.

3. The sum is multiplied by a factor (0.581) derived from the formula for the volume of an ellipsoidal cylinder and a correction factor for x-ray divergence. This product is the total thoracic volume (TTV).

The non-gas volume (NGV) must be subtracted from the TTV. The volume under the right and left diaphragms is calculated separately, as follows:

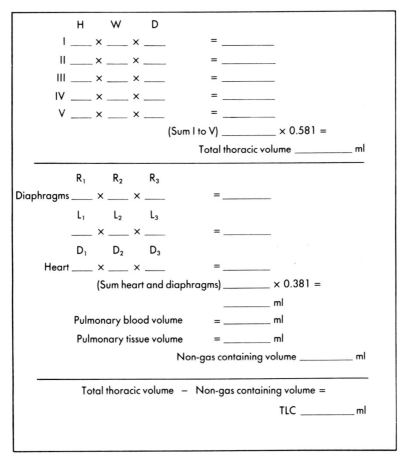

FIG 1–7.
Typical data record sheet for radiologic estimation of total lung capacity *(TLC)*. The height *(H)*, width *(W)*, and depth *(D)* of each of the five thoracic segments *(I* to *V)* are multiplied; these five products are added and multiplied by a factor derived from the equation for the volume of an ellipsoid (see text). A similar procedure is used for the two hemidiaphragms and heart; their volumes are added to those for the pulmonary blood and tissue. The difference between the total thoracic volume and the nongas volume is the TLC.

1. R_1 equals half the length of line #5; R_2 is the height of the right diaphragm; and R_3 is the length of line #5 on the lateral film.
2. L_1, L_2, and L_3 are measured similarly for the left side.
3. The product of these measurements is multiplied by 0.381, a factor for their volumes.
4. The heart dimensions D_1, D_2, and D_3 are treated similarly (see Fig. 1–7).

Pulmonary tissue and blood volumes are derived from body measurements (see Appendix). These volumes and the heart and diaphragm volumes are all subtracted from the TTV to derive the TLC (in milliliters). It is important to note that both the P-A and lateral films should be taken with the subject at TLC; the subject should specifically be instructed to inspire as deeply as possible so that TLC is accurately estimated.

Significance and Pathophysiology

Total lung capacity values determined radiologically correlate well with plethysmographic determinations in healthy persons and in subjects who have obstruction. Radiologic techniques produce more accurate TLC values than the gas dilution techniques in subjects who have moderate to severe obstruction. Radiologic determination of TLC offers a means of double checking volumes determined by other methods, and may be available where the equipment for gas dilution or plethysmographic measurements is not. Additionally, radiologic determination of TLC may provide lung volume information in subjects in whom other methods are impractical, such as those with tracheotomy. Chest radiograph determination of TLC may be used in infants or children who are unable to perform the breathing maneuvers required by gas dilution or plethysmography.

As noted previously, subjects must hold their breath at TLC when each film is exposed or the TLC may be underestimated. The presence of space-occupying lesions, such as masses or atelectasis, may confound the ellipsoid method, but more than five segments may be created in order to subdivide around a well-defined lesion. In such instances, methods employing a planimeter to measure the areas of the lung fields may produce a more accurate estimate of lung volumes than the ellipsoidal segment method. Diffuse space-occupying lesions, such as pneumonia or pulmonary edema, and diseases that increase pulmonary tissue/blood volume, may reduce the accuracy of the radiologic lung volume determination because it is difficult to correct for the discrepancy between lung areas on the film and the actual lung volume.

TOTAL LUNG CAPACITY (TLC) AND RESIDUAL VOLUME/TOTAL LUNG CAPACITY RATIO (RV/TLC × 100)

Description

The TLC is the volume of gas contained in the lungs at the end of a maximal inspiration. It is measured in liters or milliliters, and is corrected to BTPS. The RV/TLC ratio is a statement of the fraction of the TLC that can be defined as RV, expressed as a percentage.

Technique

The TLC is normally calculated by a combination of other specific lung volume measurements. The two most common are addition of the FRC plus IC, and addition of the VC plus RV. The TLC can be calculated by the radiologic method described earlier. In addition, TLC can be calculated using one of several single-breath techniques (i.e., single-breath He dilution or single-breath N_2 washout). These techniques are commonly used in conjunction with other measurements when a lung volume determination is required for the calculation of a particular parameter (i.e., alveolar volume for the calculation of $D_{L_{CO}}$ discussed in Chapter 5). Although single-breath lung volume determinations correlate well with multiple-breath techniques in healthy subjects, single-breath lung volume values tend to be lower than true values in the presence of moderate to severe obstruction.

The RV/TLC ratio is calculated by dividing the RV by the TLC and multiplying by 100 to express the ratio as a percentage. Either ambient temperature, pressure, saturated with water vapor (ATPS), or BTPS values may be used in the ratio, but both RV and TLC must be expressed in the same units before performing the division.

Significance and Pathophysiology

The TLC may be decreased by processes which occupy space in the lungs, such as edema, atelectasis, neoplasms, or fibrotic lesions. Other diseases which commonly result in decreased TLC include pulmonary congestion, pleural effusions, pneumothorax, or thoracic deformities. Pure restrictive defects show proportional decreases in most lung compartments (Fig. 1–8) as described previously in this chapter for FRC and RV, although it is possible for one lung volume subdivision to be reduced more than others. When the TLC value is less than 80% of that predicted or less than the 95% confidence limit, a restrictive process should be suspected. A reduction in VC with a normal or increased FEV_1/FVC ratio (see Chapter 3) is suggestive of restriction; if there is a contradiction between VC and TLC in defining restriction, the classification should be based on the TLC.

Total lung capacity may be either normal or increased in obstructive processes such as asthma, chronic bronchitis, bronchiectasis, cystic fibrosis, and emphysema. (see Table 1–1 and Fig. 1–8.) A normal or increased TLC does not mean that ventilation or surface area for diffusion is normal. A normal TLC in conjunction with an increased RV value is consistent with air trapping (i.e., the RV increased at the expense of the VC). When the TLC is greater than 120% of that predicted or above the 95% confidence limit as a result of increased RV, hyperinflation is present and the work of breathing is usually increased. For predicted normal values, see the Appendix.

In healthy young adults, the RV/TLC ratio may vary from 20% to 35%. Because this is a ratio, values greater than 35% may result from absolute increases of the

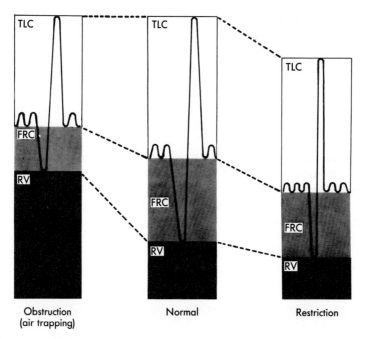

Obstruction (air trapping)	Normal	Restriction

FIG 1–8.
Lung volume changes in obstructive and restrictive patterns. A comparison of the changes in lung volume compartments in obstruction and restriction shows the following: in obstruction (with air trapping) functional residual capacity *(FRC)* and residual volume *(RV)* are both increased at the expense of the vital capacity (VC), and so total lung capacity (TLC) remains relatively unchanged; similar increases in RV and FRC may occur without loss of VC, in which case the TLC increases (not shown). In restrictive patterns, the FRC, RV, and VC are all decreased proportionately, resulting in a decrease in the TLC, which defines restriction (see text).

RV, as in emphysema, or from a decrease in the TLC because of a loss of VC. Values greater than 35% do not indicate dysfunction but are of greatest diagnostic value when correlated to the absolute values of RV and TLC. A large RV/TLC ratio in the presence of an increased TLC is often indicative of hyperinflation, while an increased RV/TLC ratio with a normal TLC indicates that air trapping is present.

SELF-ASSESSMENT QUESTIONS

1. Which of the following correctly describes the measurement of FRC by the nitrogen washout method:
   I. Alveolar N_2 is assumed to be 65% at the beginning of the test
   II. The test is continued until alveolar N_2 is reduced to 1%
   III. Some N_2 is released from the blood and tissues
   IV. A fast response O_2 analyzer is required
   a. I, II, IV
   b. I, III only
   c. II, III only
   d. II, IV only

2. A subject has these lung volumes measured using a body plethysmograph:

	Measured	**Predicted**
VC	4.2	4.4
FRC	3.9	3.7
RV	2.2	2.1
TLC	6.3	6.5

   These values are consistent with:
   a. An obstructive pattern such as emphysema
   b. A restrictive pattern such as sarcoidosis
   c. Normal lung volumes
   d. A calculation error involving the FRC

3. Calculate the FRC from the closed-circuit method using the following data (refer to the Appendix):

   $$He \text{ added} = 0.5 \text{ L}$$
   $$\%He \text{ initial} = 9.0\% \ (0.090 \text{ as a fraction})$$
   $$\%He \text{ final} = 7.1\% \ (0.071 \text{ as a fraction})$$
   $$He \text{ absorption correction} = 0.1 \text{ L}$$
   $$Temperature = 24° \text{ C}$$

   FRC = _____ (BTPS)

4. A patient with emphysema has his FRC measured using the closed-circuit method and by plethysmography with the following results obtained:

FRC (He dilution) = 4.1 L

V_{TG} = 4.6 L

FRC predicted = 3.6 L

Which of the following best explains these results?
a. This is a normal pattern for the patient's diagnosis
b. The FRC by He dilution is erroneously low
c. The V_{TG} is erroneously high
d. The predicted FRC is incorrect

5. Which of the following are characteristic of obstructive lung diseases when measured values are compared with predicted normals:
I. The VC is increased
II. The FRC is increased
III. The RV is increased
IV. The RV/TLC ratio is increased
a. I, II, IV
b. II, III, IV
c. II, III only
d. I, IV only

6. In order to measure FRC in a body plethysmograph, the V_{TG} must be measured by:
a. Closing the shutter at a point of zero flow
b. Having the patient pant rapidly and deeply
c. Closing the shutter at end-expiration
d. Performing a combined Raw/V_{TG} maneuver

7. The following raw data is obtained from spirometry and an He dilution FRC test (all values have been corrected to BTPS):

VC = 3.4 L

IC = 2.1 L

ERV = 1.3 L

FRC = 3.9 L

Calculate the:
RV _____ L
TLC _____ L
RV/TLC % _____ %

9. A subject has the following results from spirometry and N_2 washout FRC determination:

	Measured	Predicted	% Predicted
VC	4.6	4.7	98
FRC	8.2	3.8	216
TLC	10.2	7.5	136
RV/TLC%	55	37	—

Which of the following best explains these findings:
a. The subject has normal lung volumes
b. The subject has severe air trapping
c. A leak occurred during the VC test
d. A leak occurred during the FRC test

10. A subject with an RV that is 60% of that predicted and an RV/TLC ratio of 20% would be most likely to have:
a. An obstructive disease pattern
b. A restrictive diease disease pattern
c. Combined obstruction and restriction
d. Normal lung function

11. Alveolar pressure is measured in the body plethysmograph by:
a. Integrating the flow signal during panting
b. Plotting box pressure changes when the shutter is closed
c. Recording mouth pressure when the shutter is closed
d. Deriving the slope of mouth flow/box pressure

12. In addition to a spirometer, which of the following pieces of equipment are needed to perform a closed-circuit FRC determination:
   I. CO_2 and H_2O absorbers
   II. an O_2 source
   III. an He analyzer
   IV. an N_2 analyzer
a. I, II, III
b. I, II, IV
c. I, III only
d. II, IV only

13. Which of the following methods of lung volume determination correlates best with body plethysmography in subjects with moderate or severe obstruction:
a. N_2 washout
b. He dilution
c. single-breath washout
d. radiologic estimation

SELECTED BIBLIOGRAPHY

GENERAL REFERENCES

American Thoracic Society: Lung function testing: selection of reference values and interpretive strategies. *Am Rev Respir Dis* 144:1202, 1991.

Briscoe WA: Lung volumes. In Fenn WO, Rahn H, editors: *Handbook of physiology: respiration II.* Washington, 1965, Am Physiological Society.

Forster RE: *The lung: clinical physiology and pulmonary function tests,* ed 3. Chicago, 1988, Year Book Medical Publishers.

Crapo RO, Morris AH, Clayton PD, et al: Lung volumes in healthy nonsmoking adults. *Bull Eur Physiopathol Respir* 18:419, 1982.

Goldman HI, Becklake MR: Respiratory function tests: normal values at median altitudes and the prediction of normal results. *Am Rev TB Pulmon Dis* 79:457, 1959.

Grimby G, Soderholm B: Spirometric studies in normal subjects. III: Static lung volumes and maximal voluntary ventilation in adults with a note on physical fitness. *Acta Med Scand* 173:199, 1964.

Hibbert ME, Lanigan A, Raven J, et al: Relation of armspan to height and the prediction of lung function. *Thorax* 43:657, 1988.

Pare PD, Wiggs BJR, Coppin CA: Errors in the measurement of total lung capacity in chronic obstructive lung disease. *Thorax* 38:468, 1983.

West JB: *Pulmonary pathophysiology: the essentials,* ed 4. Baltimore, 1992, Williams and Wilkins.

West JB: *Respiratory physiology: the essentials,* ed 4. Baltimore, 1992, Williams and Wilkins.

RADIOLOGIC TLC

Barnhard JH, Pierce JA, Joyce JW, et al: Roentgenographic determination of total lung capacity. *Am J Med* 28:51, 1960.

Barrett WA, Clayton PD, Lambson CR, et al: Computerized roentgenographic determination of total lung capacity. *Am Rev Respir Dis* 113:239, 1976.

Bencowitz HZ: Program for calculation of radiographic total lung capacity. *Am Rev Respir Dis* 128:576, 1983.

Campbell SC: Estimation of total lung capacity by planimetry of chest radiographs in children 5 to 10 years of age. *Am Rev Respir Dis* 127:106, 1983.

O'Brien RJ, Drizd TA: Roentgenographic determination of total lung capacity: normal values from a national population survey. *Am Rev Respir Dis* 128:949, 1983.

Wehr KL, Masferrer R: Clinical usefulness of planimetric estimation of total lung capacity. *Respir Care* 20:966, 1975.

THORACIC GAS VOLUME

Begin P, Peslin R: Influence of panting frequency on thoracic gas volume measurements in chronic obstructive pulmonary disease. *Am Rev Respir Dis* 130:121, 1984.

Bohadana AB, Peslin R, Hannhart B, et al: Influence of panting frequency on plethysmographic measurements of thoracic gas volume. *J Appl Physiol* 52:739, 1982.

Brown R, Hoppin FG, Ingram RH Jr, et al: Influence of abdominal gas on the Boyle's law determination of thoracic gas volume. *J Appl Physiol* 44:469, 1978.

Dubois AB, Bothelo SY, Bedell GH, et al: A rapid plethysmographic method for measuring thoracic gas volume: a comparison with a nitrogen washout method for measuring functional residual capacity. *J Clin Invest* 35:322, 1956.

Habib MP, Engel LA: Influence of the panting technique on the plethysmographic measurement of thoracic gas volume. *Am Rev Respir Dis* 117:265, 1978.

Leith DE, Mead J: Principles of body plethysmography. DLD-NHLBI, November 1974.

Lourenco RV, Chung SYK: Calibration of a body plethysmograph for measurement of lung volume. *Am Rev Respir Dis* 95:687, 1967.

Rodenstein DO, Stanescu DC, Francis C: Demonstration of failure of body plethysmography in airway obstruction. *J Appl Physiol* 52:949, 1982.

Shore SA, Huk O, Mannix S, et al: Effect of panting frequency on the plethysmographic determination of thoracic gas volume in chronic obstructive pulmonary disease. *Am Rev Respir Dis* 128:54, 1983.

FOREIGN GAS LUNG VOLUMES

Hathirat S, Renzetti AD, Mitchell M: Measurement of the total lung capacity by helium dilution in a constant volume system. *Am Rev Respir Dis* 102:760, 1970.

Hickham JB, Blair E, Frayser R: An open circuit helium method for measuring functional residual capacity and defective intrapulmonary gas mixing. *J Clin Invest* 33:1277, 1954.

McMichael J: A rapid method of determining lung capacity. *Clin Sci* 4:167, 1939.

Meneely GR, Ball CO, Kory RC, et al: A simplified closed circuit helium dilution method for the determination of the residual volume of the lungs. *Am J Med* 28:824, 1960.

Rodenstein DO, Stanescu DC: Reassessment of lung volume measurements by helium dilution and by body plethysmography in chronic airflow obstruction. *Am Rev Respir Dis* 126:1040, 1982.

Schaaning CG, Gulsvik A: Accuracy and precision of helium dilution technique and body plethysmography in measuring lung volume. *Scand J Clin Invest* 32:271, 1973.

2

Ventilation and Ventilatory Control Tests

TIDAL VOLUME (V_T), RESPIRATORY RATE (f), AND MINUTE VENTILATION ($\dot{V}_E$)

Description

The V_T is the volume of gas inspired or expired during each respiratory cycle, usually measured in milliliters and corrected to BTPS (see Fig. 1–1). Conventionally, the volume expired is expressed as the V_T. The respiratory rate or frequency of breathing (f) is the number of breaths per unit of time, usually per minute. The total volume of gas expired per minute ($\dot{V}_E$) includes both the alveolar and dead space ventilation, and is recorded in liters per minute, BTPS. Conventionally, the minute volume is termed as the $\dot{V}_E$.

Technique

The V_T can be measured directly by simple spirometry (see Fig. 1–1). The subject breathes into a volume displacement or flow-sensing spirometer. The volume change is measured directly from the excursions or integrated from the flow signal, and may be recorded as a spirogram either on paper or on a computer graphic screen. Because no two breaths are identical, the V_T inhaled or exhaled should be measured for at least 1 minute and then divided by the rate to determine the average volume:

$$V_T = \frac{\dot{V}}{f}$$

where:

$\dot{V}$ = volume expired or inspired over a given interval, usually the $\dot{V}_E$

f = number of breaths for same interval (i.e., the respiratory rate)

The $\dot{V}_I$ and V_T (inhaled) are normally slightly greater than the $\dot{V}_E$ and V_T (exhaled) because the body at rest produces a slightly lower volume of CO_2 than the volume of O_2 consumed. This exchange difference is termed *the respiratory exchange ratio* (RER). The RER is calculated as the $\dot{V}_{CO_2}/\dot{V}_{O_2}$, where $\dot{V}_{CO_2}$ is the volume of CO_2 produced, and $\dot{V}_{O_2}$ is the volume of O_2 consumed per minute. The RER is usually assumed to be about 0.8 at rest. For most clinical purposes, the expired volume is measured to calculate V_T.

The V_T may also be estimated by means of respiratory inductive plethysmograph (RIP), discussed in Chapter 9. The RIP uses coils of wire as transducers that respond to changes in the cross-sectional area of the rib cage and abdominal compartments. With appropriate calibration, inductive plethysmography can be used to measure V_T without connections to the airway.

The respiratory rate may be determined by counting the chest movements, or the excursions of spirometer. Counting the rate for several minutes and taking an average produces a more accurate value than shorter measurements.

The $\dot{V}_E$ may be determined by allowing the subject to breathe either into or out of a volume displacement or flow-sensing spirometer or similar metering device for at least 1 minute. Measuring expired gas volume for a period of several minutes and dividing by the time gives an average $\dot{V}_E$. Because it is measured from expired gas, the $\dot{V}_E$ is usually slightly smaller than the $\dot{V}_I$ because of the respiratory exchange ratio. In most clinical situations, this difference is negligible; BTPS corrections should be made.

Significance and Pathophysiology

Average V_T for healthy adults ranges between 400 and 700 mL, but there is considerable variation even from these values. Decreases in V_T occur in many types of pulmonary disorders, such as severe restrictive patterns, pulmonary fibrosis, and neuromuscular diseases such as myasthenia gravis. Decreased tidal breathing caused by mechanical changes in the lungs or chest wall (i.e., compliance and/or resistance) is almost always accompanied by increased respiratory rate, which is required to maintain alveolar ventilation. Decreases in both V_T and respiratory rate are usually associated with respiratory center depression, and typically result in alveolar hypoventilation. Some subjects who have pulmonary disease may exhibit increased V_T, particularly at rest. The V_T alone is not an adequate indicator of alveolar ventilation, and should never be considered outside the context of rate and $\dot{V}_E$. A rapid rate and small V_T may suggest increased dead space or hypoventilation, but must be correlated with arterial pH and P_{CO_2} values to be definitive. Many subjects who have little or no pulmonary disease display increased V_T as a result of breathing into the pulmonary function apparatus with the nose occluded. Resting ventilation may be spuriously increased when measured during pulmonary function testing.

The normal respiratory rate ranges from 10 to 20 breaths per minute. Increased demand for ventilation, such as that during exercise, usually results in increases in both the rate and depth of breathing; thus, respiratory frequency is often a good indicator of the stimulus to ventilate. Increases or decreases in the respiratory rate are indications of a change in the ventilatory status. Breathing frequency, when evaluated with the V_T, may be used as an index of ventilation. Hypoxia, hypercapnia, metabolic acidosis, conditions that cause decreased lung compliance, and exercise all result in increases in respiratory rate, in the presence of a normal respiratory drive. Decreased breathing frequency is common in central nervous system depression and in CO_2 narcosis. As with measurement of V_T, respiratory rate may be falsely elevated in subjects breathing through mouthpieces and other unfamiliar breathing circuits, and/or using a nose clip.

Normal $\dot{V}_E$ ranges from 5 to 10 L/min, with wide variations in normal subjects. The $\dot{V}_E$ is the primary index of ventilation when used in conjunction with blood gas values. Because the $\dot{V}_E$ is the sum of both the dead space and effective alveolar ventilation, absolute values for $\dot{V}_E$ do not necessarily indicate either hypoventilation or hyperventilation.

A large $\dot{V}_E$ at rest (i.e., greater than 20 L/min) may result from an enlarged dead space volume, as an increase in total ventilation is required to maintain adequate alveolar ventilation. The $\dot{V}_E$ increases in response to hypoxia, hypercapnia, metabolic acidosis, anxiety, and exercise. Decreased ventilation may result from hypocapnia, metabolic alkalosis, respiratory center depression, or neuromuscular disorders which involve the ventilatory muscles.

Hypoventilation is defined as inadequate ventilation to maintain a normal arterial P_{CO_2}, and the respiratory acidosis that results. Hyperventilation is ventilation in excess of that needed to maintain adequate CO_2 removal, with a resulting respiratory alkalosis. The diagnosis of either hyperventilation or hypoventilation requires blood gas analysis (see Chapter 6).

VENTILATORY RESPONSE TESTS FOR CO_2 AND O_2

Description

Ventilatory response to CO_2 is the measurement of the increase or decrease in $\dot{V}_E$ caused by breathing various concentrations of CO_2 under normoxic conditions (Pa_{O_2} = 90 to 100 mm Hg). It is recorded as L/min/mm Hg P_{CO_2}.

Ventilatory response to O_2 is the measurement of the increase or decrease in $\dot{V}_E$ caused by breathing various concentrations of O_2 under isocapnic conditions (Pa_{CO_2} = 40 mm Hg). The change in ventilation (L/min) may be recorded in relation to changes in Pa_{O_2} or saturation as monitored by oximetry.

Occlusion pressure (P_{100}) is the pressure generated at the mouth during the first 100 msec of an inspiratory effort while breathing against an occluded airway. Changes in P_{100} are related to changes in the ventilatory stimulant (hypercapnia or hypoxemia). It is usually measured in centimeters of water (cm H_2O).

Technique

Carbon dioxide response can be measured in two ways:

1. *Open-circuit technique.* When using this method, various concentrations (1% to 7%) of CO_2 in air or oxygen are breathed from a demand valve or reservoir until a steady state is reached. Measurements of end-tidal P_{CO_2} ($P_{ET_{CO_2}}$), arterial P_{CO_2}, P_{100}, and $\dot{V}_E$ may be made at each concentration.

2. *Closed-circuit or rebreathing technique.* The subject rebreathes from a one-way circuit containing a reservoir of 7% CO_2 in O_2 (Fig. 2–1). Valves and

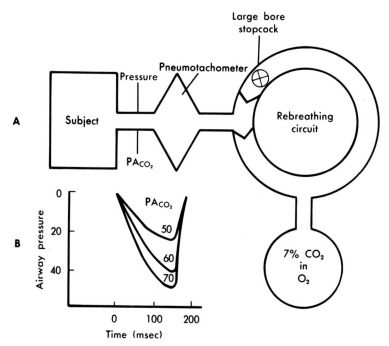

FIG 2–1.

A, apparatus for measurement of occlusion pressure (P_{100}). A rebreathing circuit is diagrammed, which can be used for measurement of P_{100} and ventilation during a CO_2 response test. Hypercapnia is produced at full arterial saturation by rebreathing 7% CO_2 in O_2 from a reservoir approximately equal to the subject's vital capacity plus 1 L. Ventilation is measured by integration of the signal from the pneumotachometer. The $P_{A_{CO_2}}$ is estimated from exhaled CO_2 wave form, and pressure is monitored from taps at the mouthpiece. A large-bore stopcock, shutter, or similar device is placed in the inspiratory line to occlude flow during at the beginning of a breath. One-way valves allow the large-bore stopcock to be closed during expiration so that the next inspiration occurs against the occluded airway at functional residual capacity. **B,** representative tracings of the airway pressure developed during occlusion at various levels of hypercapnia ($P_{A_{CO_2}}$, 50, 60, 70) for the first 100 msec. A rapid recording device, oscilloscope, or computer display may be used to obtain the curves.

pressure taps for monitoring P_{100} and ports for extracting gas samples for $P_{ET_{CO_2}}$ determinations are included in the circuit. A pneumotachometer (see Chapter 9) is placed in line to record $\dot{V}_E$. Similarly, the gas reservoir bag may be placed in a rigid container or box, and volume change measured by connecting a spirometer to the container (i.e., "bag-in-box" setup). The subject rebreathes until the concentration of $P_{ET_{CO_2}}$ exceeds 9%, or until 4 minutes have elapsed. The rebreathed gas also is analyzed to ascertain that the $F_I O_2$ remains above 0.21. The subject's oxygen saturation (Sa_{O_2}) may also be monitored by means of a pulse oximeter (see Chapter 9). Changes in $\dot{V}_E$ are monitored and plotted against $P_{ET_{CO_2}}$ to obtain a response curve.

The O_2 response can be measured by either open- or closed-circuit techniques:

1. *Open-circuit technique.* The subject breathes gas mixtures containing oxygen concentrations from 12% to 20% to which CO_2 is added to maintain alveolar P_{CO_2} ($P_{A_{CO_2}}$) at a constant level. Once a steady state is reached, Pa_{O_2}, $\dot{V}_E$, and P_{100} can be measured. This procedure, often called a step test, is repeated with decreasing O_2 concentrations to produce the response curve. Continuous monitoring of $P_{ET_{CO_2}}$ is necessary to titrate the addition of CO_2 to the system to maintain isocapnia (Fig. 2–2). Pa_{O_2} should be monitored, as it often varies from the alveolar P_{O_2} ($P_{A_{O_2}}$). Pulse oximetry may be used to monitor changes in saturation. The CO_2 response curves sometimes are measured at widely varying Pa_{O_2} values, and the subsequent difference in ventilation or P_{100} at any particular P_{CO_2} is attributed to the response to hypoxemia.

2. *Closed-circuit technique (progressive hypoxemia).* The subject rebreathes from a system similar to that used for the closed-circuit CO_2 response, but that contains a CO_2 scrubber. Carbon dioxide can be added to the inspired gas to maintain isocapnia or a variable blower may be used to direct a portion of the rebreathed gas through the scrubber to maintain isocapnia (see Fig. 2–2). Response to decreasing inspired P_{O_2} is monitored by recording $\dot{V}_E$ and/or P_{100}, and the Pa_{O_2} or saturation is measured either directly by indwelling catheter or by pulse oximetry.

The P_{100} (or $P_{0.1}$, *occlusion pressure*) is measured using a system similar to that in Fig. 2–1 and Fig. 2–2. A port at the mouth records pressure changes vs. time on a storage oscilloscope, high-speed recorder, or by computer. A large-bore stopcock or electronic shutter mechanism is included in the inspiratory line so that inspiratory flow can be randomly occluded. The stopcock or shutter can be closed so that inspiration occurs against a complete occlusion at or close to FRC. The entire apparatus is usually hidden from the subject so that he or she is unaware of the impending airway occlusion. A pressure-time curve is recorded either from the oscilloscope or by means of a high-speed (i.e., 50 to

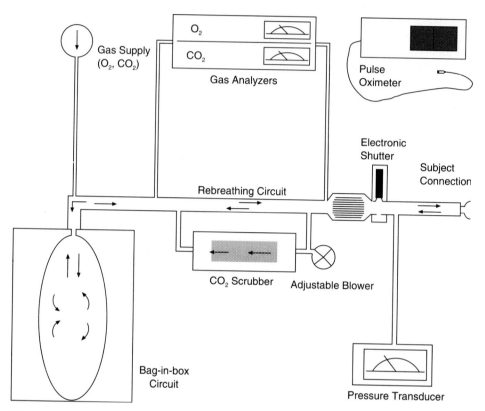

FIG 2–2.
Closed-circuit system for the rebreathing O_2 response test. The circuit allows the subject to rebreathe into a bag to which CO_2 and/or O_2 can be added. Gas analyzers allow continuous monitoring of gas concentrations in the circuit during testing. Ventilation is measured by integrating flow from the pneumotachometer or attaching a spirometer to the bag-in-box setup. A pressure transducer and mouth shutter allow the measurement of P_{100}, while a pulse oximeter provides data on the subject's saturation. A CO_2 scrubber with an adjustable blower allows the level of CO_2 in the system to be maintained at baseline levels. By scrubbing just enough of the exhaled CO_2 to maintain a near normal alveolar P_{CO_2}, increases in ventilation resulting from the gradual consumption of the O_2 in the circuit can be measured.

100 mm/sec) recorder. The P_{100} is usually measured at varying $P_{ET_{CO_2}}$ values or levels of desaturation to assess the effect of changes in the stimuli to ventilation. P_{100} and $\dot{V}_E$ are usually graphed against $P_{ET_{CO_2}}$ (Fig. 2–3), or $P_{A_{CO_2}}$ vs. O_2 saturation (O_2 response).

Significance and Pathophysiology

The response to an increase in $P_{A_{CO_2}}$ in the normal individual is a linear increase in $\dot{V}_E$ of approximately 3 L/min/mm Hg P_{CO_2}. The normal range of response varies from 1 to 6 L/min/mm Hg Pco_2, and some variation is present in repeated testing of the same individual. The response to CO_2 in subjects who have obstructive disease may be reduced. This reduction is partially attributable to increased airway resistance, which has been shown to reduce ventilatory response in healthy individuals. It is not yet clear why some subjects who have obstructive disease increase ventilation to maintain a normal $Paco_2$ while others tolerate an increased $Paco_2$. A plot of $\dot{V}E$ vs. PET_{CO_2} may be used to determine a slope or response curve.

The normal response to a decrease in Pao_2 appears to be exponential once the Pao_2 has fallen to the range of 40 to 60 mm Hg. Again, there are wide variations in responses among individuals. The hypoxic response is increased in the presence of hypercapnia and decreased in hypocapnia. Subjects who have severe chronic obstructive lung disease and chronic CO_2 retention receive their primary respiratory stimulus from the hypoxemic response. This group of subjects may suffer severe or even fatal respiratory depression if that response is obliterated by uncontrolled oxygen therapy.

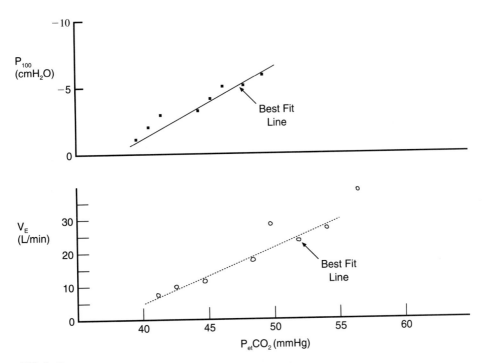

FIG 2–3.
A, P_{100} plotted against end-tidal CO_2 (PET_{CO_2}), as might be obtained during a CO_2 rebreathing study. **B,** minute ventilation plotted against PET_{CO_2} during the same study. Individual points may be plotted and a "best-fit" line constructed by statistical methods. The slope of the best-fit line is the rate at which ventilation or occlusion pressure increases with increasing stimulation from the rebreathed CO_2.

Some subjects with minimal intrinsic lung disease show markedly decreased response to hypoxemia or hypercapnia. These include subjects with myxedema, obesity-hypoventilation syndrome, obstructive sleep apnea, and idiopathic hypoventilation. The CO_2 and O_2 response measurements, along with tests of pulmonary mechanics, may be particularly valuable in the evaluation and treatment of these subjects.

The P_{100} ($P_{0.1}$) has been suggested as a measurement of ventilatory drive, independent of the mechanical properties of the lungs. Because no airflow occurs during occlusion of the airway, significant interference from mechanical abnormalities, such as increased resistance or decreased compliance, is omitted. Reflexes from the airways and chest wall are also of little influence during the first 100 ms of the occluded breath. Therefore, the pressure generated can be viewed as proportional to the neural output of the medullary centers that drive the rate and depth of breathing. This proportionality may be influenced by other factors, however, such as body position and the contractile properties of the respiratory muscles.

Subjects whose Pa_{CO_2} values are normal have P_{100} values in the range of 1.5 to 5 cm H_2O. The P_{100} has been shown to increase in hypercapnia and hypoxia and appears to correlate well with the observed ventilatory responses. Increasing P_{CO_2} (hypercapnia) in healthy subjects typically results in an increase in the occlusion pressure of 0.5 to 0.6 cm H_2O/mm Hg P_{CO_2}, with as much as 20% variability. Some subjects who have chronic airway obstruction demonstrate little or no increase in P_{100} in response to an increase in their P_{CO_2}, even with increased airway resistance. Normal subjects experience an increase in their P_{100} when breathing through artificial resistance on challenge with high P_{CO_2} or low P_{O_2}. This failure to respond to increased resistance in the airways may predispose individuals with chronic obstructive pulmonary disease (COPD) to respiratory failure when lung infections occur. Similarly, subjects maintained on mechanical ventilation may experience difficulty in weaning if their ventilatory drive is compromised, as demonstrated by failure to increase the P_{100} when challenged with increased P_{CO_2}. Determination of the P_{100} may prove helpful in determining the effects of treatment in subjects who have abnormal ventilatory responses.

RESPIRATORY DEAD SPACE (V$_D$)

Description

Respiratory dead space (V$_D$) is that volume of the lungs that is ventilated but not perfused by pulmonary capillary blood flow. The dead space can be divided into the conducting airways, or anatomic dead space, and the nonperfused alveoli, or alveolar dead space. The combination of alveolar and anatomic dead space volumes is the respiratory, or physiologic, dead space. The V$_D$ is recorded in milliliters or liters, BTPS.

Technique

Anatomic dead space may be estimated from an individual's body size but the total wasted ventilation, or respiratory dead space, is of greater importance clinically. The V_D can be calculated in two ways. The first uses Bohr's equation defining V_D:

$$V_D = \frac{(F_{A_{CO_2}} - F_{E_{CO_2}})}{F_{A_{CO_2}}} V_T$$

where:

$$V_T = \text{tidal volume}$$

$$F_{A_{CO_2}} = \text{fraction of } CO_2 \text{ in alveolar gas}$$

$$F_{E_{CO_2}} = \text{fraction of } CO_2 \text{ in expired gas}$$

Because the concentration of CO_2 in the alveoli is difficult to measure, the partial pressures of the component gases may be substituted and the equation written thus:

$$V_D = \frac{(Pa_{CO_2} - P_{E_{CO_2}})}{Pa_{CO_2}} V_T$$

where:

$$Pa_{CO_2} = \text{arterial } P_{CO_2}$$

$$P_{E_{CO_2}} = P_{CO_2} \text{ of expired gas sample}$$

Note that the arterial P_{CO_2} is substituted for the alveolar P_{CO_2}; this presumes that equilibration is perfect between the alveoli and pulmonary capillaries, which may not be true in certain diseases. The test is based on the assumption that there is very little CO_2 in the atmosphere, and therefore the partial pressure of CO_2 in the expired gas is inversely proportional to the physiologic dead space, or V_D. By collecting gas over several respiratory cycles and obtaining simultaneous Pa_{CO_2}, all the variables are supplied and a reasonably accurate physiologic dead space calculation can be made by applying the previous equation. The estimate becomes more accurate as more expired gas is collected. The accuracy depends on the measurement of $\dot{V}_E$, as well as the partial pressures of CO_2 in both the expired gas and in the arterial sample. The mixed expired gas sample is usually collected in a bag or balloon after filling and emptying it several times with expired gas to "wash out" room air from the valves, tubing, and bag itself. The volume of gas in the bag can be measured either during collection, by inclusion of an appropriate volume transducer, or by emptying the contents into a suitable spirometer (such as a Tissot). If $\dot{V}_E$ and rate are recorded during collection, the absolute volumes of the V_D and V_T can be determined. Without

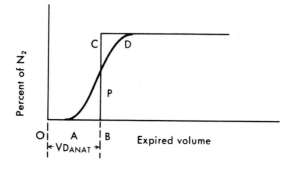

FIG 2–4.
Anatomic dead space determination. The rise in concentration of nitrogen during a single expiration after a breath of 100% O_2 is illustrated. Only the initial portion of the breath is included. As the subject expires, the N_2 concentration rises slowly at first as pure dead space gas is exhaled; then as bronchial air is expired, the N_2 concentration rises abruptly. Since different parts of the lungs empty at different rates, the change from pure dead space air to alveolar gas appears as an S-shaped curve. By constructing a square wave front *(BC)* so that the areas *ABP* and *DCP* are equal, the anatomic dead space can be estimated as equal to the volume expired up to point *B.*

measuring the actual volume expired, only the dilution ratio can be determined; this is referred to as the V_D/V_T ratio.

A second method available calculates the anatomic dead space from the single-breath analysis method (Fig. 2–4), or Fowler's method (see also Chapter 4). This technique requires continuous analysis of the concentration of N_2 in the expired gas plus simultaneous measurement of the V_E. After inhalation of 100% O_2, the subject breathes out through the recording apparatus (see Fig. 1–4, B). During the first part of the breath, pure O_2 is exhaled and the N_2 concentration remains 0 (see Fig. 2–4) until a volume equal to the anatomic dead space has been exhaled. Then the N_2 concentration rises rapidly to the level of alveolar N_2, diluted with O_2. Because the conducting airways have different lengths and volumes, the curve depicting the change in N_2 concentration does not present a "square front." By numerical methods, a square front can be constructed and the anatomic dead space is the volume expired up to the square front. Bohr's equation can be modified to apply to the data obtained from a single-breath analysis as follows:

$$V_D = \frac{(F_{A_{N_2}} - F_{E_{N_2}})}{F_{A_{N_2}}} V_E$$

where:

$$V_E = \text{expired volume}$$

$F_{A_{N_2}}$ = fraction of N_2 in alveolar gas (read from an N_2 meter at end of breath)

$F_{E_{N_2}}$ = fraction of N_2 in expired sample (computed by measuring area under %N_2 curve and dividing by V_E)

The difficulty in obtaining the $F_{E_{N_2}}$ restricts this type of calculation to more sophisticated laboratory setups.

Significance and Pathophysiology

The measurement of V_D, although difficult, yields important information regarding the ventilation/perfusion characteristics of the lungs. *Anatomic dead space* is larger in men than in women because of differences in body size; it increases along with the V_T during exercise as well as in certain forms of pulmonary disease such as bronchiectasis. It may be decreased in asthma or in diseases characterized by bronchial obstruction or mucus plugging. Because of the difficulty in measuring the anatomic dead space, estimates based on age, sex, FRC, or body size may be used. For clinical purposes, the anatomic dead space in milliliters is sometimes equated with the subject's ideal body weight in pounds.

Of greater clinical significance is the measurement of *respiratory dead space,* which is accomplished reasonably well by applying Bohr's equation. The volume of ventilation wasted on the conducting airways and poorly perfused alveoli is usually expressed as a fraction of the tidal volume, V_D/V_T, and is considered normal if the derived value is 0.2 to 0.4. Expressing dead space in this way eliminates the necessity of measuring the volume of expired gas in the application of Bohr's equation. Physiologic dead space measurements are a good index of ventilation/blood flow ratios, because all CO_2 in expired gas comes from perfused alveoli (see Chapter 6). The V_D/V_T ratio decreases in normal subjects during exercise because of increases in the cardiac output and the increased perfusion of alveoli at the lung apices. This occurs despite absolute increases in the V_D itself. Increased dead space, and V_D/V_T ratio, may be observed in pulmonary embolism and pulmonary hypertension. In pulmonary embolism, large numbers of arterioles may be blocked, resulting in little or no CO_2 removal in the associated alveoli. In pulmonary hypertension, increased pulmonary arterial pressure causes most alveoli to be perfused, so there is little or no "recruitment" of under-perfused gas exchange units. This is most notable during exercise, when the V_D/V_T normally falls.

ALVEOLAR VENTILATION ($\dot{V}_A$)

Description

The $\dot{V}_A$ is that volume of gas that participates in gas exchange in the lungs and can be considered equal to the $\dot{V}_E$ minus the dead space ventilation per minute ($\dot{V}_D$). For a single breath, the $\dot{V}_A$ equals the V_T minus the V_D. The $\dot{V}_A$ is usually expressed as volume per unit time, normally liters per minute, BTPS.

Technique

The $\dot{V}_A$ can be calculated in two ways. First, the following equation can be used:

$$\dot{V}_A = f(V_T - V_D)$$

where:

$$V_T = \text{tidal volume}$$

$$V_D = \text{respiratory dead space}$$

$$f = \text{respiratory rate}$$

Often, for the sake of convenience, the V_D is estimated as equal to the anatomic dead space. This method is valid only when there is little or no alveolar dead space, such as in individuals who do not have pulmonary disease.

Second, because atmospheric gas contains almost no CO_2, $\dot{V}_A$ can be calculated on the basis of CO_2 elimination from the lungs. A volume of expired gas is collected in a bag, balloon, or spirometer and analyzed to determine the volume of CO_2 contained (see Chapter 7). The following equation can then be utilized:

$$\dot{V}_A = \frac{\dot{V}_{CO_2}}{F_{A_{CO_2}}}$$

where:

$$\dot{V}_{CO_2} = \text{volume of } CO_2 \text{ produced in liters per minute (STPD)}$$

$$F_{A_{CO_2}} = \text{fractional concentration of } CO_2 \text{ in alveolar gas}$$

If an end-tidal CO_2 monitor is used, a close approximation of the concentration of alveolar CO_2 is easily obtained and the equation simplified as follows:

$$\dot{V}_A = \frac{\dot{V}_{CO_2}}{\% \text{ alveolar } CO_2} \times 100$$

End-tidal CO_2 may not equal alveolar CO_2 in subjects with grossly abnormal patterns of ventilation/perfusion (see Chapter 6).

The same equation can be used with a substitution of the arterial P_{CO_2} for the alveolar P_{CO_2} (i.e., $P_{A_{CO_2}}$), again presuming that arterial blood and alveolar gas are in equilibrium. The equation then becomes:

$$\dot{V}_A = \frac{\dot{V}_{CO_2}}{Pa_{CO_2}} \times 0.863$$

where:

$\dot{V}_{CO_2}$ = CO$_2$ production in mL/min (STPD)

Pa_{CO_2} = partial pressure of arterial CO$_2$

0.863 = factor for converting from concentration to partial pressure and correcting $\dot{V}_{CO_2}$ to BTPS

Significance and Pathophysiology

Both methods are suitable for calculating the $\dot{V}_A$. The CO$_2$ elimination method is more accurate than the equation $\dot{V}_A = f(V_T - V_D)$, when anatomic dead space is used in place of V_D. The differences become more apparent in situations where there are pronounced ventilation/blood flow imbalances. The $\dot{V}_A$ at rest is about 4 to 5 L/min, with large variations in healthy individuals. The adequacy of the $\dot{V}_A$ can only be determined by arterial blood gas studies. Low $\dot{V}_A$ associated with acute respiratory acidosis (i.e., Pa_{CO_2} greater than 45 and pH less than 7.35) defines *hypoventilation*. Excessive $\dot{V}_A$ (i.e., Pa_{CO_2} less than 35 and pH greater than 7.45) defines *hyperventilation*. Chronic hypoventilation and hyperventilation are associated with abnormal Pco_2 values, but near-normal pH values. Decreased $\dot{V}_A$ can result from absolute increases in dead space as well as decreases in total ventilation ($\dot{V}_E$).

SELF-ASSESSMENT QUESTIONS

1. A subject performing a closed-circuit hypoxic response test abruptly stops the test and complains of dizziness; this is most likely because of:
   a. Inadequate scrubbing of CO$_2$
   b. Failure to maintain isocapnia
   c. Incomplete gas mixing in the circuit
   d. Excessive resistance in the circuit

2. A subject has the following results after 4 minutes of a CO$_2$ rebreathing test:

	Time 0	**4 Minutes**
$P_{ET_{CO_2}}$ (mm Hg)	40	56
$\dot{V}_E$ (L/min)	6	48

These findings are consistent with a ventilatory response that is:
   a. Markedly reduced
   b. Slightly reduced

   c. Normal

   d. Extremely high

Questions 3, 4, and 5 refer to the following case:

A subject's exhaled gas is collected in a meteorologic balloon for 5 minutes, then analyzed for P_{O_2}, P_{CO_2}, and volume expired. Blood gases are drawn simultaneously, and the following data are recorded:

Room temperature:	25° C	PB:	750 mm Hg
Volume expired:	27.5 L (ATPS)	Fe_{CO_2}:	0.046 (4.6%)
Respiratory rate:	12/min (average)		
pH: 7.38	P_{CO_2}: 44	P_{O_2}: 71	

3. What is this subject's:

   $\dot{V}_E$ _____ L/min (BTPS)

   V_T _____ mL (BTPS)

4. What is the subject's:

   V_D/V_T _____ %

5. Calculate the subject's:

   $\dot{V}_A$ _____ L/min (BTPS)

6. In order to calculate respiratory dead space (V_D), which of the following are required:

   I. V_T

   II. $\dot{V}_E$

   III. Pa_{CO_2}

   IV. Pe_{CO_2}

   a. I, III

   b. II, IV

   c. I, III, IV

   d. III, IV only

7. Hyperventilation can be defined by:

   I. Respiratory rate greater than 25/min

   II. Ventilation greater than 15 L/min (BTPS)

   III. Pa_{CO_2} less than 35 mm Hg

   IV. pH greater than 7.45

   a. I, II

   b. III, IV

   c. I, II, III

   d. II, IV

8. Which of the following parameters should be measured to assess the adequacy of the output of the respiratory centers:
   a. Pa_{CO_2}
   b. Pa_{O_2}
   c. V_D/V_T
   d. P_{100}

9. Which of the following tests require a variable CO_2 scrubbing device in the breathing circuit:
   a. Dead space determination
   b. Closed-circuit O_2 response test
   c. Closed-circuit CO_2 response test
   d. Open-circuit CO_2 response test

10. A subject has the following data recorded during a rebreathing CO_2 response test:

Time (min)	0	1	2	3	4
PET_{CO_2} mm Hg)	38	41	48	54	61
$\dot{V}E$ (L/min)	5.1	5.2	5.5	5.4	5.5

These findings are consistent with:
   a. A decreased ventilatory response
   b. A normal ventilatory response
   c. An improperly calibrated pneumotachometer
   d. A malfunctioning end-tidal CO_2 analyzer

SELECTED BIBLIOGRAPHY

GENERAL REFERENCES

Forster RE: *The lung, clinical physiology and pulmonary function tests,* ed 3. Philadelphia, 1986, Yearbook Medical Publishers.

West JB: *Pulmonary pathophysiology: the essentials,* ed 4. Baltimore, 1992, Williams and Wilkins.

West JB: *Respiratory physiology: the essentials,* ed. 4. Baltimore, 1991, Williams and Wilkins.

VENTILATION

Gray JS, Gracius FS, Carter ET: Alveolar ventilation and dead space problem. *J Appl Physiol* 2:307, 1956.

Riley RL, Cournand A: 'Ideal' alveolar air and the analysis of ventilation-perfusion relationships in the lungs. *J Appl Physiol* 1:825, 1949.

Severinghaus JW, Stipfel M: Alveolar dead space as an index of distribution of blood flow in pulmonary capillaries. *J Appl Physiol* 10:335, 1957.

CONTROL OF VENTILATION

Cherniack NS, Lederer DH, Altose MD, et al: Occlusion pressure as technique in evaluating respiratory control. *Chest* 70(suppl):137, 1976.

Read DJC: A clinical method for assessing the ventilatory response to carbon dioxide. *Australas Ann Med* 16: 20, 1967.

Rebuck AS, Campbell EJM: A clinical method for assessing the ventilatory response to hypoxia. *Am Rev Respir Dis* 109:345, 1974.

Shaw RA, Schonfeld SA, Whitcomb ME: Progressive and transient hypoxic ventilatory drive tests in healthy subjects. *Am Rev Respir Dis* 126:37, 1982.

3

Spirometry and Pulmonary Mechanics

FORCED VITAL CAPACITY (FVC)

Description

The forced vital capacity (FVC) is the maximum volume of gas that can be expired, when the subject tries as forcefully and rapidly as possible, after a maximal inspiration to total lung capacity. A maneuver performed similarly beginning at maximal expiration and inspiring as forcefully as possible is called forced inspiratory vital capacity (FIVC). The FVC and FIVC maneuvers are often performed in sequence to provide a continuous flow-volume loop (see section on "Significance and Pathophysiology"). Both the FVC and FIVC are recorded in liters, BTPS.

Technique

The FVC is measured by having the subject, after inspiring maximally to TLC, expire as forcefully and rapidly as possible into a volume-displacement or flow-sensing spirometer. The volume expired may be read directly from a volume-time tracing such as that produced on a kymograph (Fig. 3–1), or derived from the integration of a flow signal. A spirometer that produces a hard-copy tracing (either volume-time or flow-volume) is essential for clinical laboratory purposes to allow visual inspection of the maneuver. Devices providing numerical data alone may be helpful for simple screening, but the results should be correlated with data obtained from a spirometer that meets the criteria proposed by the American Thoracic Society (see Chapter 11). Because the FVC maneuver is an effort-dependent test, not all subjects will be able to perform it acceptably. Criteria for judging the validity of spirometric data are detailed in Chapter 11. The reported volumes should be corrected to BTPS.

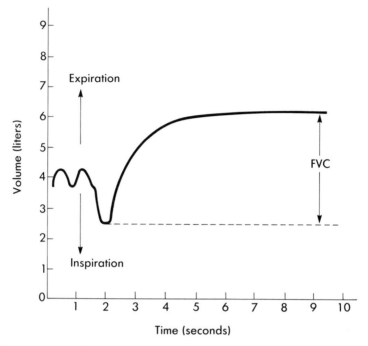

FIG 3–1.
Forced vital capacity *(FVC)*. Typical spirogram plotting volume against time as the subject exhales forcefully. In this tracing, expiration causes an upward deflection; in some systems the tracing is inverted. The subject inspires to the maximal inspiratory level *(dashed line)* at which point the lungs are close to total lung capacity. The subject then expires as forcefully and rapidly as possible to the maximal expiratory level, at which the lungs contain only the residual volume (see text).

Significance and Pathophysiology

The FVC is normally equal to the slow vital capacity (VC) (see Chapter 1). In subjects without obstruction, the FVC and VC should be within 5% of each other. The FVC and VC may differ substantially if the subject's effort is variable, or in the presence of severe *airway obstruction*. The FVC may be lower than the VC in some subjects with obstructive diseases if the forced expiration causes bronchiolar collapse from which air trapping results. The FVC may be reduced in emphysema because of loss of support for the small airways (i.e., airways less than 2 mm in diameter). The large pressure across the walls of the airways during a forced expiration results in collapse of the terminal portions of the airways. Gas is trapped in the alveoli and cannot be expired, causing the FVC to appear smaller than the VC. The FVC also may be reduced by mucus plugging and bronchiolar narrowing, as found in chronic bronchitis, chronic or acute asthma, bronchiectasis, and in cystic fibrosis. Reduced FVC also may be seen in some subjects with large airway obstructive processes such as tumors or diseases affecting the patency of the trachea and mainstem bronchi.

Not all subjects with airways obstruction exhibit a reduction in FVC in relation to their predicted values. However, the time required to expire the FVC (forced expiratory time [FET]) is often prolonged. Normal subjects can expire their FVC within 4 to 6 seconds. Subjects who have severe obstruction (such as in emphysema) may require 20 seconds or longer to expire their FVC. Accurate measurement of the FVC in severely obstructed subjects may be limited by the interval over which the spirometer accumulates volume. Many spirometers allow only 10 seconds of volume recording. The FVC and flows derived from it may be inaccurate if the subject continues to exhale for a longer time. An accurate diagnosis of obstruction, however, usually can be made from 10 seconds of recording (see Chapter 11).

Decreased FVC is also a common feature of *restrictive diseases.* A lower than predicted FVC in subjects with restriction may result from an increase in fibrotic tissue as in pulmonary fibrosis. Fibrotic changes most often result from inhalation of dust or other toxins which directly damage pulmonary tissue. Fibrosis may also result from the toxic effects of some drugs or from radiation (used in treating lung cancer). Restriction may also result from congestion of the pulmonary blood vessels as in pneumonias, pulmonary hypertension, or pulmonary edema. Space-occupying lesions such as tumors or pleural effusions also may reduce the FVC by compressing the surrounding lung tissue. Neuromuscular disorders such as myasthenia gravis, or chest deformities such as scoliosis limit chest wall movement. Any disease which affects the bellows action of the chest or the distensibility of the lung tissue itself tends to result in a reduced FVC. Obesity and pregnancy are common causes of reduced FVC because they interfere with movement of the diaphragm and excursion of the chest wall.

Interpretation of the FVC in obstructive diseases requires correlation with flows. Significant differences between the FVC and VC should be noted. The VC may be used to calculate the $FEV_{1\%}$ (see FEV_1 in this chapter) if it is larger than the FVC. In restrictive patterns, the FVC should be considered in relation to other lung volumes, particularly the TLC. A reduced FVC (or VC) is a nonspecific finding. If there is a contradiction between the FVC and the TLC in defining restriction, the TLC should be used to assess the severity of the disorder. Forced vital capacity values less than 80% of predicted, or less than the 95% confidence limit, are considered abnormal in both obstruction and restriction. Clinical interpretation of FVC values which are close to the lower limit of normal require consideration of the disease states being investigated. An FVC of 80% of predicted would be interpreted differently in a healthy subject with no symptoms than it would in a subject with a history of cough or wheezing. Values much lower than expected denote a marked reduction of FVC, and are often accompanied by a patient's complaint of exertional dyspnea.

The validity of the FVC maneuver depends largely on the subject's effort and cooperation, as well as on the instruction and coaching supplied by the technologist. Many subjects require several attempts before they perform the maneuver acceptably. In most instances, a demonstration by the technologist will assist the subject in giving a maximal effort. Placement of the mouthpiece between the teeth and lips, maximal inspiration, a slight pause, and maximal expiration may all be demonstrated. Emphasis should be placed on the initial burst of air, and on continuing expiration for at least 6 seconds. Because of its central role in routine spirometry, the acceptability of the FVC should be evaluated according to specific criteria (see Chapter 11).

FORCED EXPIRATORY VOLUME (FEV$_T$)

Description

The FEV$_T$ is the volume of gas expired over a given time interval (T) from the beginning of an FVC maneuver. The time interval is stated as a subscript to FEV. Those intervals in common use are FEV$_{0.5}$, FEV$_{1.0}$, FEV$_{2.0}$ and FEV$_3$. The FEV$_T$ is normally stated in liters, and T is expressed as seconds (Fig. 3–2). Of the various FEV measurements, the FEV$_{1.0}$ is the most widely used.

Technique

The FEV$_T$ may be measured by introducing a means of timing an FVC maneuver over the described intervals. Normally this is done by recording the FVC spirogram on graph paper moving at a fixed speed. The forced expired volume at any interval can be read from the graph as seen in Figure 3–2. Because accurate measurement of the FEV intervals depends on determination of the *start-of-test* (FVC), the spirometer should provide a tracing or printout. A graph allows direct measurement of both volume and time, and permits *back-extrapolation* when necessary (see Chapter 11). Computerized spirometers detect the start-of-test as a change in flow or volume above a certain threshold. The computer then stores volume and flow data points in memory and generates a representation of the volume-time graph. If only the expiratory data is presented, assessing the start-of-test values may be difficult. Inaccurate FEV values may result if the subject began the FVC maneuver slowly or with hesitation. Some portable spirometers report FEV$_T$ by integration of the expiratory flow without a spirogram. Such measurements should be used with caution because it may be difficult to determine if the maneuver was performed adequately (see Chapter 11). All FEV$_T$ values should be corrected to BTPS.

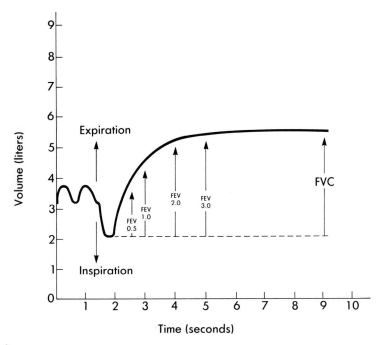

FIG 3–2.
Forced expiratory volume *(FEV)* maneuver. A spirogram of an FEV_T maneuver, with the subject exhaling as forcefully and rapidly as possible just as for the forced vital capacity. *Arrows* indicate the FEV at intervals of 0.5, 1.0, 2.0, and 3.0 seconds. Precise timing and acceptable "start-of-test" are required in order to determine the FEV_T accurately (see text and Chapter 11).

Significance and Pathophysiology

Because FEV_T maneuvers measure the volume of gas expired over various units of time, they are, in reality, measures of the average flow over their respective intervals. Decreased values for FEV_T are common in both obstructive and restrictive patterns. FEV_T values also may be reduced by poor effort or cooperation by the subject.

An obstructive ventilatory defect is characterized by a reduction in the maximal airflow from the lung with respect to the maximal volume (FVC or VC) that can be expired. Airflow is limited by airway narrowing during forced expiration. Airway obstruction may result from mucus secretion, bronchospasm, and inflammation, which are consistent with asthma or bronchitis. Airflow limitation may also result from loss of elastic support for the airways themselves, as in emphysema. The earliest changes in obstructive patterns is thought to occur in the terminal portion of the spirogram. Abnormal flows in the small airways may be detected even before the FEV_1 decreases. These changes in the flows at the terminal part of the spirogram are not specific for small airway disease.

The FEV_1 may also be decreased in the presence of obstruction to the large airways (trachea and bronchi). Tumors or foreign bodies that limit airflow cause the FEV_1 to be reduced, but these defects are better characterized by flow reductions across the entire forced expiration (see Flow-Volume Curves in this chapter).

The FEV_1 and the FEV_1/FVC ratio (see below) are the most widely used and best standardized indices of obstructive disease. Reduction of the FEV_1 in the presence of a reduced FEV_1/FVC ratio defines an obstructive impairment. The severity of obstructive disease may be gauged by the extent to which the FEV_1 is reduced. The ability to work and function in daily life is related to the FEV_1 and FVC. Morbidity (likelihood of dying) from respiratory disease is similarly related to the degree of obstruction as measured by the FEV_1. Subjects with markedly reduced FEV_1 values are much more likely to die from chronic obstructive pulmonary disease or from lung cancer. Although the FEV_1 correlates with prognosis and severity of symptoms in many forms of obstructive lung disease, the outcomes for individual patients cannot be accurately predicted.

Restrictive processes such as fibrosis, edema, space-occupying lesions, neuromuscular disorders, obesity, and chest wall deformities may all cause FEV_T values to be decreased. The reduction in the volume expired in the first second ($FEV_{1.0}$) occurs in much the same way as the reduction in FVC. Unlike the pattern seen in obstructive disorders where the FVC is preserved and FEV_T values reduced, in restriction the FVC and FEV_T values are proportionately decreased. In many subjects with moderate or severe restriction, the FEV_1 may nearly equal the FVC. The entire FVC, because it is reduced, is exhaled in the first second. Distinction between obstructive and restrictive causes for reduced FEV_T values is made by relating the FEV_T to the FVC as the FEV_T/FVC ratio (see below), and to other flow measurements. Further definition of obstruction vs. restriction may require measurement of lung volumes (FRC, TLC, etc.).

Of all the FEV parameters, the FEV_1 is the most widely used spirometric parameter, particularly for assessment of airway obstruction. The FEV_1 is used in conjunction with the FVC for simple screening, for assessment of response to bronchodilators, for inhalation challenge studies, and for detection of exercise-induced bronchospasm (see Chapters 7 and 8).

The validity of the FEV_1 measurement depends largely on the cooperation and effort of the subject. Adequate instruction and demonstration of the forced expiratory maneuver by the technologist is essential. This is true of all the FEV_T parameters commonly recorded ($FEV_{0.5}$, FEV_1, FEV_2, and FEV_3), as each of these includes the effort-dependent early portion of the forced exhalation. Reproducibility of the FEV_T should be within 5% for the two best of at least three acceptable maneuvers. Accurate measurement of the FEV requires an acceptable spirometer, preferably one that allows inspection of the volume-time curve and back extrapolation (see Chapter 11).

FORCED EXPIRATORY VOLUME/FORCED VITAL CAPACITY RATIO (FEV$_T$/FVC OR FEV$_{T\%}$)

Description

The FEV$_{T\%}$ is the ratio of FEV$_T$ to the FVC expressed as a percentage, where T is the interval from the start of the FVC maneuver up to a specific time (see FEV$_T$ above). The FEV$_{1\%}$ (FEV$_1$/FVC) is by far the most widely used of the various FEV$_T$ parameters. The slow VC (either inspiratory or expiratory) may be used in place of the FVC if the VC is significantly larger (see below).

Technique

The subject performs the FVC maneuver and the FVC and FEV$_T$ are computed. The ratio is then derived with this equation:

$$FEV_{T\%} = \frac{FEV_T}{FVC} \times 100$$

The reported values for FEV$_T$ and FVC should be the maximal values obtained from at least three acceptable FVC maneuvers. The FEV$_1$/FVC ratio based on these values may be different than the ratio obtained on any single maneuver (see Chapter 11). If both slow and forced VC maneuvers have been performed, it is preferable to use the largest VC in the calculation. Many computerized spirometers, however, calculate only the ratio obtained from a series of FVC maneuvers. If other measurements of flow (i.e., either instantaneous or averaged) are to be reported, they should be obtained from the single forced expiratory maneuver with the largest sum of FVC and FEV$_1$ (see Chapter 11).

Significance and Pathophysiology

A healthy young adult can expire 50% to 60% of the FVC in 0.5 second, 75% to 85% in 1 second, 94% in 2 seconds, and 97% in 3 seconds. The actual expected ratio in an individual subject may be derived by taking the ratio of predicted FEV$_T$ to predicted FVC, although many studies of normals have derived regression equations for the ratio itself. The FEV$_1$/FVC ratio tends to decrease with increasing age. Older healthy adults may have FEV$_1$/FVC ratios in the 65% to 75% range. The FEV$_1$ decreases with age presumably because of changes in the elastic properties of the lung itself.

Subjects without airways obstruction can expire their entire FVC within 4 seconds. Conversely, subjects who have obstructive disease will show a reduced FEV$_{T\%}$ ratio for the typical intervals (i.e., 1 second, 2 seconds, etc.). The FEV$_1$/FVC ratio is the most important measurement for distinguishing an obstructive impairment. An FEV$_1$/FVC lower than 65% is the hallmark of obstructive disease. Because the FEV_1/FVC is a ratio, mild to moderate obstructive disease can be identified without reference to absolute predicted values. If the ratio is less than 65% (except in the oldest subjects) then some degree of obstruction is present. The $FEV_{1\%}$ may be as low as 30% in severe obstructive disease.

Diagnosis of an obstructive pattern based on spirometry should focus on the three primary variables: FVC, FEV_1, and FEV_1/FVC. Other expiratory flow measurements (such as $FEF_{25\%-75\%}$ later in this chapter) should be considered only after the presence and severity of obstruction has been determined using the primary variables above. If the FEV_1/FVC is borderline abnormal, additional flow measurements may confirm the presence of an obstructive pattern. Care should be taken when interpreting the FEV_1/FVC ratio in subjects who have FVC and FEV_1 values greater than predicted. The FEV_1/FVC ratio may appear to indicate an obstructive pattern because of the variability of the greater than normal FVC and FEV_1 values. *cannot get air in*

Subjects who have restrictive disease, such as pulmonary fibrosis, often have normal or increased $FEV_{T\%}$ values. Because air flow may be minimally affected in restrictive diseases, the FEV_1 and FVC are usually reduced in equal proportion. If the restriction is severe, the FEV_1 may approach the FVC value, and the $FEV_{1\%}$ appears to be higher than normal. The FEV_1/FVC may be 100% if the FVC is severely reduced. The presence of a restrictive disorder may be suggested by a reduced FVC and a normal or increased FEV_1/FVC ratio. Further studies, such as measurement of the TLC, should be employed to confirm the diagnosis of restriction.

Validity of the $FEV_{T\%}$ depends on the subject's effort and cooperation on the specific FEV_T and the FVC measurements. Because the values used to derive the ratio may be taken from separate maneuvers, both the FEV_T and FVC should be reproducible within 5% (see Chapter 11). Poor effort on the FVC may result in an overestimate of the $FEV_{T\%}$. If the subject exhales for less than 6 seconds, the FVC (the denominator of the ratio) will appear smaller than it actually is. The $FEV_{1\%}$ in this case will then appear larger than it actually is. Some clinicians prefer to use the largest slow VC to calculate the $FEV_{T\%}$ (see Chapter 12, Case Studies). This may be necessary if the slow VC is significantly larger than the FVC because of airway compression during maximal effort.

Patients who have moderate or severe obstruction may require more than 10 seconds to completely exhale. Even though continuing to exhale will increase the FVC measured, the diagnosis of obstruction can be made with a less than complete expiration. In some cases, a prolonged effort may difficult for the subject. The large transpulmonary pressure generated by the forced expiratory maneuver often reduces cardiac output. Subjects may complain of dizziness, seeing "spots," ringing in the ears, or numbness of the extremities. Occasionally a subject may faint as a result of the decreased cerebral blood flow. This complication may be serious if it causes the subject to fall, either from a standing or sitting position.

FORCED EXPIRATORY FLOW 25%–75% (FEF$_{25\%-75\%}$)

Description

The FEF$_{25\%-75\%}$ is the average flow during the middle half of an FVC maneuver. It is usually recorded in liters per second. This test was formerly designated the maximum midexpiratory flow rate (MMFR). Other measures of average flow over specific intervals of the FVC are usually expressed as FEF$_X$, where the subscript X describes the interval. Other FEF values that are sometimes reported include the FEF$_{200-1200}$ (the 200 to 1200 mL portion of the FVC), and the FEF$_{75\%-85\%}$.

Technique

The FEF$_{25\%-75\%}$ is measured from an FVC maneuver. The time required for the subject to expire the middle 50% of the FVC is divided into 50% of the FVC. To calculate the FEF$_{25\%-75\%}$ manually, a volume-time spirogram is used. The points at which 25% and 75% of the VC has been expired are marked on the curve (Fig. 3–3). A straight line connecting these points is extended so that it intersects two time lines 1 second apart. The flow rate (in liters per second) can be read directly as the vertical distance between the points of intersection.

Computerized measurement of the FEF$_{25\%-75\%}$ requires storage of flow and volume data points for the entire maneuver. Calculation of the average flow over the middle portion of the exhalation is simply the volume expired divided by the time required to get from the 25% point to the 75% point. The FEF$_{25\%-75\%}$ is dependent on the FVC. Large FEF$_{25\%-75\%}$ values may be derived from maneuvers that produce small FVC measurements because the "middle half" of the volume is actually gas expired at the beginning of expiration. This effect may be particularly evident if the subject terminates the FVC maneuver before reaching RV. When the FEF$_{25\%-75\%}$ is used for assessing the response to bronchodilator or inhalation challenge, the effect of changes in the absolute lung volumes must be considered. Measuring the FEF$_{25\%-75\%}$ at the same lung volumes in the comparison tests is referred to as the "isovolume" technique, and is typically applied when the FVC changes by more than 10% (indicating a change in TLC or RV). The isovolume technique may also be used with other flow measurements that are FVC dependent.

The largest FEF$_{25\%-75\%}$ is not necessarily the value reported. The FEF$_{25\%-75\%}$ is recorded from the maneuver with the largest sum of FVC and FEV$_1$ according to the American Thoracic Society's criteria for the "best test" (see Chapter 11). Flows must be corrected to BTPS.

Significance and Pathophysiology

The FEF$_{25\%-75\%}$ measures the average flow over a given interval (volume), which is based on a segment of the FVC that includes flow from medium and

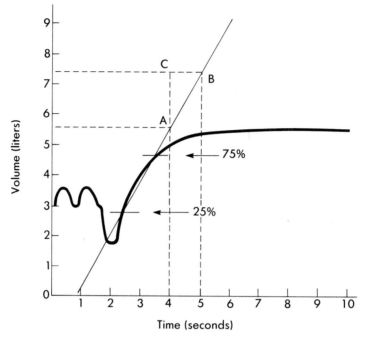

FIG 3–3.
FEF$_{25\%-75\%}$. A forced vital capacity (FVC) spirogram showing the points at which 25% and 75% of the FVC have been expired; these points may be determined by multiplying the FVC by 0.25 and 0.75, respectively. A line connecting these points is extended to intersect two time lines 1 sec apart, points A and B. The flow rate in liters per sec can be read as the vertical distance between the points of intersection *(AC)*—in this case, approximately 2 L/sec. Alternatively, the slope of the line connecting the 25% and 75% points can be determined by dividing half of the FVC by the actual time interval between the points.

small airways. Typical values for a healthy young adult average 4 to 5 L/sec. These values decrease with age. The FEF$_{25\%-75\%}$ is quite variable, even in normal subjects with 1 standard deviation approximately equal to 1 L/sec. Values as low as 65% of predicted normal may be statistically within normal limits. This variability requires guarded interpretation of the FEF$_{25\%-75\%}$.

The FEF$_{25\%-75\%}$ is indicative of the status of the medium- to small-sized airways. Decreased flow rates are common in the early stages of obstructive disease. Abnormalities in these mid-range flow measurements, however, are not specific for small airways disease. Though the FEF$_{25\%-75\%}$ may suggest changes in the small airways, it should not be used to diagnose small airways disease in individual patients. In the presence of a borderline value for FEV$_1$/FVC, low results for the FEF$_{25\%-75\%}$ may help confirm the presence of airways obstruction. When the FEV$_1$ and FEV$_1$/FVC are within normal limits the FEF$_{25\%-75\%}$ should not be graded regarding severity. Assessment of the FEF$_{25\%-75\%}$ following bronchodilator must take changes in the FVC into consideration. Volume adjustment (as described previously) has been used to allow the $FEF_{25\%-75\%}$ to be considered in bronchodilator studies. The inherent variability of the $FEF_{25\%-75\%}$ and its dependence on the FVC make it less useful than the FEV_1 for interpreting postbronchodilator changes.

Reduced $FEF_{25\%-75\%}$ is sometimes seen in cases of moderate or severe restrictive patterns, when the restrictive lesion causes a decrease in the cross-sectional area of the small airways. Figure 3–4 shows typical abnormal spirograms comparing obstructive and restrictive patterns. Case study examples

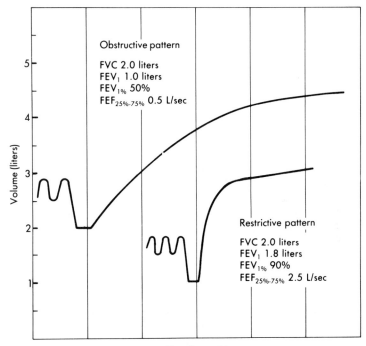

Obstructive pattern

FVC 2.0 liters
FEV_1 1.0 liters
$FEV_{1\%}$ 50%
$FEF_{25\%-75\%}$ 0.5 L/sec

Restrictive pattern

FVC 2.0 liters
FEV_1 1.8 liters
$FEV_{1\%}$ 90%
$FEF_{25\%-75\%}$ 2.5 L/sec

Volume (liters)

Time (seconds)

FIG 3–4.
Obstructive vs. restrictive spirograms. The *obstructive pattern* shows a decreased FVC as well as reduced flow rates. The volume expired in the first second *(FEV₁)* is only 50% of the forced vital capacity *(FVC)* (i.e., FEV_1/FVC or $FEV_{1\%}$). The $FEF_{25\%-75\%}$ is also markedly reduced. The *restrictive pattern* also shows a reduced FVC, approximately equal to that observed in the obstructive defect, but the FEV_1/FVC ratio is increased. In contrast to the obstructive pattern, almost all of the VC is expired in the first second. The $FEF_{25\%-75\%}$ is not decreased as in the obstructive pattern. The FVC alone cannot be used to distinguish obstructive from restrictive disease patterns. Flow rates are typically decreased in obstructive patterns, and are only decreased significantly in restrictive disease when the lung volumes are markedly reduced. The FEV_1/FVC ratio, used in conjunction with the actual measured values for FEV_1 and FVC, is the most useful parameter for differentiating obstruction from restriction (see text).

of spirometric measurements in both obstructive and restrictive disease patterns are included in Chapter 12. The general descriptions of FVC, FEV_T, and FEF_X measurements in this section may be used to help interpret the numerical data of the case studies.

The $FEF_{25\%-75\%}$ is somewhat dependent on subject effort because it depends on the FVC exhaled. Subjects who perform the FVC maneuver inadequately often show widely varying mid-expiratory flows. There is little evidence that the $FEF_{25\%-75\%}$ is more reliable than instantaneous flow measurements obtained from flow-volume curves, although it is more commonly used.

PEAK EXPIRATORY FLOW (PEF)

Description

The PEF is the maximum flow rate attained during an FVC maneuver. It is usually recorded in liters per second, but may be reported in liters per minute, BTPS.

Technique

The PEF can be measured by drawing a tangent to the *steepest* part of a volume-time spirogram. Even with a fast recording device, measurement of this slope is difficult, particularly in subjects with normal peak flows. The PEF may be measured more accurately by means of a device that senses flow directly (see Chapter 9) or by deriving flow from the rate of volume change in a volume displacement spirometer. With either method, PEF is usually represented on a flow-volume display (Fig. 3–5). The peak inspiratory flow (PIF) is measured similarly. Many portable devices are available to measure maximal flow during a forced expiration. Many of these sense flow as bulk movement of gas against a turbine or through an orifice, and record only the PEF. The PEF and PIF, whether reported in liters per second or per minute, should be corrected to BTPS.

Significance and Pathophysiology

The PEF attainable by healthy young adults may exceed 10 L/sec (600 L/min) BTPS. Even when measured using an accurate pneumotachometer, the value of PEF measurements may be limited because they are effort dependent and primarily measure large airway function. Decreased peak flows should be evaluated for reproducibility before a diagnostic interpretation is made. This same effort dependence, however, also makes the PEF a good index of subject effort. Maximal transpulmonary pressures correlate well with maximal PEF. Subjects who exert variable efforts during the FVC maneuver are seldom able to

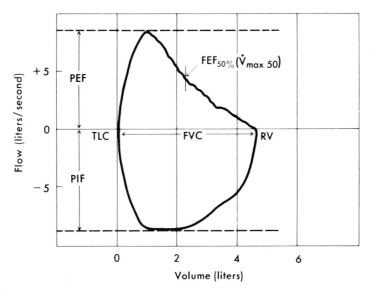

FIG 3–5.
Flow-volume loop. A flow-volume recording in which a forced vital capacity *(FVC)* and an FIVC maneuver are recorded in succession. Flow, in liters per second, is plotted on the *vertical axis* and volume, in liters, on the *horizontal axis*. The FVC can be read from the tracing as the maximal horizontal deflection along the zero flow line. Peak flows for inspiration and expiration (PEF and PIF) can be read directly from the tracing as the maximal deflections on the flow axis (positive and negative). The instantaneous flow ($\dot{V}_{max}$) at any point in the FVC can also be measured directly. Plotting devices that are capable of interjecting time marks or tics in the tracing allow the FEV_T to be read directly as well (not shown here). Phenomena such as small or large airway obstruction show up as characteristic changes in the maximal flow rates (see Fig. 3–6).

reproduce their PEF. Many clinicians now use PEF in addition to the FVC and FEV_1 to gauge maximal effort during spirometry.

Subjects with early small airways obstruction may develop an initially high flow rate before airway closing occurs, and show relatively normal PEF values. The PEF measurements, when performed with a good effort, correlate well with the FEV_1 as measured by spirometry. Severe obstruction in the small airways is accompanied by a decrease in PEF, although the reduction is often less than in the flows in the small airways themselves.

Uniformly decreased PEF is often associated with upper or large airway obstruction but is nonspecific. Assessing PEF from flow-volume loops, (along with the PIF), helps to define both the severity and site of large airway obstruction (Fig. 3–6).

Small, inexpensive devices that measure PEF as described above are becoming widely used. The PEF measured via such portable devices is most useful for following gross changes in airway function in outpatients, or for making bedside assessment of response to bronchodilators. Peak flow meters, whether the office variety or inexpensive portable type, are employed in the management of asthma. PEF measurements help to assess the degree of airway obstruction in physicians' offices, emergency rooms, and by patients at home. Alone, however, PEF measurements are not sufficient to indicate a diagnosis of asthma, or to evaluate fully the associated physiologic impairment. Daily monitoring of PEF helps to detect onset of airway obstruction. Assessing

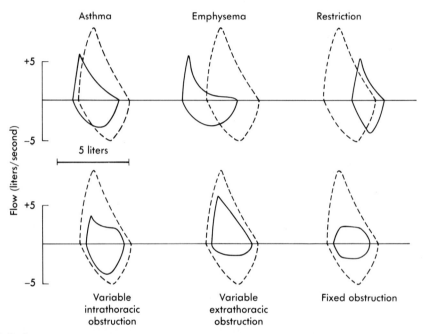

FIG 3–6.

Normal and abnormal flow-volume loops. Six curves are shown plotting flow in liters per second against the forced vital capacity (FVC). In each example, the expected curve is shown by the *dashed lines,* while the curve illustrating the particular disease pattern is superimposed. In patients who have asthma and emphysema, the portion of the expiratory curve from the peak flow to residual volume is characteristically concave. Both the total lung capacity (TLC) and residual volume (RV) points are displaced toward higher lung volumes (to the left of the expected curves in this diagram). These patterns are indicative of hyperinflation and/or air trapping. In restrictive patterns, the shape of the loop is preserved but the FVC is decreased. The TLC and RV displaced toward lower lung volume (to the right of the expected curves). The *bottom* three examples depict types of large airway obstruction. Variable intrathoracic obstruction shows reduced flows on expiration despite near normal flows on inspiration, resulting from flow limitation in the large airways during a forced expiration. Variable extrathoracic obstruction shows an opposite pattern. Inspiratory flow is reduced while expiratory flow is relatively normal. Fixed large airway obstruction is characterized by equally reduced inspiratory and expiratory flows. Comparison of the $FEF_{50\%}$ with the $FIF_{50\%}$ may be helpful in differentiating large airway obstructive processes. Because the magnitude of inspiratory flow is effort dependent, low inspiratory flows should be carefully evaluated.

day-night (circadian) variations in lung function provide objective measures for planning, initiating, or terminating therapy. The presence of changes in PEF during the day and night correlate with the degree of airway hyperresponsiveness. Peak expiratory flow measurements are most useful in following serial changes within individual subjects. Changes in PEF should be interpreted in relation to the subject's personal best value after maximum therapy.

Because simple peak flow meters may not be accurate (see ATS Standards, Chapter 11), and because of the effort dependence of the PEF, measurements should be compared with spirometry done under laboratory conditions.

FLOW-VOLUME CURVES

Description

The flow-volume curve is a graphic analysis of the flow generated during the FVC maneuver plotted against volume change; it is usually followed by a forced inspiratory volume (FIV) maneuver, plotted similarly (see Fig. 3–5). Flow is usually recorded in liters per second and the volume in liters, BTPS. The maximal expiratory flow-volume (MEFV) curve is the expiratory portion of the curve from TLC to RV. The inspiratory component is the maximal inspiratory flow-volume (MIFV), and is plotted from RV to TLC. When both the MEFV and MIFV curves are plotted together, the resulting figure is referred to as a "flow-volume loop."

Technique

The subject performs a standard FVC maneuver inspiring fully to TLC and then exhaling as rapidly as possible to RV. To complete the loop, the FVC maneuver is followed by an FIV maneuver, with the subject inspiring as rapidly as possible from RV to TLC. Volume is plotted on the X axis while flow is plotted on the Y axis. This type of spirogram must be done either with a recorder capable of plotting flow and volume from their respective analog inputs (see Fig. 9–27), by a storage oscilloscope, or by computer-generated graphics. From the loop, PIF and PEF can be read, as well as the FVC. Commonly used recording sensitivities are 2 L/sec per unit distance on the flow axis vs. 1 L per unit distance on the volume axis, though other scaling factors are sometimes used. The instantaneous flow at any lung volume (over the VC) can be read directly from the MEFV tracing. Flows at 75%, 50%, and 25% of the VC are commonly reported as the $\dot{V}_{max75}$, $\dot{V}_{max50}$, and $\dot{V}_{max25}$, respectively, with the subscript referring to the lung volume (VC) remaining. Flows at the same intervals are also reported as the $FEF_{25\%}$, $FEF_{50\%}$, and $FEF_{75\%}$ with the subscript in this scheme referring to portion of the lung volume (VC) which has been exhaled. If automatic timing is available on the graphing device or computer, the FEV_T and $FEV_{T\%}$ can be determined for specific intervals. Plotting of stored data points allows manipulation of the flow-volume tracings. Comparisons of a series of MEFV curves is achieved by superimposing the tracings or plotting with contrasting colors. Computer-generated plots permit bronchodilator or inhalation challenge studies to be presented similarly. A predicted MEFV curve can also be depicted by plotting the points for PEF, and maximal flows at 75%, 50%, and 25% of the VC. The subject's flow-volume curve can then be superimposed directly over the expected values.

Significance and Pathophysiology

All of the parameters measured from a standard volume-time tracing of the FVC maneuver can be obtained from a flow-volume curve, provided a timing mechanism is incorporated as described in the previous section. In addition, instantaneous flows at any point in either the forced expiration or forced inspiration can be easily measured. Significant decreases in either flow (indicating obstruction) or volume (indicating restriction) are easily discernable from a single graphic display.

The shape of the expiratory limb of the MEFV tracing from about 75% of the FVC down to RV is largely independent of subject effort. Flow over this segment is determined by two properties of the lung: elastic recoil and flow resistance. The lung is stretched to its maximum by inspiration to TLC. Elastic recoil determines the pressure which can be transmitted to the gas in the lung by the chest wall and expiratory muscles during a forced expiration. Resistance to flow in the airways is the second factor affecting the shape of the flow-volume curve. Flow limitation occurs in the large- and medium-sized airways during the early part of a forced expiration. The site of flow limitation migrates "upstream" rapidly during forced expiration. Resistance to flow in the small (less than 2 mm) airways is determined primarily by their cross-sectional area. In healthy subjects, flow ($\dot{V}_{max}$) over the effort-independent segment decreases in a linear pattern with decreasing volume. The pressures surrounding the airways are balanced by the gas pressure in the airways so that flow is limited at an "equal pressure point." As the lung continues to empty, the equal pressure point moves upstream into smaller and smaller airways. This continues until the lung is almost completely empty. Finally, the small airways begin to close, trapping some gas in the alveoli (the RV).

Because of this pattern of airflow limitation in the healthy lung, the expiratory curve has a "straight line" or slightly concave appearance (see Fig. 3–5). In subjects who have obstruction in the small airways, flow is decreased, particularly at lower lung volumes. The effort-independent segment of the flow-volume curve takes on a more concave or "scooped out" appearance (see Fig. 3–6). Values for $\dot{V}_{max50}$ and $\dot{V}_{max25}$ are characteristically decreased. Decreases in $\dot{V}_{max50}$ correlate well with the reduction in $FEF_{25\%-75\%}$ in subjects with small airway obstructive disease.

Because both elastic recoil *and* resistance in the small airways determine the shape of the expiratory limb of MEFV tracing, quite different lung diseases can result in similarly decreased flows. Emphysema destroys terminal lung units with a loss of elastic recoil and support for the small airways. Flow in the small airways is decreased mainly by the collapse of the unsupported walls. In contrast, bronchitis, asthma, and similar inflammatory processes increase the resistance in the small airways by edema, mucus production, and smooth muscle constriction. Flow limitation in these processes primarily results from a reduction in the cross-sectional area of the small airways. Clinically, emphysema and chronic bronchitis are often found in the same individual because of their common cause, cigarette smoking. The MEFV curve presents a picture of the extent of obstruction without necessarily determining its cause.

Obstruction of the upper airway, trachea, and mainstem bronchi show characteristic limitations to either expiratory flow, inspiratory flow, or both. The flow-volume curve is extremely useful in diagnosing these types of large airway abnormalities (see Fig. 3–6). Comparison of expiratory and inspiratory flows at 50% of the FVC is helpful in distinguishing the site of the obstruction. Fixed large airway obstructions typically result in reduced, but approximately equal, flow at 50% of the VC for both inspiration and expiration (Fig. 3–6). Obstructive processes which vary with the phase of breathing also produce characteristic patterns. Variable extrathoracic obstruction usually shows normal expiratory flows with diminished inspiratory flows. Because the obstructive process is outside the thorax, the MEFV portion of the curve appears as it would in a healthy individual. The inspiratory portion of the loop is flattened. The flow developed is dependent on how much obstruction is present. In variable intrathoracic obstruction, the PEF is usually reduced and expiratory flow is limited until the site of flow limitation reaches the smaller airways. This gives the expiratory limb a squared-off appearance. The inspiratory portion of the loop is typically normal.

Airway obstruction associated with abnormality of the muscular control of the posterior pharynx and larynx sometimes produces a ''saw-toothed'' pattern visible on the inspiratory and expiratory limbs of the MEFV curve. This pattern is sometimes observed in subjects suspected of having sleep apnea.

The PIF rate and the pattern of flow during inspiration are largely effort dependent. Poor subject effort may result in inspiratory flow patterns similar to those in variable extrathoracic obstruction. Careful instruction by the technologist should include emphasis on maximal effort during the inspiratory phase as well as the expiratory portion. However, if the inspiratory flow pattern is reproducible over repeated efforts, a true obstructive process should be suspected.

Restrictive disease processes may show normal or above-normal PEF values along with linear decreases in flow vs. lung volume. The lung volume itself as displayed on the X axis is decreased. Moderate or severe restriction demonstrates equally reduced flows at all lung volumes. Reduced flows primarily result from the decreased cross-sectional area of the small airways at low lung volumes. Simple restriction causes the flow-volume loop to appear as a miniature of the normal curve (see Fig. 3–6).

Before- and after-bronchodilator MEFV curves can be superimposed to facilitate measurement of relative increases in flow at each lung volume. The curves are usually positioned by superimposing at TLC. If postbronchodilator lung volume measurements are performed, the curves may be superimposed on an absolute volume scale. This type of presentation displays the effects of bronchodilators not only on expiratory flows, but on changes in lung volumes as well (see Fig. 3–6 for a similar plot of measured vs. predicted curves). Inhalation challenge studies (see Chapter 8) can be manipulated in a like manner to assess the reduction in flows at specific lung volumes. Tidal breathing curves or maximum voluntary ventilation (see later in this chapter) curves can also be superimposed on the flow-volume curve (inspiratory and expiratory curves). By comparing the areas enclosed under each of the curves, the subject's ventilatory reserve can be assessed. Subjects who have severe obstructive lung disease may generate maximal flow-volume curves of only slightly greater dimensions than their tidal breathing curves. In severe obstruction, flow during tidal breathing may exceed flow during a forced expiration because of collapse of the small airways. These patterns are consistent with limited ventilatory reserve and usually associated with dyspnea on exertion.

The ability to measure both flow and volume from a single graphic representation of the FVC maneuver is responsible for the widespread popularity of the flow-volume curve. Reproducible MEFV curves, particularly the PEF, are good indicators of adequate subject effort. It may be difficult, however, to gauge the validity of the start-of-test and whether exhalation was continued for at least 6 seconds from the flow-volume plot. Many spirometers allow the user to display flow-volume and/or volume-time curves. Although most computerized systems employ algorithms to calculate the back-extrapolated volume, a simultaneous volume-time tracing may be necessary to perform manual back extrapolation (see Chapter 11).

LOW DENSITY GAS SPIROMETRY

Description

Low-density gas spirometry refers to the measurement of air flow from the lungs using gases less dense than air. Maximal expiratory flow volume maneuvers may be performed using a gas mixture of 80% helium and 20% oxygen, and then comparing changes in flow in reference to the MEFV performed while the subject breathes air. Two primary parameters are derived using this technique: the change in maximal flow at specific points in the VC, usually 50% and 25% ($\Delta \dot{V}_{maxX}$), and the volume of isoflow (Viso$\dot{V}$). The Viso$\dot{V}$ is the volume of the VC remaining in the lungs when gas flow becomes independent of gas density. The VisoV̇ is normally expressed as a percentage of the FVC or VC. The $\Delta\dot{V}_{maxx}$ is recorded as the percent of change in flow at the specific point in the VC.

Technique

The MEFV curves are obtained as described previously with the subject first breathing air. Then the MEFV maneuver is repeated after the subject has breathed the He-O_2 mixture. The subject may either breathe the mixture for 10 minutes (i.e., tidal breathing) or take three slow VC breaths of the mixture before performing the maneuver. Both of these techniques yield similar results. The He-O_2 and air curves are then superimposed and matched at RV if the FVC values are different. The point at which the expiratory curves meet determines VisoV̇, the lung volume at which gas flow becomes independent of gas density (Fig. 3–7).

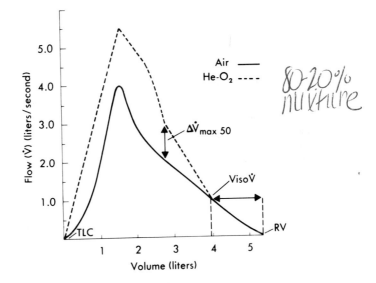

FIG 3–7.
Helium-air maximal expiratory flow volume (MEFV) curves. The subject performs two MEFV maneuvers. The first effort is a simple MEFV maneuver breathing air. The second MEFV maneuver is performed after the subject has breathed a mixture of 80% He and 20% O_2 for several minutes, or for several vital capacity breaths. The two curves are then superimposed by matching at residual volume. The $\dot{V}_{max50}$ (or $\dot{V}_{max}$ at any other lung volume) can then be read directly from each of the tracings. Decreases in the $\dot{V}_{max50}$ are consistent with diseases causing increased resistance in the small airways (i.e., less than 2 mm in diameter). There is apparently little change in $\dot{V}_{max50}$ if the primary disorder is loss of elastic recoil. The point at which both curves converge is the volume of isoflow (VisoV̇). At this lung volume, maximum expiratory flow becomes independent of the gas density of the expirate. Diseases that compromise the small airways, either by increased resistance or loss of elastic recoil, tend to increase the VisoV̇. The curves converge earlier (that is, at a higher lung volume) during the expiratory maneuver in the presence of small airways obstruction.

From the same superimposed tracing, the increase in maximal flow at 50% of the VC ($\dot{V}_{max50}$) can be determined. Because flow in larger airways depends on gas density, the amount of increase in $\dot{V}_{max50}$ while breathing the He-O_2 mixture is relatively specific for changes in airway caliber. The increase in $\dot{V}_{max50}$ while breathing the He-O_2 mixture is expressed as a percentage of the $\dot{V}_{max50}$ while breathing air and is called the $\Delta\dot{V}_{max50}$.

It can be computed using the following equation:

$$\Delta\dot{V}_{max50} = \frac{\dot{V}_{max50}He - \dot{V}_{max50}Air}{\dot{V}_{max50}Air} \times 100$$

where:

$\dot{V}_{max50}He$ = flow at 50% of the VC when breathing He-O_2 mixture

$\dot{V}_{max50}Air$ = flow at 50% of the VC when breathing air

Significance and Pathophysiology

Normal values for Viso$\dot{V}$ as a percentage of the FVC appear to be in the range of 10% to 20% for subjects 20 to 50 years of age. In the absence of obstruction in the small airways (i.e., less than 2 mm in diameter), laminar air flow, which is independent of the density of the gas being breathed, occurs near the very end of a forced expiration.

An increase in the Viso$\dot{V}$ (i.e., flow limitation in the small airways occurring earlier in the forced expiration) is consistent with obstruction of small airways. During forced expiration in normal subjects, the site of flow limitation is in the large airways until low lung volumes are reached. Breathing a gas of low density improves flow in these larger airways because the pattern of flow is turbulent. At the point that flow limitation shifts to the smaller airways at the end of a forced expiration, air flow becomes laminar and is independent of gas density. This is the point at which the He-O_2 and air curves converge. Therefore, in diseases of the small airways in which there is increased resistance (i.e., asthma) or in which there is a loss of elastic recoil (i.e., emphysema), flow limitation occurs at a higher lung volume and Viso$\dot{V}$ is increased.

The $\Delta\dot{V}_{max50}$ may be reduced in diseases that cause increased resistance. As airway diameter is compromised, flow becomes laminar at higher lung volumes and less dependent on gas density. Loss of elastic recoil does not appear to influence $\dot{V}_{max50}$. Therefore, measurement of the $\Delta\dot{V}_{max50}$ may be a relatively specific test for changes in the caliber of small airways. A subject who has early small airways disease would typically have an increased volume of isoflow. If the $\Delta\dot{V}_{max50}$ is also decreased, then a process causing primarily changes in resistance would be suspected. If, however, the $\Delta\dot{V}_{max50}$ is relatively normal despite of the abnormal Viso$\dot{V}$, then loss of elastic recoil might be the cause of the small airway abnormality. The Viso$\dot{V}$ appears to be a sensitive test for small airways obstruction. It may be abnormal even before the FEV_1 or $FEF_{25\%-75\%}$ drop below the lower limits of normal.

Low-density gas spirometry is relatively simple to perform. A means of supplying the He-O_2 mixture to the subject is the only additional equipment required. Flow-based spirometers should not be used for low-density gas spirometry unless a means of correcting for the differences in gas density and viscosity are provided. Low-density gas spirometry is primarily a research tool for evaluating the pathology causing early small airways disease.

MAXIMUM VOLUNTARY VENTILATION (MVV)

Description

The maximum voluntary ventilation (MVV) is the largest volume that can be breathed into and out of the lungs during a 10- to 15-second interval with voluntary effort. It is recorded in liters per minute, BTPS, by extrapolating the 10- to 15-second accumulated volume to 1 minute.

Technique

The MVV is measured by having the subject breathe deeply and rapidly for a 10- to 15-second interval. The subject should set the rate, and should move a volume greater than the V_T but less than the VC on each breath. The test is conducted for a specific interval, usually 10, 12, or 15 seconds. The volume expired (or inspired) may be measured by a suitable spirometer. The spirometer should have an adequate frequency response in order to accommodate a wide variety of flows (see Chapter 11). The volume may be read from a volume-time spirogram, or from a recording of accumulated volume (Fig. 3–8). Manual calculation requires measurement and summing of each volume-time deflection, which can be quite time consuming. By incorporating a one-way valve in the breathing circuit, either the volume exhaled or inhaled can be isolated. If a volume displacement spirometer is used, it must have a sufficient volume to accumulate the gas for the 10- to 15-second interval. Most spirometers have volume ranges of 7 to 10 liters, and are not suitable for collecting the accumulated volume, even for 10 seconds. Some older systems use a mechanical pen system that records only expired volume vs. time. This type of recording system allows the total volume to be read directly from the tracing, similar to the computer-generated graphic in Figure 3–8. The absolute volume of gas moved determined by any of these methods is extrapolated from 10, 12, or 15 seconds to 1 minute. The result is recorded as a flow rate in liters per minute, as follows:

$$MVV = \frac{Vol_x}{X} \times 60$$

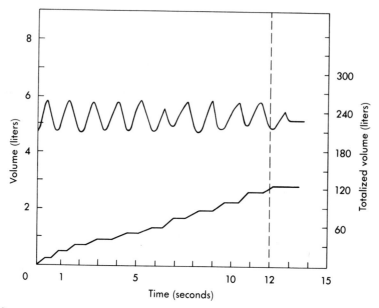

FIG 3–8.
Maximum voluntary ventilation (MVV). A composite MVV spirogram on which breath-by-breath volume change and totalized volume are plotted against time. The *top tracing* shows the actual volume moved during each breath over a 12-second interval. In order to calculate MVV, the volumes of individual breaths are added and multiplied by a factor of 5 (i.e., 60 seconds/12 seconds = 5). Because the MVV is stated as a flow rate in liters per minute, the values for 12 seconds must be extrapolated to 1 minute. The *lower tracing* is computer generated and depicts the totalized volume, in liters, per minute, exhaled during the 12-second maneuver. In this example, the volume is approximately 120 L/min, as read from the right-hand scale. Healthy subjects can maintain the same MVV flow throughout the maneuver. Subjects who have pulmonary disease will show decreased absolute values. The MVV will often decrease significantly as the maneuver progresses because of fatigue of the respiratory muscles, increased work of breathing, or because of air trapping.

where:

Vol_X = the volume in liters inspired or expired in X seconds

X = duration of the maneuver in seconds (usually 10, 12, or 15 seconds)

60 = factor for extrapolation from seconds to minutes

The volumes must be corrected to BTPS.

Significance and Pathophysiology

The maximum voluntary ventilation is a test of the overall function of the respiratory system. It is influenced by the status of the respiratory muscles, the compliance of the lung-thorax system, the condition of the ventilatory control mechanisms, and the resistance offered by the airways and tissues. Maximum voluntary ventilation values in healthy young men average between 150 and 200 L/min. Values are slightly lower in healthy females and decrease with age in both men and women. MVV values are quite variable in healthy subjects. Normal values may vary by as much as 30% from the mean, so only large reductions in MVV are usually considered significant.

The MVV is typically decreased in subjects with moderate or severe obstructive disease. This may be the result of the increased airway resistance caused by bronchospasm or secretion of mucus, as in asthma. Reduction of the MVV may also occur because of hyperinflation, as found in emphysema. The MVV maneuver exaggerates air trapping and airflow limitation. Volume-time tracings made with a volume displacement device may show a shift in the tracing as gas is removed from the spirometer and trapped in the lungs. A slight shift is usually noted during the first few breaths even in healthy subjects. These breaths are sometimes discarded because the subject is adjusting to a lung volume that allows maximal air flow.

The MVV maneuver also places a load on the respiratory muscles. Because both inspiratory and expiratory muscles are utilized in the MVV maneuver, weakness or decreased endurance of either system may result in low values. Similarly, poor coordination of the respiratory muscles because of a neurologic deficit may also cause low values for the MVV. Disorders affecting the control of the respiratory muscles, such as paralysis or nerve damage, may also reduce the MVV.

A markedly reduced MVV is correlated with postoperative risk for patients undergoing abdominal or thoracic surgery. Subjects who have low preoperative MVV values have an increased incidence of complications when the respiratory system is compromised by thoracic or upper abdominal surgery. Reduced strength or endurance of the respiratory muscles may be the factor making the MVV a predictor of postoperative problems.

Maximum voluntary ventilation may be helpful in estimating the level of ventilation that can be expected during exercise testing. Subjects who have moderate or severe obstruction and who have MVV values less than 50 L/min usually exhibit ventilatory limitation during exercise. Maximal ventilation during exercise is usually less than 70% to 80% of the MVV in healthy subjects. In subjects who have obstruction, the maximal ventilation during exercise may approach or even exceed their MVV. This pattern occurs in part because the MVV itself is typically reduced in obstruction. Highly conditioned healthy subjects also may reach their MVV during maximal exercise. Aerobic training allows a sufficiently high cardiac output, so ventilation becomes the factor limiting further exercise (see Chapter 7).

The MVV may remain within normal limits in some subjects who have restrictive pulmonary disease. Limitation of lung or thoracic expansion may not interfere significantly with flow. Subjects who have restrictive disease often compensate by performing the MVV maneuver with low tidal volumes (V_T) and high breathing rates.

The MVV maneuver is largely dependent on subject effort and cooperation. Low MVV values should always be weighed to ascertain whether the reduction is a result of obstruction, muscular weakness, defective ventilatory control, or poor subject performance. An indirect index of subject effort on the MVV maneuver may be obtained by multiplying the FEV_1 by a factor of 35. For example, a subject with an FEV_1 of 2 L might be expected to ventilate about 70 L/min (35 × 2 L) during the MVV test. If the measured MVV is much less than 70 L/min, then subject effort may be suspect. If the MVV exceeds 70 L/min by a large volume, the FEV_1 may be erroneous. Criteria for acceptability of the MVV maneuver are outlined in Chapter 11.

COMPLIANCE

Description

Compliance is the volume change per unit of pressure change for the lungs (C_L), the thorax (C_T), or the lungs-thorax system (C_{LT}). The compliance for all three is recorded in liters or milliliters per centimeter of water. The elastic recoil pressure is the force generated by the lungs (or thorax) at a particular lung volume. Elastic recoil pressure is recorded in centimeters of water (cm H_2O) and the reported value is usually measured at TLC.

Technique

The compliance of the lungs-thorax system (C_{LT}) may be measured as a unit. Measurement of C_{LT} is cumbersome, as it requires the subject to be completely relaxed or anesthetized with an artificial airway in place. The C_{LT} is measured by inflating the lungs of a subject in a sealed chamber by reducing the pressure around the thorax (as in an iron lung); a volume-pressure curve is then plotted. The subject likewise may be intubated with an endotracheal tube and have the lungs inflated by positive pressure. The pressure changes at various volumes above the end-expiratory level are then plotted to obtain a pressure-volume curve. This technique normally requires that the subject be anesthetized.

A similar technique is sometimes utilized for patients receiving mechanically supported ventilation with positive pressure. By inflating the lungs-thorax system with different volumes and recording the pressure during periods of no flow (usually by occluding the expiration valve of the ventilator), a pressure-volume curve can be constructed.

Both of these techniques (in anesthetized subjects and in ventilated patients) may be influenced by the position of the subject or by any contribution from the respiratory muscles. For this reason, C_{LT} is not routinely measured in clinical practice. C_L alone is determined as described below, C_T can be calculated by subtraction.

Alternatively, a subject may be allowed to breathe tidally from a spirometer before and after weights are added. The pressures used to calculate compliance are the system pressures when different weights are added. The volumes used are the changes in the end-expiratory levels (from the spirogram) that occur in response to the different pressures. Each of the techniques for measuring C_{LT} presents difficulties which limit their usefulness for clinical studies.

Measurement of C_L is accomplished by passing a catheter with a 10-cm long balloon fixed to the end into the esophagus. The catheter is advanced to mid-thorax level and then connected to a suitable pressure transducer. Serial pressure measurements are recorded at various volumes and plotted to produce a compliance curve (Fig. 3–9). Normally, the subject inspires to TLC before the measurements to standardize the lung volume history. Lung compliance increases slightly after a full inspiration. Then the subject inspires again, and pressure and volume points are measured at points of zero flow. The subject may hold the breath with the glottis open, or flow may be interrupted by means of a shutter. If the latter technique is used, mouth pressure should be subtracted from esophageal pressure to obtain the recoil pressure of the lungs. Similar measurements are recorded during the subsequent expiration.

The C_L is usually taken from the slope of the pressure-volume curve over the segment from FRC to FRC + 0.5 L. Because of the effects of a previous deep inspiration on the measured compliance, measurements are usually recorded from the exhalation half of the curve. Maximum static elastic recoil pressure (Pst) is recorded as the most negative pressure recorded at the maximum lung volume attained, normally TLC.

The optimal method of presenting compliance data is to plot the entire pressure curve (inflation and deflation) against either absolute lung volume or percent of TLC. The entire compliance curve then can be displayed together with the normal ranges for purpose of comparison.

Thoracic compliance can be derived if C_{LT} and C_L are known:

$$\frac{1}{C_{LT}} - \frac{1}{C_L} = \frac{1}{C_T}$$

Significance and Pathophysiology

Measurements of compliance determine the elasticity of the lungs, the thorax, and the combination of the two. The average C_L in a normal adult is

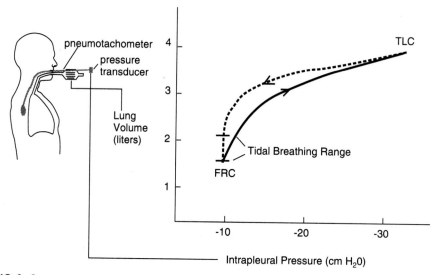

FIG 3–9.

Measurement of pulmonary compliance (C_L) using the esophageal balloon technique. Determination of C_L requires measurement of intrapleural pressure during periods of no flow at various lung volumes. A pressure transducer is connected to an esophageal balloon containing a small amount of air and located in the mid-thorax. The balloon reflects changes in intrapleural pressure (ΔP). A pneumotachometer is used to measure inspired or expired gas volumes (ΔV). Static C_L is the slope of the line defined by:

$$\frac{\Delta V \text{ (liters)}}{\Delta P \text{ (cm } H_2O)}$$

and is normally recorded from the tidal breathing range (FRC + 500 mL). The C_L varies with the lung volume history, as illustrated by the steeper expiratory pressure-volume curve. Compliance measurements are often performed with the subject in the body plethysmograph to facilitate determination of absolute lung volumes.

approximately 0.2 L/cm H_2O. The C_T has been measured as 0.2 L/cm H_2O in normal subjects. In series, the *total compliance* is calculated using the following equation:

$$\frac{1}{C_L} + \frac{1}{C_T} = \frac{1}{C_{LT}}$$

or substituting the usual values:

$$\frac{1}{0.2} + \frac{1}{0.2} = 10$$

where the reciprocal of 10 is the total compliance, (or C_{LT}):

$$\frac{1}{10} = 0.1 \text{ L/cm H}_2\text{O}$$

The total compliance is less than either of its two components because the forces act in series resulting in the counterbalancing forces of the lung parenchyma and the thorax.

The C_L varies with the volume of the lungs at the end-expiratory level (i.e., the FRC). To compare the compliance of diseased lungs with that of normal lungs, the FRC in each case should be known. Plotting the entire compliance curve against absolute lung volume (or percent of predicted lung volume) facilitates relating compliance and lung volume. This relationship is sometimes reported as the compliance/FRC ratio. Lung compliance is normally decreased (that is, the lungs themselves are stiffer) in diseases that result in congestion of the pulmonary vasculature, such as edema. The same is true in diseases in which the airways become filled with fluid or blocked, as in atelectasis, pneumonia, or loss of surfactant. Diseases that alter the normal elasticity of the lung tissue also result in lowered compliance. These include pulmonary fibrosis resulting from silicosis, asbestosis, or sarcoidosis. Decreases in compliance may also result from a pathologic reduction of FRC resulting from tumors or other space-occupying lesions. When compliance is severely reduced from any cause, clinical findings typically include increased work of breathing and dyspnea on exertion. Lung compliance normally decreases with age, presumably because of the changes in the connective tissues of the lung.

Emphysema is often accompanied by an increase in lung compliance, as elastic tissue is lost with the destruction of alveolar septa. As a result of the decreased elastic recoil of the lungs, the balance of forces between the lungs and thorax is altered, with the lungs containing a larger volume at end-expiration (FRC). Hyperinflation results from the imbalance between chest wall (tending to spring outward) and the highly compliant lungs (with reduced recoil pressure). The actual compliance of the chest wall (C_T) also may be modified in obstructive diseases because of the chronic hyperinflation. Although the lung tissue is more easily distended, the chest wall does not operate in its usual position and tends to be less compliant. Subjects with severe air trapping typically have abnormal breathing patterns and markedly increased work of breathing.

Chest wall compliance (C_T) may be decreased as a result of thoracic diseases such as kyphoscoliosis (curvature of the spine) or pectus excavatum ("pigeon breast"). Abdominal disorders such as obesity also sometimes interfere with the distensibility of the chest wall. In moderate or severe cases of thoracic deformity, gas exchange may be compromised. Gas exchange abnormalities may be exaggerated during exertion.

Lung compliance measurement requires cooperation on the part of the patient. If a mouth shutter is not used to interrupt flow, the subject must hold the breath with the glottis open so that the pressure and volume can be recorded. The compliance and elastic recoil pressure measurements themselves are largely independent of effort, provided the subject is cooperative.

AIRWAY RESISTANCE (RAW) AND CONDUCTANCE (GAW AND SGAW)

Description

Airway resistance (Raw) is the pressure difference developed per unit flow as gas flows into or out of the lungs; it is measured as the difference in pressure between the mouth (i.e., atmospheric) and that in the alveoli, related to gas flow at the mouth. This pressure difference is created primarily by the friction of gas molecules coming in contact with the conducting airways. Airway resistance is recorded in centimeters of water per liter per second (cm H_2O/L/sec).

Airway conductance (Gaw) is the flow generated per unit of pressure drop across the airways. It is the reciprocal of Raw (i.e., 1/Raw) and is recorded in liters per second per centimeter of water (L/sec/cm H_2O). Airway conductance is not commonly reported because it is dependent on lung volume. In clinical practice, specific conductance (SGaw) is usually reported. Specific conductance is the conductance per liter of lung volume, reported in liters per second per centimeter of water per liter of lung volume (L/sec/cm H_2O/L).

Technique

The Raw is the ratio of alveolar pressure (PA) to air flow ($\dot{V}$). Gas flow at the mouth can be easily measured with a pneumotachograph, and PA is measured in the body plethysmograph (Fig. 3–10). For gas to flow into the lungs during inspiration, PA must fall below atmospheric pressure; the opposite occurs during expiration. Changes in $\dot{V}$ are plotted simultaneously against plethysmograph pressure changes (which are proportional to alveolar volume changes) on a storage oscilloscope or on a computer screen. The subject pants with a small VT and a rate of 1 to 2 breaths per second. This produces an S-shaped pressure-flow curve (see Fig. 3–10, B). A tangent is measured through the zero flow point of this curve, with points at $+0.5$ L/sec and -0.5 L/sec flow defining the ends of the tangent. The slope of this line is $\dot{V}/P_{BOX}$, where $\dot{V}$ is airflow and P_{BOX} is the plethysmograph pressure.

Immediately after this measurement, an electronic shutter at the mouthpiece is closed, and changes in plethysmograph pressure (P_{BOX}) are plotted

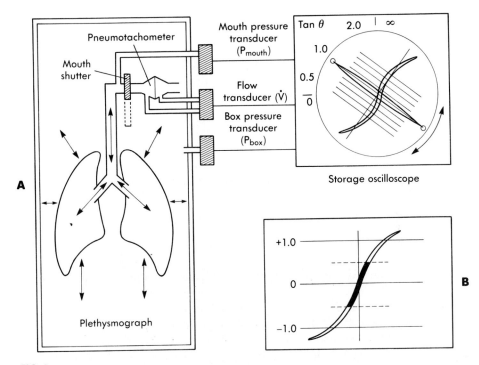

FIG 3–10.
Measurement of airway resistance (Raw) using the body plethysmograph. **A,** diagrammatic representation of the measurement of airway resistance:

$$Raw = \frac{Atmospheric\ pressure - Alveolar\ pressure}{Flow}$$

Flow ($\dot{V}$) is measured directly by means of the pneumotachometer. As the subject pants with the shutter open, flow is plotted against box pressure ($\dot{V}/P_{box}$) as an S-shaped curve on the oscilloscope. A shutter occludes the airway momentarily, usually at end-expiration, and a sloping line representing the ratio of mouth pressure to box pressure (P_{mouth}/P_{box}) is recorded in a manner similar to that used for measurement of V_{TG}. In this example, the flow tracing (shutter open) and volume tracing (shutter closed) are superimposed. The P_{mouth}/P_{box} tangent is measured as for the V_{TG}. **B,** the flow tangent is measured from the steep portion of the flow tracing, from about -0.5 L/sec to $+0.5$ L/sec. Airway resistance is then calculated as the ratio of these two tangents using appropriate calibration factors (see text and Appendix.)

against airway pressure at the mouth (P_{MOUTH}), just as is done for measurement of the V_{TG}. Because there is no air flow into or out of the lungs, mouth pressure approximates P_A. The slope of this line is P_A/P_{BOX}, where P_A equals alveolar pressure. This step serves to calibrate changes in P_A to changes in P_{BOX} for each subject.

The Raw is then calculated by taking the ratio of these two slopes in the following equation:

$$\text{Raw} = \frac{P_A/P_{BOX}}{\dot{V}/P_{BOX}} \times \frac{\text{mouth cal}}{\text{flow cal}}$$

where:

$\dot{V}$ = air flow

P_A = alveolar pressure

P_{BOX} = plethysmographic pressure, measured with the shutter open and closed

mouth cal = calibration factor for the mouth pressure transducer

flow cal = calibration factor for the pneumotachometer

Calibration factors for the flow and mouth pressure transducers are included in the previous equation (see sample calculations in the Appendix). Panting eliminates a number of artifacts from the tracing. Small rapid breaths (1 or 2 per second) reduce thermal drift. Panting also helps the subject keep the glottis open, and allows measurements to be made at or near FRC. Corrections for the resistance of the mouthpiece and flowmeter are usually made. Conductance (Gaw) can be calculated as the reciprocal of Raw.

Lung volume determinations can be easily made at the same time, using the plethysmographic method (see Chapter 1). Computerized plethysmograph systems permit V$_{TG}$, Raw, and SGaw to be measured from a combined maneuver. The subject breathes through the pneumotachometer with the plethysmograph sealed. Tidal breathing is recorded until a stable end-expiratory level (i.e., the subject is breathing near FRC) is observed. The computer stores this end-expiratory level or volume as a reference point. The subject then pants, and the open-shutter slope of $\dot{V}/P_{BOX}$ is recorded. The mouth shutter is then closed and the slope of P_{MOUTH}/P_{BOX} is recorded as described previously. Because the shutter is closed at a volume different from the FRC, the V$_{TG}$ in this maneuver does not equal the FRC. However, the change in volume from the tidal breathing level, which was stored at the beginning of the maneuver, can be used to correct the V$_{TG}$ so that the FRC can be determined. Most subjects pant above their FRC, so the V$_{TG}$ in this method is usually slightly greater. The combined maneuver allows lung volume and airway resistance to be determined quickly in a single sitting.

Both the Raw and Gaw may be expressed per liter of lung volume, specific resistance and specific conductance (SRaw and SGaw, respectively). Expressing Raw and Gaw in this way allows comparisons between subjects with different lung volumes, or in the same subject when lung volume increases or decreases.

Significance and Pathophysiology

Normal values of Raw in panting adults, using the plethysmograph method, range from 0.6 to 2.4 cm $H_2O/L/sec$. The Gaw normally varies as the reciprocal between 0.42 and 1.67 L/sec/cm H_2O. The SGaw varies in a manner similar to Gaw, even after correction for lung volume. Specific conductance values less than 0.10 to 0.15 L/sec/cm H_2O/L are typically consistent with obstructed airways. Measurements are normally standardized at flow rates of 0.5. L/sec, as described previously.

Resistance in the normal adult is distributed across the airways thus:

Nose, mouth, and upper airway $\cong$ 50%

Trachea and bronchi $\cong$ 30%

Small airways $\cong$ 20%

Because the small airways (i.e., airways less than 2 mm in diameter) contribute only about a fifth of the total resistance to flow, significant obstruction can occur in them with relatively little increase in Raw or decrease in SGaw. Early or mild obstructive processes usually are not identified by abnormalities of Raw or SGaw. Airway resistance may be increased in asthma during an acute episode by as much as three times the normal values. Swelling, mucus secretion, and bronchospasm all increase the resistance to air flow in the small- and medium-sized airways. Airway resistance is increased in advanced emphysema because of airway narrowing and collapse in some of the larger airways as well as the more distal bronchioles. Other obstructive diseases, such as bronchitis, may cause increases in Raw proportionate to the degree of obstruction in medium and small airways.

Lesions obstructing the larger airways, such as tumors, traumatic injuries, or foreign bodies, may cause a significant increase in Raw. Large airway obstructions are often accompanied by increased work of breathing, along with symptoms such as dyspnea on exertion. Because air flow in the trachea and mainstem bronchi is predominantly turbulent, breathing low-density gas mixtures reduces Raw and the work of breathing.

Measurement of Raw may be useful in distinguishing between restrictive and obstructive diseases. Airway resistance is decreased at increased lung volume because the airways (particularly the large- and medium-sized airways) are distended slightly and their cross-sectional area increases. It is often advantageous to ascertain the FRC (i.e., the V$_{TG}$ as noted previously) in conjunction with Raw measurements. To use Gaw or Raw for comparative study, these values are often expressed per unit of lung volume. Specific conductance is particularly useful for assessing changes in airway caliber following bronchodilator therapy or inhalation challenge. The SGaw may change significantly following either bronchodilator or inhalation challenge, even though other measures of flow (i.e., FEV_1) vary only slightly. The primary site of airway obstruction (i.e., large vs. small airways) may play a role in determining which parameters reflect changes in airway caliber.

Airway resistance and conductance measurements are objective insofar as the subject cannot influence results by degree of effort. For this reason, they may be useful for determining airway status in patients who are unable or unwilling to exert maximum effort. Acceptable performance of the panting maneuvers in the plethysmograph does require a certain degree of subject coordination, and not all subjects may be able to perform these maneuvers. Subjects with moderate or severe obstruction may produce pressure-flow curves during panting from which the accurate measurement of slopes is quite difficult, whether done manually or by computer.

In addition to resistance caused by $\dot{V}$ through the conducting airways, some of the total pulmonary resistance results from the friction caused by the displacement of the lungs, rib cage, and diaphragm. In healthy subjects, this "tissue" resistance is only about a fifth of the total resistance, and therefore total pulmonary resistance is approximately 20% greater than the measured Raw.

MAXIMAL INSPIRATORY PRESSURE (MIP) AND MAXIMAL EXPIRATORY PRESSURE (MEP)

Description

The MIP is the greatest subatmospheric pressure that can be developed during inspiration against an occluded airway; it normally is measured at RV. MEP is the highest pressure that can be developed during a forceful expiratory effort against an occluded airway; it usually is measured at TLC. Both MIP and MEP are sometimes measured at FRC. Both are recorded in either cm H_2O or mm Hg.

Technique

The subject is connected to a three-way valve, or shutter apparatus, with a flanged mouthpiece and nose clip in place. The airway is occluded by switching the valve to one port which is blocked, or by closing the shutter. In either method, a small leak is introduced between the occlusion and the mouth in order to negate any influence of the cheek muscles. The leak (usually a large bore needle or similar opening) allows a small amount of gas to enter the oral cavity, but does not significantly influence the lung volume or pressure measurement. For MIP, the subject is instructed to expire maximally to RV. It is helpful to monitor expiratory flow, or have the subject signal, to determine when maximal expiration has been achieved. Then the airway is occluded and the subject inspires maximally and maintains the inspiration for 1 to 3 seconds. The maximal subatmospheric pressure may be measured using a manometer, aneroid-type gauge, or pressure transducer. The pressure-monitoring device should be linear and capable of recording pressures from − 10 to approximately − 200 cm H_2O. The most negative value from at least three efforts is reported. The first second of each maneuver is discarded because it may include transient pressure changes that occur initially.

The MEP is recorded similarly, except that the subject inspires to TLC and then expires maximally against the occluded airway for 1 to 3 seconds. Longer efforts should be avoided because of the possibility of reduction of cardiac output by the high thoracic pressures (i.e., Valsalva maneuver) that are sometimes developed. Because MEP is typically larger than MIP, the pressure-monitoring device should be able to accommodate the higher pressure developed. The best of three MEP efforts is reported, again disregarding any initial pressure transients. These tests require subject cooperation and low values may reflect lack of understanding or insufficient effort.

Significance and Pathophysiology

The MIP primarily measures inspiratory muscle *strength*. The normal adult can generate inspiratory pressures in excess of − 60 cm H_2O. (For prediction regressions, see the Appendix.) Decreased MIP is seen in subjects with neuromuscular disease, or diseases involving the diaphragm, intercostals, or accessory muscles. Because the diaphragm is flattened by the increased volume of trapped gas in the lungs, MIP may also be decreased in patients with hyperinflation, such as in emphysema. The intercostals and other accessory muscles also may be compromised by alteration of the chest wall configuration. Patients with chest wall or spinal deformities, such as kyphoscoliosis, also may exhibit reduced inspiratory pressures. The MIP is sometimes used to assess subject response to training of the strength of the respiratory muscles. As a measure of respiratory muscle strength, MIP is often employed in the assessment of respiratory muscle function in subjects who require ventilatory support (see also Chapter 8, Bedside Testing).

The MEP measures the pressure generated during maximal expiration, and depends on the function of the accessory muscles of respiration and the abdominal muscles, as well as the elastic recoil of the lungs and thorax. Normal adults can generate MEP values in excess of 80 to 100 cm H_2O. Adult males may develop pressures greater than 200 cm H_2O. The MEP may be decreased in neuromuscular disorders, particularly those which result in generalized muscle weakness. The other common group of disorders that result in reduction of expiratory pressures is high cervical spine fractures. Damage to the nerves controlling the abdominal and other accessory muscles of expiration can dramatically reduce the MEP, even though the MIP is somewhat preserved.

Reduced MEP may be related to increased RV and may accompany decreased expiratory flows on simple spirometry or flow-volume maneuvers. Decreased MEP is associated with inability to cough effectively and may complicate chronic bronchitis, cystic fibrosis, or other diseases resulting in excessive mucus secretion.

Because of the effort dependence of both the MIP and MEP, it is essential to carefully instruct the subject in the performance of the maneuver. Low values may result if the subject does not inspire or expire completely before beginning the occluded airway maneuver. At least three maximal efforts should be recorded and the best efforts should be reproducible. Widely varying pressures, on either the MIP or MEP, should be considered carefully before any interpretation is made.

SELF-ASSESSMENT QUESTIONS

1. A subject has an FVC of 1.8 L (39% of predicted); the same individual has a slow VC of 2.7 L. Which of the following might explain these findings:
   I. Normal findings in severe restrictive disease
   II. Airway compression in obstructive lung disease
   III. Poor effort or early termination of the FVC
   IV. Representative findings in early small airways disease
   a. I, III, IV
   b. II, III only
   c. I, IV only
   d. II only

2. A subject has these results from simple spirometry:

	Measured	**Predicted**
FVC (L, BTPS)	4.5	4.0
FEV_1 (L, BTPS)	3.6	3.2

   These findings are consistent with:
   a. Combined obstruction and restriction
   b. Moderate obstructive disease
   c. Normal lung function
   d. Incorrectly selected predicted values

3. A subject referred for pulmonary function tests because of shortness of breath has an $FEV_{1\%}$ of 98%. This finding is suggestive of:
   a. Restrictive lung disease
   b. Obstructive lung disease
   c. Normal lung function
   d. Upper airway abnormality

4. The $FEF_{25\%-75\%}$ depends on which of the following:
   a. FVC
   b. PEF
   c. FEV_1
   d. $FEV_{1\%}$

5. In diseases that cause obstruction of the small airways, the MEFV curve may assume a concave appearance because of:
   I. Loss of elastic recoil
   II. Turbulent gas flow patterns
   III. Increased specific conductance
   IV. Increased airway resistance
   a. I, II, III, IV
   b. I, IV
   c. II, III
   d. III, IV

6. A patient has spirometry performed with the following results reported:

	Measured	Predicted
FVC (L)	4.0	4.1
FEV_1(L)	2.0	3.3
MVV (L/min)	45	110

   These findings indicate that:
   I. Obstruction is present
   II. Restriction is present
   III. The FEV_1 is overestimated
   IV. The MVV is underestimated
   a. I, II, III
   b. II, III, IV
   c. I, IV only
   d. II, III only

7. A patient with pulmonary fibrosis has a compliance study performed. Which of the following results are consistent with the diagnosis:
   a. 0.055 L/cm H_2O
   b. 1.95 L/cm H_2O
   c. 2.75 L/cm H_2O
   d. 4.00 L/cm H_2O

8. In addition to the FEV_1 and FVC, which of the following are useful in gauging subject effort during spirometry:
   a. PEF
   b. MVV
   c. $FEF_{25\%-75\%}$
   d. $\dot{V}_{max25}$

9. A 20-year-old subject performs MEFV maneuvers breathing air and then again breathing an 80% helium–20% air mixture. When the curves are superimposed, they coincide at approximately 10% of the FVC above RV. This finding is consistent with:
   a. Obstruction of small airways
   b. Normal lung function
   c. Large airway obstruction
   d. A restrictive disease process

10. When performing a determination of the MIP, the pulmonary technologist introduces a small leak at the mouthpiece:
    a. To assist the subject in maintaining the pressure
    b. To negate the influence of the cheek muscles
    c. To correct for pressure transients during the first second
    d. To allow the subject to hold the breath at TLC

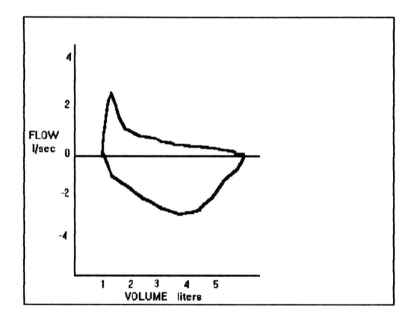

11. Which of the following is consistent with the flow-volume curve shown above:
    a. Normal forced expiratory flow pattern
    b. Variable intrathoracic obstruction
    c. Small airways obstruction
    d. Fixed extrathoracic obstruction

12. By performing a combined Raw and V_{TG} maneuver in a plethysmograph, a subject has the following values determined:

Raw (cm H_2O/L/sec) = 2.00

V_{TG} (L) = 3.00

This subject's SGaw (specific conductance) would be:

a. 0.04 L/sec/cm H_2O/L
b. 0.17 L/sec/cm H_2O/L
c. 0.67 L/sec/cm H_2O/L
d. 1.50 L/sec/cm H_2O/L

SELECTED BIBLIOGRAPHY

GENERAL REFERENCES

American Thoracic Society: Lung function testing: selection of reference values and interpretative strategies. *Am Rev Respir Dis* 144:1202, 1991.

Bates DV, Macklem PT, Christie RV: *Respiratory function in disease,* ed 2. Philadelphia, 1971, WB Saunders.

Becklake MR, Permutt S: Evaluation of tests of lung function for "screening" for early detection of chronic obstructive lung disease. In Macklem PT, Permutt S, editors: *The lung in transition between health and disease.* New York, 1979, Marcel Dekker.

Forster RE: *The lung: clinical physiology and pulmonary function tests,* ed 3. Chicago, 1986, Yearbook Medical Publishers.

Kanner RE, Morris AH, editors: *Clinical pulmonary function testing,* ed 2. Salt Lake City, 1984, Intermountain Thoracic Society.

West JB: *Pulmonary pathophysiology: the essentials,* ed 4. Baltimore, 1992, Williams and Wilkins.

FLOW-VOLUME CURVES

Acres J, Kryger M: Clinical significance of pulmonary function tests: upper airway obstruction. *Chest* 80:207, 1981.

Bass H: The flow volume loop: normal standards and abnormalities in chronic obstructive pulmonary disease. *Chest* 63:171, 1973.

Despas PJ, Leroux M, Macklem PT: Site of airway obstruction in asthma as determined by measuring flow breathing air and a helium-oxygen mixture. *J Clin Invest* 51:3235, 1972.

Gelb AF, Klein E: The volume of isoflow and increase in maximal flow at 50 percent of forced vital capacity during helium-oxygen breathing as tests of small airway. *Chest* 71:396, 1977.

Haponik EF, Blecker ER, Allen RP, et al: Abnormal inspiratory flow-volume curves in patients with sleep disordered breathing. *Am Rev Respir Dis* 124:571, 1981.

Hyatt RE, Black LF: The flow volume curve. *Am Rev Respir Dis* 107:191, 1973.

Ingram RH, Schilder DP: Effect of thoracic gas compression on the flow-volume curve of the forced vital capacity. *Am Rev Respir Dis* 94:56, 1966.

Knudson RJ, Slatin RC, Lebowitz MD, et al: The maximal expiratory flow-volume curve: normal standards, variability and effects of age. *Am Rev Respir Dis* 113:587, 1976.

Knudson RJ, Lebowitz MD, Holberg CJ, et al: Changes in the normal maximal expiratory flow-volume curve with growth and aging. *Am Rev Respir Dis* 127:725, 1983.

Miller RD, Hyatt RE: Evaluation of obstructing lesions of the trachea and larynx by flow volume loops. *Am Rev Respir Dis* 108:475, 1973.

Owens GR, Murphy DMF: Spirometric diagnosis of upper airway obstruction. *Arch Intern Med* 143:1331, 1983.

MAXIMAL RESPIRATORY PRESSURES

Arora NS, Rochester DF: Respiratory muscle strength and maximal voluntary ventilation in undernourished patients. *Am Rev Respir Dis* 126:5, 1982.

Black LF, Hyatt RE: Maximal static respiratory pressure in generalized neuromuscular disease. *Am Rev Respir Dis* 103:641, 1971.

Gilbert R, Auchincloss JH Jr, Bleb S: Measurement of maximum inspiratory pressures during routine spirometry. *Lung* 155:23, 1978.

Vincken GH, Cosio MG: Maximal static respiratory pressures in adults: normal values and their relationship to determinants of respiratory function. *Bull Eur Physiopathol Respir* 23:435, 1987.

COMPLIANCE AND AIRWAYS RESISTANCE

Baydur A, Behrakis PK, Zin WA, et al: A simple method for assessing the validity of the esophageal balloon technique. *Am Rev Respir Dis* 126:788, 1982.

Behrakis PK, Baydur A, Jaeger MJ, et al: Lung mechanics in sitting and horizontal body positions. *Chest* 83:643, 1983.

Dubois AB, Bothello SV, Comroe JH: A new method for measuring airway resistance in man using a body plethysmograph: values in normal subjects and in patients with respiratory disease. *J Clin Invest* 35:327, 1956.

Gillespie DJ: Comparison of intraesophageal balloon pressure measurements with a nasogastric-esophageal balloon system in volunteers. *Am Rev Respir Dis* 126:583, 1982.

Woolcock AJ, Vincent NJ, Macklem PT: Frequency dependence of compliance as a test for obstruction in the small airways. *J Clin Invest* 48:1099, 1969.

SPIROMETRY

American Thoracic Society: Standardization of spirometry: 1987 update. *Am Rev Respir Dis* 136:1285, 1987.

Knudson RJ, Lebowitz MD: Maximal mid-expiratory flow (FEF_{25-75}):normal limits and assessment of sensitivity. *Am Rev Respir Dis* 117:609, 1978.

Krowka MJ, Enright PL, Rodarte JR, et al: Effect of effort on measurement of forced expiratory volume in one second. *Am Rev Respir Dis* 136:829, 1987.

Leuallen EC, Fowler WS: Maximal midexpiratory flow. *Am Rev Tuberculosis* 72:783, 1955.

Morris JF, Koski A, Johnson LC: Spirometric standards for healthy non-smoking adults. *Am Rev Respir Dis* 107:57, 1971.

Nowak RM, Pensler MI, Sarkar DD, et al: Comparison of peak expiratory flow and FEV$_1$: admission criteria for acute bronchial asthma. *Ann Emerg Med* 11:64, 1982.

Sackner MA, Rao ASV, Birch S, et al: Assessment of time-volume and flow-volume components of forced vital capacity. *Chest* 82:272, 1982.

Smith AA, Gaensler EA: Timing of forced expiratory volume in one second. *Am Rev Respir Dis* 112:882, 1975.

Townsend MC, DuChene AG, Fallat RJ: The effects of underrecording forced expirations on spirometric lung function indexes. *Am Rev Respir Dis* 126:734, 1982.

4

Gas Distribution Tests

SINGLE-BREATH NITROGEN WASHOUT (SBN₂), CLOSING VOLUME (CV), AND CLOSING CAPACITY (CC)

Description

The single-breath nitrogen washout test (SBN$_2$), also referred to as the SBO$_2$ or Fowler's test, measures the distribution of ventilation. Distribution is analyzed by measuring the change in N$_2$ concentration during expiration of the vital capacity following a single breath of 100% O$_2$. The evenness of distribution is assessed by two parameters: the $\Delta\%N_{2_{750-1250}}$, and the slope of Phase III. Each of these indices is recorded as percent of change per unit of lung volume.

Closing volume (CV) is that portion of the VC that can be expired from the lungs following the onset of airway closure. The CV is usually expressed as a percentage of the VC. A related measurement, closing capacity (CC), is the sum of the CV and RV (see Chapter 1). Closing capacity is expressed as a percentage of the TLC.

Technique

The test is performed with the subject connected to spirometer with a N$_2$ analyzer in line (see Fig. 1–2) similar to the equipment used for the open-circuit FRC determination. The subject expires to RV, then inspires a measured breath of 100% O$_2$, usually from a reservoir or demand flow system. Without holding the breath, the subject expires slowly and evenly at a flow rate of 0.3 to 0.5 L/sec. The N$_2$ analyzer monitors the N$_2$ concentration of the expired gas while the exhaled volume is measured by the spirometer. The volume expired is plotted against N$_2$

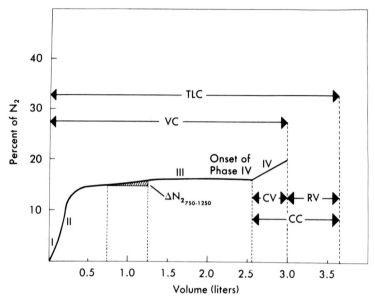

FIG 4–1.

Single-breath nitrogen elimination (SBN$_2$). A plot of the increasing nitrogen concentration on expiration following a single vital capacity *(VC)* breath of 100% O$_2$. The curve is divided into four phases: *Phase I* is the extreme beginning of the expiration when only O$_2$ is being exhaled. *Phase II* shows an abrupt rise in N$_2$ concentration as mixed bronchial and alveolar air is expired. *Phase III* is the alveolar gas plateau, and nitrogen concentration changes slowly as long as ventilation is uniformly distributed. *Phase IV* is an abrupt increase in N$_2$ concentration as basal airways close and a larger proportion of gas comes from the nitrogen-rich lung apices. Several useful parameters are derived from the SBN$_2$ tracing. Anatomic dead space can be calculated (see Chapter 2). The $\Delta N_{2750-1250}$ and slope of Phase III are indexes of the evenness of ventilation distribution. Closing volume *(CV)* can be read directly from the onset of Phase IV until residual volume *(RV)* is reached; VC can also be read directly. RV, total lung capacity *(TLC)*, and closing capacity *(CC)* can be calculated if the area under the curve is determined either by planimetry or electronic integration (see text).

concentration on a suitable graph (Fig. 4–1). This washout curve can be divided into four phases:

Phase I   is extreme upper airway gas (from the anatomic dead space) consisting of 100% O$_2$.

Phase II   is mixed V_D gas in which the relative concentrations of O$_2$ and N$_2$ change abruptly as the anatomic V_D volume is expired.

Phase III   is a plateau caused by the exhalation of alveolar gas, in which relative O$_2$ and N$_2$ concentrations change slowly and evenly.

Phase IV   is marked by an abrupt increase in the concentration of N$_2$ that continues until RV is reached.

The initial 750 mL of expired gas contains mostly dead space gas from Phases I and II and is not used in the analysis of distribution of ventilation. The difference in N_2 concentration between the 750 mL and 1250 mL points is called the delta N_2 ($\Delta\%N_{2_{750-1250}}$).

The slope of Phase III is the change in N_2 concentration from the point at which 30% of the VC remains up to the onset of Phase IV, and is recorded as $\Delta\%N_2$ per liter of lung volume.

The volume expired from the onset of Phase IV up to the termination of the breath is called the closing volume (CV). The CV may be added to the RV, if the RV has been determined, and expressed as the CC. The CV is normally recorded as a percentage of the VC:

$$\frac{CV}{VC} \times 100$$

Closing capacity is recorded as a percentage of the TLC:

$$\frac{CC}{TLC} \times 100$$

The TLC can be determined from the SBN_2 test by measuring the area under the washout curve, either by electronic integration or planimetry, using a dilution equation to calculate RV, and then adding it to the measured VC. The RV is calculated as follows:

$$RV = VC \times \frac{F\bar{E}_{N_2}}{FA_{N_2} - F\bar{E}_{N_2}}$$

where:

$F\bar{E}_{N_2}$ = mean expired N_2 concentration determined by a planimeter or electronic integration of the area under the curve

FA_{N_2} = N_2 concentration in the lungs at the beginning of inspiration, approximately 0.75 to 0.79

This method is accurate only in subjects who do not have significant obstructive disease or dead space–producing disease.

Significance and Pathophysiology

$\Delta\%N_{2_{750-1250}}$. The normal $\Delta\%N_{2_{750-1250}}$ is 1.5% or less for healthy young adults and slightly higher for healthy older adults (up to approximately 3%). Increases in $\Delta\%N_{2_{750-1250}}$ are found in diseases characterized by uneven distribution of gas during inspiration and/or unequal emptying rates during expiration. In subjects with severe emphysema, $\Delta\%N_{2_{750-1250}}$ may exceed 10%.

Slope of Phase III.   A best-fit line is drawn through the Phase III segment of the tracing from the point where 30% of the VC remains above RV to the onset of Phase IV. The slope of this line is used as an index of gas distribution, in a manner similar to the $\Delta\%N_{2_{750-1250}}$. Values in healthy young adults range from 0.5% to 1.0% N_2/L of lung volume, with wide variability. Very slow expiratory flow rates may cause oscillations in the tracing of Phase III, making the accurate measurement of $\Delta\%N_{2_{750-1250}}$ difficult. These oscillations are attributed to changes in alveolar N_2 concentrations as blood pulses through the pulmonary capillaries during cardiac systole. Increasing the expiratory flow rate slightly eliminates this common artifact. Subjects who have small VC values may have difficulty exhaling enough gas to make the $\Delta\%N_{2_{750-1250}}$ or slope of Phase III meaningful.

CV and CC.   Phase IV of the SBN_2 test can be explained by the fact that after a maximal expiration in an upright subject, more RV gas remains at the apices of the lungs than at the bases, resulting from the effects of gravity. When a test gas such as O_2 is inspired, the apices receive the gas occupying the subject's dead space which consists largely of N_2. The test gas (O_2 in this case) goes preferentially to the bases of the lungs. Gas concentrations in the lungs become widely different, because the apices contain RV gas plus dead space gas (mostly N_2), while the bases contain predominantly test gas (O_2 in this case). Compression of the airways during the subsequent expiration causes airways to narrow, and then close, as lung volume approaches RV. The airways at the base of the lungs close first because of gravity and the weight of the lung in subjects sitting upright. As airways at the bases of the lung close, proportionately more gas comes from the apices, the concentration of N_2 rises, and Phase IV begins.

The onset of Phase IV indicates the lung volume at which airway closure begins. The point in the VC maneuver at which Phase IV begins depends on the caliber of the small airways. In healthy young adults, closing volume occurs near the end of the VC, after 80% to 90% of the VC has been expired. The closing capacity in healthy young adults usually occurs at about 30% of the TLC, again with wide variations. The CV and CC may be increased, indicating earlier onset of airway closure in the following conditions:

- Increase in age of the subject
- Restrictive disease patterns in which the FRC becomes less than the CV
- In smokers and other subjects with early obstructive disease of small airways
- Congestive heart failure when the caliber of the small airways is compromised by edema.

Subjects with moderate or severe obstructive disease may display no sharp inflection separating Phases III and IV of the SBN_2. This lack of a clear point of airway closure results from grossly uneven distribution of gas in the lungs. Subjects who have airway obstruction typically show $\Delta\%N_{2_{750-1250}}$ values and slopes of Phase III greater than normal.

Closing volume and CC measurements may be erroneous if the subject does not perform a true VC maneuver. The inspired and expired VCs should be within 5%. The VC during the SBN_2 should match the FVC or SVC within 5%. Expiratory flow should be maintained between 0.3 and 0.5 L/sec. In some individuals who have no pulmonary disease, the onset of Phase IV cannot be accurately determined. Because of the variability in both the CV and CC, the mean of three tests is usually reported. Because of its poor reproducibility, the closing volume test is not widely used. Although it appears to be a sensitive indicator of abnormalities in the small airways, particularly in smokers, an increased CV/VC ratio is not highly predictive of which individuals will go on to develop chronic airways obstruction. To calculate normal values for CV and CC according to age and sex, see the Appendix.

NITROGEN WASHOUT TEST (7 MINUTE)

Description

The N_2 washout test measures the concentration of N_2 in alveolar gas at the end of 7 minutes of 100% O_2 breathing. The N_2 washout test value is recorded as a percentage of alveolar N_2. A graph of the breath-by-breath washout curve may be used to assess the distribution of ventilation.

Technique

The simplest method of calculating the degree of N_2 washout from the lungs is by having the subject breathe 100% O_2 for 7 minutes, then measuring the N_2 concentration of a sample of alveolar gas collected at the end of a forced expiration. The distribution of ventilation determines whether the concentration of N_2 will be reduced to a low level within 7 minutes. Alternatively, the duration of oxygen breathing required to reduce the $\%N_2$ to less than 1% can be used as an index of gas distribution.

A more quantitative test is that in which the washout of N_2 by O_2 is graphed or displayed breath-by-breath using rapid analysis of expired gas. Normally, the percent of N_2 or its logarithm is plotted against the expired volume or number of breaths. The washout of N_2 from a normal lung is nearly exponential. The end-expiratory points of a normal washout curve appear as a straight line when the log $\%N_2$ is graphed on semilog paper (Fig. 4–2).

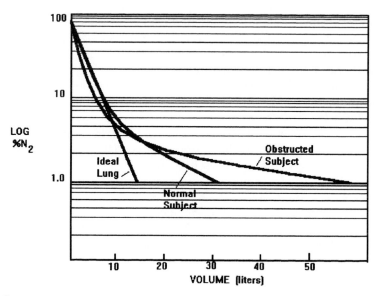

FIG 4–2.
Nitrogen washout (7 minute) patterns. The nitrogen concentration (at end-expiration) vs. expired volume is plotted on semilog paper (Y axis is logarithmic). The elimination of nitrogen from the lungs by O_2 breathing occurs exponentially. An ideal lung (i.e., a single-chambered container) would produce a J-shaped curve during washout; the percent of N_2 is plotted on semilog paper resulting in a straight line. Normal healthy subjects produce a slightly concave line because various lung units empty at slightly different rates. In subjects who have airway obstruction, there is a rapid washout initially and progressive slowing as the test proceeds. This begins as a steep curve with more and more flattening toward the end. The slope of the washout curve is determined mainly by the rate, tidal volume, functional residual capacity, and dead space. The test normally lasts 7 minutes, or until the alveolar N_2 concentration has been reduced to less than 1%, or until an expired volume limit has been reached (i.e., 60 L). The Log $\%N_2$ may also be plotted against time or number of breaths.

Significance and Pathophysiology

The normal value for the concentration of N_2 in alveolar gas after 7 minutes of O_2 breathing is less than 2.5%. The results of a 7-minute N_2 washout test are of little value without consideration of the V_T, V_D, and FRC of the individual subject during the test. Large increases in $\dot{V}_E$ (i.e., increased V_T or rate) can lower the percent of N_2 in the alveoli to near normal levels within the 7-minute limit even though there is marked unevenness of gas distribution. For this reason, some clinicians prefer to graph the $\%N_2$ against the total volume expired, rather than against time. Subjects who do not have pulmonary disease wash N_2 out of their lungs with 3 to 4 minutes of O_2 breathing. Washout times longer than 3 to 4 minutes are usually consistent with poor distribution, increased FRC, reduced alveolar ventilation, or a combination of these.

The graphic method of displaying breath-by-breath washout provides a means of quantifying the evenness of ventilation. The slope of the washout curve is determined by the FRC, V_T, V_D, and frequency of breathing. If the N_2 is washed out of the lungs evenly, the curve will appear as a straight line on semilog paper, regardless of the slope (see Fig. 4–2). Because the lung is not a perfectly symmetric organ, the curve is typically slightly concave. The deviation from a straight line is indicative of the extent to which ventilation is uneven.

Uneven distribution of gas in the lungs is characteristic of all obstructive disease patterns. Emphysema, particularly in the advanced stages, shows the greatest degree of maldistribution. Patients who have bronchitis and/or asthma show similar unevenness of ventilation, particularly during acute exacerbations. The effect of uneven distribution of ventilation is largely dependent on the matching of ventilation and perfusion. Uneven ventilation often results in blood gas abnormalities, specifically hypoxemia (see Chapter 6). When ventilation is not matched to the same lung units receiving pulmonary capillary blood flow, the arterial saturation (Sao_2) falls. If the mismatch of ventilation and perfusion is severe, the $Paco_2$ may rise. Some subjects who have marked maldistribution of ventilation, such as those who have emphysema, may have relatively normal blood gases. If the disease process destroys pulmonary capillaries along with the other alveolar structures, ventilation distribution may be poor, but matches pulmonary capillary perfusion. As a result, blood gas values appear normal, with little or no hypoxemia.

Normal washout values are often produced by subjects who have a purely restrictive pattern. This is particularly true if the restricted subject hyperventilates as a result of the restriction. However, tumors or other space-occupying lesions may impinge on the airways and cause regional differences in ventilation. Thoracic deformities, such as kyphoscoliosis and pectus excavatum, may also cause marked unevenness in the distribution of ventilation. The 7-minute washout test may or may not appear abnormal in many of these types of restrictive disorders. Ventilation and perfusion lung scans offer the best means of assessing regional gas distribution and blood flow. Other imaging techniques, including magnetic resonance imaging (MRI), positron-emission tomography (PET), and ultrasonography, may be quite useful in identifying and localizing the causes of uneven gas distribution.

The multiple-breath N_2 test is independent of subject effort, although the subject must maintain an adequate seal on the mouthpiece of the apparatus to prevent contamination of the test gas (O_2). Leaks in the breathing circuit or in the N_2 sampling device usually result in room air being mixed with the washed-out gas. A leak usually results in prolonged washout times or inability to reduce the alveolar N_2 to less than 2.5%, even in normal lungs. Leaks are usually identifiable by abrupt increases in the N_2 concentration during the maneuver.

LUNG SCANS (^{133}XE)

Description

Lung scans using ^{133}xenon (^{133}Xe), as well as techniques employing inhalation of ^{81m}krypton and ^{127}xenon, measure the regional distribution of ventilation.

Technique

1. The subject, usually in a sitting position, inhales either a V_T or a VC breath from a reservoir that contains a measured dose of ^{133}Xe (10 to 20 mCi). The subject then holds the breath for 10 to 20 seconds, during which time scintiphotos are made over the lung fields to demonstrate areas of poor ventilation (Fig. 4–3).

2. The subject is allowed to rebreathe the gas mixture containing the ^{133}Xe for 3 to 5 minutes. During this interval, serial scintiphotos are made to demonstrate the rapidity and evenness of equilibration of the ^{133}Xe. Addition of

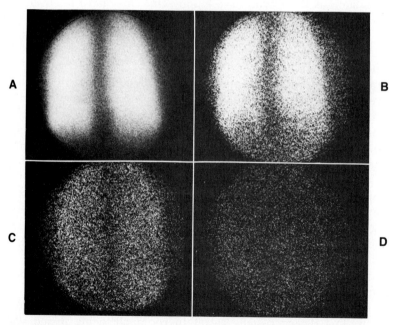

FIG 4–3.
^{133}Xe ventilation lung scan. Posterior-anterior views of normal lung fields. **A,** washin or equilibration after rebreathing radioactive Xe. **B,** 30 seconds after washout begins, breathing room air. **C,** 1 minute after breathing room air. **D,** 3 minutes after breathing air, only background radiation remains. (Courtesy of Nuclear Medicine Dept., St. Louis University Hospital, St. Louis.)

O_2 and removal of CO_2 are required because a closed circuit is used, similar to that employed in the He dilution FRC determination. Because the rebreathing period is usually short, the circuit may be flushed with 100% O_2 to provide adequate oxygen during the maneuver. If the reservoir bag is of sufficient volume ($\cong 10$ L), the addition of oxygen may be unnecessary. However, 100% oxygen breathing in subjects who have poorly ventilated lung units, even over a short interval, may cause some absorption atelectasis, resulting in greater unevenness of ventilation than might otherwise be seen.

3. During the final step, the subject is returned to breathing air to cause the ^{133}Xe to be washed out. Serial scintiphotos indicate those areas that have trapped the ^{133}Xe during the equilibration phase. Ratios of counts from various lung zones can be used to determine the relative degree of ventilation of each lung zone. This normally requires discrete counters or computerized segregation of counts from the various lung zones.

Significance and Pathophysiology

^{133}Xe is ideal for identifying regional ventilation disorders. It has a half-life of 5.27 days and requires sophisticated monitoring equipment, but is not metabolized by the body and tends to remain in the gas phase. The three types of ^{133}Xe studies described above can be done individually or as a series, and are helpful diagnostically in cases of pronounced regional differences in ventilation.

Regional distribution of inspired gas is dependent on the volume of air in the lungs before the breath and the volume of the breath itself. Differences in regional ventilation can be quantified by calculating the concentration of ^{133}Xe in each lung zone by means of external counters placed over the chest. The fractional concentration of ^{133}Xe can be derived by comparing radiation counts during an initial breath of ^{133}Xe to counts at the same lung volume after rebreathing. When the concentration of ^{133}Xe is equal in both the lung and the breathing circuit, the fractional concentration of ^{133}Xe during the initial breath can be derived. This fractional concentration can then be stated as a ventilation index, expressing it as a percentage of the simultaneous mean concentration of ^{133}Xe in the lungs. The concentration of ^{133}Xe is expressed per unit of lung volume. Similar data from different subjects can be compared in this way. Of more practical value, although less quantitative, is direct visual examination of the scintiphotos to determine the size and pattern of the ventilation defect.

^{133}Xe scans in normal upright subjects show proportionately greater ventilation at the bases of the lungs than in the apices. Because gravity causes most perfusion to be directed to the lower two thirds of the lungs, ventilation is closely matched to blood flow in healthy individuals. Despite the smaller alveolar size in the lower lung zones resulting from gravity and hydrostatic pressure, tidal ventilation is directed to the areas of gravity-dependent blood flow. In healthy subjects, a major portion of lung units have $\dot{V}/\dot{Q}$ ratios of 0.8 to 1.0.

Technical problems with ventilation lung scans may involve the breathing circuitry, with leaks posing the problem of inaccurate measurements as well as the escape of radioactive gas. Most systems, however, enclose the reservoir and the majority of the breathing circuit in a shielded container. The subject must be instructed carefully, and must keep noseclips in place during the procedure to prevent inadvertent loss of the radioactive gas.

The distribution of pulmonary blood flow may be demonstrated by intravenous injection of radioactive particles labelled with technetium (Tc). Macroaggregated albumin (MAA) labeled with ^{99m}Tc (^{99m}Tc-MAA) or human albumin microspheres (HAM) labeled with ^{99m}Tc (^{99m}Tc-HAM) are commonly used. These particles, measuring 30 to 40 μm, are injected by a venous route. The particles mix with blood passing through the right heart and lodge in the pulmonary arterioles. Their distribution matches the pulmonary blood flow at the time of injection. Scintiphotos are normally made of six views: anterior, posterior, left lateral, right lateral, left posterior oblique, and right posterior oblique (Fig. 4–4). These particles normally break up, pass through

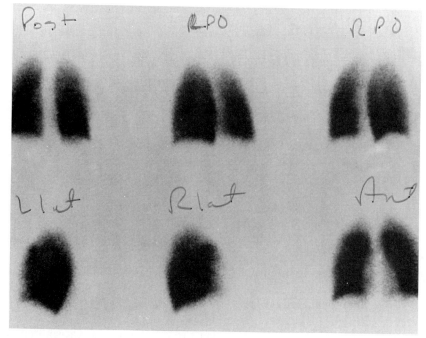

FIG 4–4.
^{99m}Tc-HAM perfusion lung scan. Normal perfusion lung scan using human albumin microspheres tagged with radioactive technetium. **A,** posterior; **B,** left posterior oblique; **C,** right posterior oblique; **D,** left lateral; **E,** right lateral; **F,** anterior. (Courtesy of Nuclear Medicine Dept., St. Louis University Hospital, St. Louis.)

the pulmonary capillaries, and are removed by the liver and spleen. When the usual dosage is used, approximately 1 of every 1000 arterioles is occluded, and no functional abnormalities can be demonstrated following injection.

Perfusion lung scanning may be contraindicated in subjects with severe pulmonary hypertension because of their reduced vascular bed, and in individuals with anatomic right-to-left shunts, because the particles pass unchanged through the lungs for embolization in the brain, kidney, heart, or other organs. Perfusion scanning routinely is combined with ventilation scans of the lung to evaluate subjects with obstructive airways disease or with suspected pulmonary emboli. Perfusion and ventilation scans may be combined by computer to provide projection of the ventilation/perfusion characteristics of various lung segments.

SELF-ASSESSMENT QUESTIONS

1. Closing volume (CV) is the volume of gas:
    a. Exhaled after the dead space
    b. Remaining in the lungs after a maximal expiration
    c. That can be exhaled after airway closure begins
    d. Remaining in the lungs when airways begin to close

2. Phase III of the SBN_2 test represents:
    a. The onset of airway closure
    b. Exhalation of alveolar gas
    c. Exhalation of dead space gas
    d. The anatomic dead space

3. A subject performs a lung volume determination and an SBN_2:

	Measured	**Predicted**
TLC (L BTPS)	6.4	6.0
RV (L BTPS)	2.0	2.1
CV (L BTPS)	0.9	-

   The CV/VC ratio is:
    a. 45%
    b. 31%
    c. 20%
    d. Cannot be determined

4. A subject performs the N_2 washout procedure; after 3 minutes, the $\%N_2$ displayed on the graph of the washout is 0.9%. This is consistent with:

a. Severe obstructive lung disease
b. An acute asthmatic episode
c. Increased intrapulmonary shunting
d. Normal distribution of ventilation

5. In healthy subjects who have no lung disease, a graph of the N_2 washout curve appears as a _____ when displayed on a semi-logarithmic graph.
   a. Straight line
   b. Convex curve
   c. J-shaped curve
   d. S-shaped curve

6. A subject with normal spirometry has an alveolar N_2 concentration of 10.2% after 7 minutes of oxygen breathing; which of the following best explain this finding:
   a. Kyphoscoliosis
   b. Chronic bronchitis
   c. Pulmonary fibrosis
   d. A breathing circuit leak

7. In subjects with obstructive lung disease, breathing air after rebreathing ^{133}Xe will show:
   a. ^{133}Xe trapped in poorly ventilated regions
   b. A rapid washout of ^{133}Xe from poorly ventilated regions
   c. Better ventilation at the bases of the lungs
   d. Areas with the greatest pulmonary blood flow

8. Ventilation scans of normal upright subjects show:
   a. Most ventilation goes to the apexes of the lungs
   b. Most ventilation goes to the bases of the lungs
   c. Ventilation is evenly distributed across all lung fields
   d. Ventilation distribution depends on respiratory rate

9. Perfusion lung scans are most useful in demonstrating:
   a. Pulmonary hypertension
   b. Anatomic right-to-left shunts
   c. Pulmonary emboli
   d. Pulmonary fibrosis

10. Which of the following is most likely to be abnormal in a healthy young smoker:
    a. CV/VC ratio
    b. FVC (percent of predicted)
    c. 7-minute N_2 washout
    d. ^{133}Xe lung scan

SELECTED BIBLIOGRAPHY

GENERAL REFERENCES

Bouhuys A: Distribution of inspired gas in the lungs. In Fenn WO, Rahn H, editors: *Handbook of physiology: respiration I.* Washington, 1964, Am Physiologic Society.

Comroe JH, Fowler WS: Lung function studies: VI. Detection of uneven alveolar ventilation during a single breath of oxygen. *Am J Med* 10:408, 1951.

Darling RC, Cournand A, Richards DW: Studies of intrapulmonary mixture of gases: V. Forms of inadequate ventilation in normal and emphysematous lungs analyzed by means of breathing pure oxygen. *J Clin Invest* 23:55, 1944.

Fowler WS: Lung function studies: III. Uneven pulmonary ventilation in normal subjects and in patients with pulmonary disease. *J Appl Physiol* 2:283, 1949.

Hathirat S, Renzetti AD, Mitchell M: Intrapulmonary gas distribution: a comparison of the helium mixing time and nitrogen single breath test in normal and diseased subjects. *Am Rev Respir Dis* 102:750, 1970.

Shinokazi T, Abajian JC Jr, Tabakin BS, et al: Theory of a digital nitrogen washout computer. *J Appl Physiol* 21:202, 1966.

CLOSING VOLUME

Abboud R, Morton J: Comparison of maximal mid-expiratory flow, flow-volume curves, and nitrogen closing volumes in patients with mild airway obstruction. *Am Rev Respir Dis* 111:405, 1975.

Becklake MR, Permutt S: Evaluation of tests of lung function for "screening" for early detection of chronic obstructive lung disease. In Maclem PT, Permutt S, editors: *The lung in transition between health and disease.* New York, 1979, Marcel Dekker.

Berend N, Glanville AR, Grunstein MM: Determinants of the slope of phase III of the single breath nitrogen test. *Bull Eur Physiolpathol Respir* 20:521, 1984.

Buist AS, Ross BB: Predicted values for closing volumes using a modified single breath nitrogen test. *Am Rev Respir Dis* 107:744, 1973.

Cormier Y, Belanger J: The role of gas exchange in phase IV of the single breath nitrogen test. *Am Rev Respir Dis* 125:396, 1982.

MacFadden ER, Holmes B, Kiker R: Variability of closing volume measurements in normal man. *Am Rev Respir Dis* 111:135, 1975.

Make B, Lapp NL: Factors influencing the measurement of closing volume. *Am Rev Respir Dis* 111:749, 1975.

Martin R, Macklem PT: Suggested standardization procedures for closing volume determinations (nitrogen method). DHD-NHLBI, 1973.

McCarthy DS, Spencer R, Greene R, et al: Measurement of closing volume as a simple and sensitive test for early detection of small airway disease. *Am J Med* 52:747, 1972.

LUNG SCANS

Bernier DR, Zangman JK, Wells LD: *Nuclear medicine technology and techniques,* ed. 2. St Louis, 1988, CV Mosby.

Dolfuss RE, Milic-Emili J, Bates DV: Regional ventilation of the lung studied with boluses of 133 Xenon. *Respir Physiol* 2:234, 1967.

Secker-Walker RH, Siegal BA: The use of nuclear medicine in the diagnosis of lung disease. *Radiol Clin North Am* 11:215, 1973.

5

Diffusion Tests

CARBON MONOXIDE DIFFUSING CAPACITY ($D_{L_{CO}}$)

Description

Carbon monoxide (CO) diffusing capacity ($D_{L_{CO}}$ or D_{CO}) measures the transfer of a diffusion-limited gas (CO) across the alveolocapillary membrane. The $D_{L_{CO}}$ is reported in milliliters of CO per minute per millimeter of mercury at 0°C, 760 mm Hg, dry (i.e., STPD).

Technique

Carbon monoxide combines with hemoglobin (Hb) about 210 times more readily than O_2 does, but otherwise acts similar to O_2. In the presence of normal amounts of Hb and normal ventilatory function, the primary limiting factor to diffusion of CO is the status of the alveolocapillary membrane. Small amounts of CO in inspired gas produce measurable changes in the concentration of inspired vs. expired gas. Because there is normally little or no CO in pulmonary capillary blood, the pressure gradient causing diffusion is basically the alveolar pressure ($P_{A_{CO}}$). There are several methods for determining the $D_{L_{CO}}$ (Table 5–1), all of which use the general equation:

$$D_{L_{CO}} = \frac{\dot{V}_{CO}}{P_{A_{CO}} - P_{C_{CO}}}$$

where:

$\dot{V}_{CO}$ = milliliters of CO transferred per minute (STPD)

$P_{A_{CO}}$ = mean alveolar partial pressure of CO

$P_{C_{CO}}$ = mean capillary partial pressure of CO, assumed to be 0

97

TABLE 5–1

Advantages and Disadvantages of $D_{L_{CO}}$ Testing Methods

Method	Technique	Advantages
$D_{L_{CO}}SB$ (breath-hold)	He and Co analysis relatively simple; 10 seconds breath-hold	Easy calculations, simple; fast; no COHb back pressure; can be automated
$D_{L_{CO}}SS_1$ (Filey technique)	CO, CO_2, O_2 analysis; arterial blood sample; relatively simple	Most accurate steady-state method; good for exercise testing
$D_{L_{CO}}SS_2$ (end-tidal CO)	End-tidal sample, $F_{U_{CO}}$ simultaneously; CO analysis only	No arterial puncture or breath-hold; easy calculation
$D_{L_{CO}}SS_3$ (assumed V_D)	CO analysis (slow or fast); large V_T improves accuracy	Relatively simple calculations; good for exercise studies
$D_{L_{CO}}SS_4$ (mixed venous P_{CO_2})	CO, CO_2 analysis (rapid); rebreathing required	No arterial puncture; easy calculations; slow CO analysis acceptable
$D_{L_{CO}}RB$ (rebreathing)	He and CO analysis (rapid); rebreathing required	Less sensitive to V_A than $D_{L_{CO}}SB$; less sensitive to $\dot{V}/\dot{Q}$ abnormalities
$D_{L_{CO}}SS_{He}$ (washout equilibration)	CO, He analysis (rapid); sequencing required	Eliminates V_A, $\dot{V}/\dot{Q}$, and distribution problems
$D_{L_{CO}}IB$ (intrabreath)	Rapid responding CO, CH_4 analyzers required	Breath-holding not required
$F_{U_{CO}}$ (fractional CO uptake)	CO analysis; may be done with $D_{L_{CO}}SS_2$	Simple; CO analysis of inspired and expired gas only
$1/Dm + 1/\theta Vc$ (membrane and red blood cell resistance)	$D_{L_{CO}}SB$ repeated before and after O_2 breathing	Differentiates membrane from red cell components; calculates Vc

Diffusing capacity is essentially a measure of transfer of CO across the alveolocapillary membranes. The $D_{L_{CO}}$ is expressed as milliliters of gas per minute per unit of driving pressure. An additional method of quantifying diffusing capacity, fractional uptake of CO ($F_{U_{CO}}$), simply relates the inspired and expired CO concentrations during normal breathing.

Modified Krogh technique — single breath ($D_{L_{CO}}SB$). The subject inspires a VC breath from a spirometer or reservoir (Fig. 5–1). The spirometer/reservoir contains a gas mixture of 0.3% CO, 10% He, 21% O_2, and the balance, N_2. The subject holds the breath at TLC for approximately 10 seconds. The subject then expires, and a sample of alveolar gas is collected in a small volume

Disadvantages	Application
Sensitive to distribution of ventilation and $\dot{V}/\dot{Q}$; "non-physiologic"; not practical for exercise	Screening and clinical application; good standardization
Aterial puncture and blood gas analysis; sensitive to uneven $\dot{V}/\dot{Q}$	Clinical application; exercise studies
COHb back pressure; V_T must be maintained high; very sensitive to $\dot{V}/\dot{Q}$	Fast, easy screening and clinical method; not used for exercise studies
Large error if V_T is too small; sensitive to COHb	Screenings and clinical applications; exercise studies
Sensitive to COHb; rebreathing must be controlled closely	Not yet widely used clinically
Complex calculations; rapid CO and He analyzers required; sensitive to COHb	Clinically applicable; provides most accurate $D_{L_{CO}}$
Complex calculations (computerized)	Research applications
Complex calculations (computerized); flow must be controlled; sensitive to uneven $\dot{V}/\dot{Q}$	Screening; may be useful in subjects who cannot breathhold
Sensitive to $\dot{V}_E$, $\dot{V}/\dot{Q}$, and V_D/V_T	Screening or correlation to $D_{L_{CO}}SS_2$
Complex calculations; estimates of alveolar PO_2 critical	Research with limited clinical applications

bag ($\cong$ 500 mL) after a suitable washout volume (750 to 1000 mL) has been discarded (Fig. 5–2). The sample is analyzed to obtain the fractional CO and He concentrations in alveolar gas, $F_{A_{CO_T}}$ (where T is the time of the breath-hold) and $F_{A_{He}}$, respectively. The concentration of CO in the alveolar gas at the beginning of the breath-hold ($F_{A_{CO_0}}$) is computed thus:

$$F_{A_{CO_0}} = F_{I_{CO}} \times \frac{F_{A_{He}}}{F_{I_{He}}}$$

where:

$F_{A_{CO_0}}$ = fraction of CO at the beginning of the breath-hold (time = 0)

$F_{I_{CO}}$ = fraction of CO in the reservoir (usually 0.003)

$F_{A_{He}}$ = fraction of He in alveolar gas in the end-tidal sample

$F_{I_{He}}$ = fraction of He in inspired gas (usually 0.10)

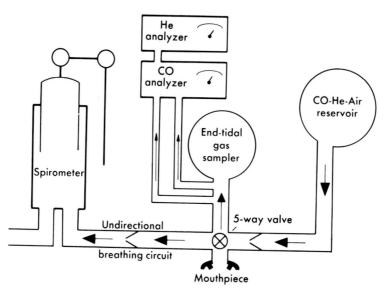

FIG 5–1.

$D_{L_{CO}}$ apparatus. The basic equipment for performing the $D_{L_{CO}}$ test (specifically the $D_{L_{CO}}$SB) is illustrated. Included is a reservoir containing 0.3% CO, 10% He, 21% O_2, and the balance, N_2. The reservoir may be a large volume bag, a sealed spirometer, or a demand valve system connected directly to a tank of special gas mixture. A multidirectional valve that may be automatic or manual allows rapid switching of the breathing gases and directs exhaled gas to the end-tidal sampler or spirometer or both. A method of measuring the inspired volume is also required, and is usually accomplished by using a bag-in-box or similar apparatus for the diffusion mixture reservoir. A spirometer (or pneumotachometer) is required to measure the exhaled volume in order to determine the volume of dead space to be washed out. Some systems connect the spirometer to the bag-in-box to measure both inspired and expired volumes. Helium (He) and carbon monoxide (CO) analyzers are used to analyze the end-tidal sample, as well as to determine inspired gas concentrations from the CO-He-air reservoir. Most automated systems include electronic timing of the maneuver, automatic switching of the valve, and direct sampling of the end-tidal gas.

The $D_{L_{CO}}$SB is then calculated as follows:

$$D_{L_{CO}}SB = \frac{V_A \times 60}{(P_B - 47) \times (T)} \times Ln\frac{F_{A_{CO_0}}}{F_{A_{CO_T}}}$$

where:

V_A = alveolar volume (STPD)

60 = correction from seconds to minutes

P_B = barometric pressure

47 = water vapor pressure (P_H2O) at 37°C

T = breath-hold interval (usually 10 seconds)

Ln = natural logarithm

FA_{CO_0} = fraction of CO in alveolar gas at the beginning of the breath-hold, before diffusion

FA_{CO_T} = fraction of CO in alveolar gas at the end of diffusion

V_A may be calculated from the single-breath dilution of He:

$$V_A = \frac{V_I}{FA_{He}/FI_{He}} \times STPD \text{ correction factor}$$

where:

V_I = volume of test gas inspired (see Fig. 5–2)

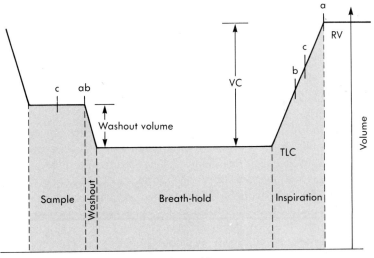

Time (seconds)

FIG 5–2.
Typical $DL_{CO}SB$ maneuver tracing. A tracing of the single-breath DL_{CO} maneuver proceeding from right to left, with inhalation causing the tracing to deflect downward. The subject, after exhaling to residual volume *(RV)*, inspires a vital capacity *(VC)* breath of the diffusion test gas rapidly to total lung capacity *(TLC)*, then holds the breath for approximately 10 seconds. At the end of the breath-hold, the subject exhales a fixed washout volume (usually 0.750 to 1.0 L). Then a sample of alveolar gas is taken (usually 0.5 to 1.0 L), and any remaining volume is exhaled. Various timing methods are illustrated. Method *a,* Ogilvie, considers diffusion to be occurring from the beginning of inspiration to the beginning of alveolar sampling; method *b,* ESP, considers diffusion to occur from the midpoint of inspiration to the beginning of alveolar sampling; method *c,* Jones, measures diffusion from two-thirds of the inspired VC to the midpoint of the alveolar sample.

$F_{A_{He}}$ = fraction of He in alveolar gas

$F_{I_{He}}$ = fraction of He in inspired gas (known)

A simplification of the above single-breath method is widely employed. If both the He and CO analyzers are calibrated to read full scale (100% or 1.000) when sampling the diffusion mixture and the analyzers are set to zero appropriately, the $F_{A_{He}}$ obtained from the end-tidal sample equals the $F_{A_{CO_0}}$. This technique assumes that both He and CO are diluted equally during inspiration. Because no He leaves the lung during the breath-hold, its concentration in the alveolar sample must equal that of the CO before any diffusion occurs. The logarithmic ratio of CO disappearance from the alveoli can then be expressed:

$$\text{Ln}\left(\frac{F_{A_{He}}}{F_{A_{CO_T}}}\right)$$

where:

$F_{A_{He}}$ = fraction of He in the alveolar sample, equal to $F_{A_{CO_0}}$

$F_{A_{CO_T}}$ = fraction of CO in the alveolar sample after the breath-hold

This technique avoids the necessity of analyzing the absolute concentrations of the two gases, but requires that both analyzers be linear with respect to each other. Analysis of CO is often done using infrared analyzers (see Chapter 9), and their output is nonlinear. Care must be taken to ensure that corrected CO readings are used in the computation. This correction is easily accomplished either electronically or via software in automated systems. Corrections must be made for anatomic V_D as well as inspired dead space in the valve and expired dead space in the sample bag. All lung volumes must be corrected from ATPS to STPD for the $D_{L_{CO}}$ calculations. The V_A, however, when used to calculate the ratio of diffusing capacity to lung volume (D_L/V_A), is normally expressed in BTPS units. Two or more tests are usually averaged, with 4 minutes of delay between repeated maneuvers to allow for washout of the test gas from the lungs. Corrections for abnormal Hb concentrations should be applied (see "Significance and Pathophysiology" in this chapter). Corrections for the presence of carboxyhemoglobin (COHb) in the subject's blood and for the effects of altitude may be necessary. Subjects should be asked to refrain from smoking for 24 hours before the test to reduce the CO back pressure in the blood. See Chapter 11 for criteria for acceptability of the $D_{L_{CO}}$SB maneuver.

Filey technique—steady state ($D_{L_{CO}}SS_1$). The subject breathes a gas mixture of 0.1% to 0.2% CO in air for 5 to 6 minutes. During the final 2 minutes, expired gas is collected in a Douglas bag and an arterial blood sample is drawn. The exhaled volume is measured and the expired gas is analyzed for CO, CO_2, and O_2. The arterial blood is analyzed for P_{CO_2}. Steady-state diffusing capacity is calculated by the equation:

$$D_{L_{CO}}SS_1 = \frac{\dot{V}_{CO}}{P_{A_{CO}}}$$

where:

$\dot{V}_{CO}$ = volume of CO transferred in milliliters per minute (STPD)

$P_{A_{CO}}$ = mean alveolar partial pressure of CO

The $\dot{V}_{CO}$ is determined from an analysis of the fractional inspired and expired CO ($F_{I_{CO}}$ and $F_{E_{CO}}$, respectively), the $\dot{V}_E$, and the fractional inspired ($F_{I_{N_2}}$), which is known, and the fractional expired N_2, ($F_{E_{N_2}}$), which is determined indirectly from the fractions of O_2, CO_2, and H_2O vapor in the exhaled gas as follows:

$$\dot{V}_{CO} = \dot{V}_E \left(F_{I_{CO}} \frac{F_{E_{N_2}}}{F_{I_{N_2}}} - F_{E_{CO}}\right)$$

The $P_{A_{CO}}$ is determined by using a form of the Bohr equation, as follows:

$$P_{A_{CO}} = P_B - 47 \frac{(F_{E_{CO}} - rF_{I_{CO}})}{1 - r}$$

where:

$$r = \frac{P_{a_{CO_2}} - P_{E_{CO_2}}}{P_{E_{CO_2}}}$$

where:

$P_{a_{CO_2}}$ = partial pressure of arterial CO_2

$P_{E_{CO_2}}$ = partial pressure of mixed expired CO_2

Estimating $P_{A_{CO}}$ in this way avoids the necessity of obtaining a direct alveolar sample.

End-tidal CO determination ($D_{L_{CO}}SS_2$). The $D_{L_{CO}}SS_2$ method is basically the same as the $D_{L_{CO}}SS_1$ in that the volume of CO transferred ($\dot{V}_{CO}$) is derived similarly. The $P_{A_{CO}}$, however, is determined by taking the average end-tidal CO tension ($P_{ET_{CO}}$) from instantaneous analysis of multiple breaths. The end-tidal value is assumed to be equal to the mean $P_{A_{CO}}$.

Assumed V_D technique ($D_{L_{CO}}SS_3$). The $D_{L_{CO}}SS_3$ method is similar to the $D_{L_{CO}}SS_1$. The $\dot{V}_{CO}$ is determined as in $D_{L_{CO}}SS_1$, but the $P_{A_{CO}}$ is measured differently. The fraction of CO in alveolar gas ($F_{A_{CO}}$) which can be used to derive $P_{A_{CO}}$ when P_B is known, is computed as follows:

$$F_{A_{CO}} = \frac{V_T\,(F_{E_{CO}}) - V_D\,(F_{I_{CO}})}{V_T - V_D}$$

where:

$$V_T = \text{tidal volume}$$

$$V_D = \text{dead space volume}$$

$$F_{E_{CO}} = \text{fraction of expired CO}$$

$$F_{I_{CO}} = \text{fraction of inspired CO}$$

The V_T is measured by averaging multiple breaths. The V_D is often assumed to be equal to 1 mL per pound of body weight. The mechanical V_D of the breathing circuit is subtracted.

Mixed venous P_{CO_2} technique ($D_{L_{CO}}SS_4$). The $\dot{V}_{CO}$ is obtained as in $D_{L_{CO}}SS_1$. The $P_{A_{CO}}$ is calculated by estimating the mixed venous P_{CO_2} from an equilibration technique and then determining the $P_{A_{CO_2}}$ from the $P\bar{v}_{CO_2}$ and the normal gradient. Once the $P_{A_{CO_2}}$ is derived, an equation similar to that used to determine $P_{A_{CO}}$ in the $D_{L_{CO}}SS_1$ technique can be employed. Using mixed venous P_{CO_2} avoids the necessity of arterial puncture.

Rebreathing technique ($D_{L_{CO}}RB$). The subject rebreathes from a reservoir containing a mixture of 0.3% CO, 10% He, and the remainder air for 30 to 60 seconds at a rate of about 30 breaths per minute. After this interval, measurements of the final CO, He, and O_2 concentrations in the reservoir are made. An equation similar to that used for the single-breath technique is used (see $D_{L_{CO}}SB$):

$$D_{L_{CO}}RB = \frac{V_S \times 60}{(P_B - 47)\,(T2 - T1)} \times Ln\,\frac{F_{A_{CO_{T1}}}}{F_{A_{CO_{T2}}}}$$

where:

$$V_S = \text{volume of the lung reservoir system (initial volume} \times F_{I_{HE}}/F_{A_{He}})$$

$$60 = \text{correction from seconds to minutes}$$

$$P_B = \text{barometric pressure}$$

$$47 = \text{water vapor pressure } (P_{H_2O})$$

$$T2 - T1 = \text{rebreathing interval}$$

$$Ln = \text{natural logarithm}$$

$F_{A_{CO_{T1}}}$ = fraction of CO in alveolar gas before diffusion

$F_{A_{CO_{T2}}}$ = fraction of CO in alveolar gas at the end of diffusion

Equilibration — washout method ($D_{L_{CO}}SS_{He}$). The subject rebreathes from a reservoir containing 0.3% CO, 10% He, and the remainder air until equilibrium is reached. Then the subject again breathes room air, and the washouts of both CO and He are recorded by a rapid gas analyzer. During the washout, CO is removed at a rapid rate by diffusion as well as by ventilation, while He is removed more slowly by ventilation alone. The difference in washout rates is caused by the rate of CO diffusion. An equation similar to the $D_{L_{CO}}SB$ equation is used to calculate $D_{L_{CO}}SS_{He}$. A logarithmic expression of the ratio of final He concentration to initial He concentration is included as a factor along with the CO concentration ratio. Representation of these washout curves in real time normally requires computerization.

Slow exhalation single breath — intrabreath method ($D_{L_{CO}}IB$). In this technique, the subject inspires a VC breath of test gas containing 0.3% CO, 0.3% methane (CH_4), 21% O_2, and the balance, N_2. The subject then exhales slowly and evenly at a rate of approximately 0.5 L per second from TLC to RV. Gas concentrations are monitored by rapidly responding infrared analyzers. The rate of disappearance of CO can be calculated in a manner similar to the washout method. Change in lung volume (V_A) is calculated from the change in concentration of the methane tracer gas. Methane is used in place of helium because it can be rapidly measured using an infrared analyzer. Multiple estimates of $D_{L_{CO}}$ can be made during a single exhalation, recording $D_{L_{CO}}$ as a function of lung volume. This is done using an equation similar to that employed for the single-breath method. Instead of one estimate of V_A (equal to the lung volume at breath-hold) multiple increments of V_A are made, and $D_{L_{CO}}$ is plotted against lung volume. A single estimate of the overall $D_{L_{CO}}$ can also be obtained.

Fractional CO uptake ($F_{U_{CO}}$). The subject first inspires a mixture of 0.1% CO in air from a reservoir to establish a steady-state breathing pattern, then expires into a spirometer or reservoir, from which an average expired CO sample is analyzed. The $F_{U_{CO}}$ is expressed as:

$$F_{U_{CO}} = \frac{F_{I_{CO}} - F_{E_{CO}}}{F_{I_{CO}}}$$

where:

$F_{I_{CO}}$ = fraction of inspired CO

$F_{E_{CO}}$ = fraction of expired CO

The resulting fraction may be multiplied by 100 and expressed as a percentage. The level of $\dot{V}_E$ is critical for a valid determination of Fu_{CO} and should be monitored closely.

Membrane diffusion coefficient (Dm) and capillary blood volume (Qc). The subject performs two $D_{L_{CO}}SB$ tests, each at a different level of alveolar Po_2. The first $D_{L_{CO}}SB$ is performed as outlined above. The subject then breathes an elevated concentration of O_2 (balance, N_2) for approximately 5 minutes, exhales to RV, and performs the second $D_{L_{CO}}SB$ maneuver. The $D_{L_{CO}}$ values are calculated for both the air- and oxygen-breathing maneuvers. The total resistance caused by the alveolocapillary membrane (Dm) and the resistance caused by the rate of chemical combination with hemoglobin (Hb) and transfer into the red blood cell (ΘQc) is calculated according to the following equation:

$$1/D_{L_{CO}} = 1/Dm + 1/\Theta Qc$$

where:

$1/D_{L_{CO}}$ = reciprocal of diffusing capacity, or resistance

$1/Dm$ = alveolocapillary membrane resistance

$1/\Theta Qc$ = resistance caused by the red blood cell membrane and rate of reaction with Hb

Θ = transfer rate of CO per milliliter of capillary blood

Qc = capillary blood volume

Because CO and O_2 compete for binding sites on Hb, measurement of diffusion of CO at different levels of Po_2 can be used to distinguish resistance caused by the alveolocapillary membrane from resistance caused by the red blood cell membrane and Hb reaction rate. The Qc is presumed to remain the same for both tests, but Θ varies in response to changes in PO_2. By plotting Θ at two points against $1/D_{L_{CO}}$ and extrapolating back to zero as if no O_2 were present, the resistance caused by the alveolocapillary membrane can be calculated.

Significance and Pathophysiology

The average $D_{L_{CO}}$ value for resting adult subjects by the single-breath method is 25 mL CO/min/mm Hg (STPD). The expected $D_{L_{CO}}$ value in a healthy subject varies directly with the subject's lung volume. Regression equations for calculation of normal values are included in the Appendix. Values derived using one of the steady-state methods are usually slightly less than the single-breath method in healthy subjects, but may vary by as much as 30%. Females have slightly lower normal values, presumably in correlation with smaller normal lung volumes. The $D_{L_{CO}}$ values can increase two to three times in healthy individuals during exercise.

Diffusing capacity is generally decreased in restrictive lung diseases. Many restrictive disorders are the result of alveolar fibrosis. Fibrotic changes in the lung parenchyma are associated with sarcoidosis, asbestosis, berylliosis, and silicosis. Many other "dust" diseases (i.e., diseases whose causes are related to inhalation of dusts) also cause fibrotic changes in lung tissue. Inhalation of toxic gases, including O_2, may result in reduction of the $D_{L_{CO}}$. These disease states are sometimes categorized as "diffusion defects." In fact, the decrease in diffusing capacity is probably more closely related to the loss of lung volume, alveolar surface area, or capillary bed.

Diffusing capacity is usually decreased when there is loss of lung tissue or replacement of normal parenchyma by space-occupying lesions such as tumors. The $D_{L_{CO}}$ may also be reduced in the presence of pulmonary edema. The reduction in diffusing capacity in edema results not only from congestion of the alveoli but also from disruption of alveolar ventilation and reduction of lung volume.

The $D_{L_{CO}}$ is sometimes reduced as a result of medical or surgical intervention for cardiopulmonary disease. Lung resection for cancer or other reasons typically results in decreased $D_{L_{CO}}$. The extent of reduction is usually directly proportional to volume of lung removed. Radiation therapy which involves the lungs almost always causes a loss of $D_{L_{CO}}$. Drugs used in chemotherapy as well as those used to suppress rejection in organ transplantation may cause reductions in $D_{L_{CO}}$. These drugs appear to directly affect the alveolocapillary membranes. The diffusing capacity is frequently used to monitor drug toxicity during a course of therapy. Some antiarrhythmic drugs used in the treatment of cardiac dysrhythmias have been shown to reduce $D_{L_{CO}}$.

The $D_{L_{CO}}$ also may be decreased in obstructive lung disease, both acute and chronic. Diffusing capacity is reduced in emphysema for several reasons. Emphysematous lungs have a reduced surface area, with the loss of both alveolar walls (septa) and their associated capillary beds. As a result of the decreased surface area, less gas can be transferred per minute, even if the remaining gas exchange units are structurally normal. However, besides the loss of surface area for gas exchange, there is an increase in the distance from the terminal bronchiole to the alveolocapillary membrane in emphysema. Again, as alveolar structures break down, the terminal lung unit becomes larger and gas must diffuse further just to reach the alveolocapillary surface. In addition, there is mismatching of ventilation and pulmonary capillary blood flow in emphysema. As the alveolar structures become disrupted, there is loss of support for the terminal airways. Airways collapse and gas is trapped in the gas exchange units resulting in $\dot{V}/\dot{Q}$ abnormalities. Other obstructive processes, such as bronchitis or asthma, may not reduce the diffusing capacity unless they result in markedly abnormal $\dot{V}/\dot{Q}$ patterns.

Because $D_{L_{CO}}$ is directly related to V_A, expression of this relationship is often useful in differentiating disease processes in which there may be decreased $D_{L_{CO}}$ as a direct result of loss of lung volume (restrictive) from those in which decreased $D_{L_{CO}}$ is caused by uneven $\dot{V}/\dot{Q}$ or uneven distribution of inspired gas (obstructive). As an index, the measured $D_{L_{CO}}$ may be divided by the lung volume at which the measurement was made to obtain an expression of diffusing capacity per unit of lung volume. This is recorded as the D_L/V_L or D_L/V_A and may be accomplished easily, as the V_A must be calculated to derive the $D_{L_{CO}}$. In normal subjects, the D_L/V_L is approximately 4 to 5 (4 to 5 mL of CO transferred per minute, per liter of lung volume). In obstruction, loss of $D_{L_{CO}}$ without reduction in lung volume results in a low ratio. In restriction, the loss of $D_{L_{CO}}$ parallels the loss of lung volume and the ratio is preserved.

$D_{L_{CO}}$ measurements at rest have been used to estimate the probability of oxygen desaturation during exercise. Although not all clinicians agree that a reduction in diffusing capacity can predict desaturation, there does appear to be a correlation between $D_{L_{CO}}$ and gas exchange during exercise. In some subjects who have chronic obstructive pulmonary disease, a $D_{L_{CO}}$ less than 50% of predicted is often accompanied by oxygen desaturation during exercise. Table 5–1 compares some of the advantages and disadvantages of the different $D_{L_{CO}}$ testing methods discussed in this chapter.

The $D_{L_{CO}}SB$ is the most widely used method because of its relative simplicity and noninvasive nature. The rapidity with which repeated maneuvers can be performed also lends to its popularity. Many automated systems utilize the $D_{L_{CO}}SB$, thus contributing a certain degree of standardization to the methodology. There is, however, a large variability in reported results between laboratories. This variability has been attributed to differing testing techniques, problems in the gas analysis involved in the test, and differences in computations. In addition, because breath-holding at TLC is not a physiologic maneuver, and the measured value of $D_{L_{CO}}$ varies with lung volume while holding the breath, the $D_{L_{CO}}SB$ may not be an entirely accurate description of diffusing capacity. The $D_{L_{CO}}SB$ is not practical for use during exercise, and some subjects have difficulty expiring fully, inspiring fully, or breath-holding. The American Thoracic Society (ATS) has published guidelines to improve standardization of the single-breath maneuver. See Chapter 11 for criteria for acceptability for $D_{L_{CO}}$ maneuvers.

The steady-state methods, $D_{L_{CO}}SS_{1-4}$, all use various methods of estimating the mean alveolar P_{CO}. The $D_{L_{CO}}SS_1$ probably has the broadest application of the steady-state methods, and the availability of arterial blood gas analysis has enabled more common usage. The $D_{L_{CO}}SS_2$ is gaining popularity because of the availability of fast-response CO analyzers (see Chapter 9) and is often done in combination with the Fu_{CO}. The $D_{L_{CO}}SS_3$ is commonly used for measurement of diffusion capacity during exercise, as small differences in the assumed V_D become less significant when the V_T increases. All of the steady-state methods can be applied to exercise testing, but $D_{L_{CO}}SS_3$ and $D_{L_{CO}}SS_3$ are most commonly employed.

The rebreathing method is more complicated in terms of the calculations involved but offers the advantage of a normal breathing pattern without arterial puncture. The $D_{L_{CO}}RB$ is less sensitive to $\dot{V}/\dot{Q}$ abnormalities and uneven ventilation distribution than either the $D_{L_{CO}}SB$ or the steady-state methods. The rebreathing method and the steady-state methods may suffer some inaccuracy because of a buildup of COHb in the capillary blood and the resultant "back pressure." Capillary P_{CO} is routinely assumed to be zero, but the actual alveolocapillary gradient at the time of testing can be estimated, though with some difficulty.

The $D_{L_{CO}}SS_{He}$ is the most sophisticated technique. It is relatively insensitive to $\dot{V}/\dot{Q}$ and ventilation abnormalities but requires computerization and is probably limited to research applications.

The measurement of $D_{L_{CO}}$ by the intrabreath method offers the advantage of not requiring a breath-hold at TLC. The subject must, however, inspire a large enough volume of test gas so that the subsequent exhalation will clear the instrument and anatomic dead space. In addition, the single-breath exhalation must be slow and even. In some systems, a flow restrictor may be necessary to limit expired flow. The single-breath slow exhalation technique produces values similar to those obtained by the breath-hold method in healthy subjects when flow is maintained at 0.5 L per second. Uneven distribution of ventilation may produce intrabreath $D_{L_{CO}}$ values that are artificially elevated. Because the evenness of distribution of ventilation can be assessed from the washout of the tracer gas, CH_4, unacceptable $D_{L_{CO}}$ values can be detected.

Measurement of the membrane and red blood cell components of diffusion resistance has revealed that each component accounts for approximately half of the total resistance. Difficulty in quantifying the partial pressure of O_2 in the lungs (pulmonary capillaries) restricts the use of the membrane diffusing capacity determination.

Numerous other factors can influence the observed $D_{L_{CO}}$:

1. *Hemoglobin (Hb) and hematocrit (Hct).* Decreased Hb and/or Hct reduces the $D_{L_{CO}}$, while increased Hb and Hct elevate the $D_{L_{CO}}$. The $D_{L_{CO}}$ may be corrected if the subject's Hb is known. For each gram of Hb, CO uptake varies approximately 7%. The measured $D_{L_{CO}}$ may be corrected so that the value reported is standardized to an Hb of approximately 14.6 g%. The adjustment factor may be calculated:

$$Hb\ correction = \frac{10.22 + Hb}{1.7 \times Hb}$$

The $D_{L_{CO}}$ then may be corrected:

$$\text{Hb adjusted } D_{L_{CO}} = \text{Hb correction} \times \text{observed } D_{L_{CO}}$$

It should be noted that when this correction is applied, the $D_{L_{CO}}$ will be reduced for hemoglobins greater than 14.6, and increased for hemoglobins less than 14.6. Both the corrected and uncorrected values should be reported. Care should be taken to use an Hb value that is representative of the subject's true hemoglobin level at the time of the $D_{L_{CO}}$ test.

2. *Carboxyhemoglobin.* Elevated COHb levels, as found in smokers, reduce $D_{L_{CO}}$. Smokers may have COHb levels of 5% to 10% or even greater, causing significant CO back pressure. Normally the diffusion gradient for CO across the alveolocapillary membrane is determined solely by the alveolar pressure of CO, as there is no CO in pulmonary capillary blood. In the presence of carboxyhemoglobinemia, CO transfer is reduced because the gradient across the membrane is reduced. In addition, COHb causes an anemia-like effect, further reducing gas transfer. In practice, each 1% increase in the COHb level in the blood causes an approximate 1% decrease in the measured $D_{L_{CO}}$. The $D_{L_{CO}}$ may be adjusted as follows:

$$\text{COHb-adjusted } D_{L_{CO}} = \text{measured } D_{L_{CO}} \times (1.00 + \frac{\%COHb}{100})$$

CO back pressure corrections also can be made by estimating the partial pressure of CO in the pulmonary capillaries and subtracting this value from the $F_{A_{CO_0}}$ and the $F_{A_{CO_T}}$.

3. *Alveolar P_{CO_2}.* Increased P_{CO_2} raises $D_{L_{CO}}$ because the alveolar P_{O_2} is necessarily decreased. Significant increases in the alveolar P_{CO_2} lower the alveolar P_{O_2}.

4. *Pulmonary capillary blood volume.* Increased blood volume in the lungs (Qc) increases $D_{L_{CO}}$. Increases in pulmonary capillary blood volume may result from increased cardiac output, such as occurs during exercise. Pulmonary hemorrhage also may cause an increase in the blood volume in the lungs. In each of these cases, the increase in $D_{L_{CO}}$ is related to the increased volume of Hb available for gas transfer.

5. *Body position.* The supine position increases $D_{L_{CO}}$. Changes in body position affect the distribution of capillary blood flow.

6. *Altitude above sea level.* The $D_{L_{CO}}$ varies inversely with changes in alveolar oxygen pressure ($P_{A_{O_2}}$). The $P_{A_{O_2}}$ changes as a function of altitude, as well as with the oxygen pressure of the test gas. The $D_{L_{CO}}$ increases approximately 0.35% for each mm Hg decrease in the $P_{A_{O_2}}$. By using test gas mixtures that produce an inspired O_2 pressure of 150 mm Hg (i.e., 21% at sea level) $D_{L_{CO}}$ values will be equivalent to those measured at sea level. Alternatively, 21% oxygen can be used in the test gas and the $D_{L_{CO}}$ corrected by adjusting either the $P_{A_{O_2}}$ or the $P_{I_{O_2}}$.

For a $P_{A_{O_2}}$ of 120 mm Hg:

Altitude-adjusted $D_{L_{CO}}$ = measured $D_{L_{CO}} \times (1.0 + 0.0035[P_{A_{O_2}} - 120])$

For a $P_{I_{O_2}}$ or 150 mm Hg (sea level):

Altitude-adjusted $D_{L_{CO}}$ = measured $D_{L_{CO}} \times (1.0 + 0.0031[P_{I_{O_2}} - 150])$

Several additional technical considerations may affect the measurement of the $D_{L_{CO}}$ (particularly the $D_{L_{CO}}SB$). Calculation of V_A from He dilution during the single-breath maneuver may result in an underestimate of the lung volume in subjects who have moderate or severe obstruction. Low estimated V_A results in low $D_{L_{CO}}$ values. Some clinicians prefer to use a separately determined lung volume to estimate V_A. The RV, as measured by one of the foreign gas techniques, or by plethysmography, can be added to the inspired volume to derive V_A. However, V_A calculated in this way is typically larger in subjects with obstruction than V_A calculated from the single-breath dilution, resulting in a larger estimate of $D_{L_{CO}}$. This approach may not be valid because the single-breath He dilution value ($F_{A_{He}}$) is also used to derive the logarithmic ratio that describes the disappearance of CO from the alveoli. Some laboratories report $D_{L_{CO}}$ calculated by both methods.

Various methods of measuring the breath-holding time may also lead to differing values for $D_{L_{CO}}$ (see Fig. 5–2). Most systems measure breath-holding time by one of three methods: 1. Ogilvie method—from the beginning of inspiration (V_I) to the beginning of alveolar sampling; 2. Epidemiology Standardization Project (ESP) method—from the midpoint of inspiration (half of the V_I) to the beginning of alveolar sampling; or 3. Jones method—from the two-thirds point of inspiration to the midpoint of the alveolar sample.

Theoretically, the breath-holding time is considered the time during which diffusion occurs. However, because some gas transfer may take place early in inspiration, $D_{L_{CO}}$ may be greater if timing starts at the mid-V_I point, as when the ESP method is used. Similarly, some diffusion may occur during alveolar sampling. If the timing period is extended into the alveolar sampling phase as is done in the Jones method, the actual time of breath-holding is increased and the additional diffusion accounted for. The exact timing method may become significant if the predicted values used for comparison were generated by one of the other methods. Rapid inspiration and rapid expiration to the alveolar sampling phase reduces the differences resulting from the timing methods.

The volume of gas discarded before collecting the alveolar sample may affect the measured $D_{L_{CO}}$. Most automated systems allow variable washout volumes, with 0.75 to 1.0 L most commonly being used. Washout volume may need to be reduced when the subject's VC is less than 2 L. In subjects who have obstructive disease, reducing the washout volume may result in an increased volume of dead space gas being added to the alveolar sample. Because dead space gas resembles the diffusion mixture, $D_{L_{CO}}$ tends to be underestimated.

Alveolar sampling technique also affects the measurement of $D_{L_{CO}}$. If alveolar gas is collected for longer than 3 seconds, $D_{L_{CO}}$ will increase if the Ogilvie timing method is used. A sample volume of 0.5 to 1.0 L is commonly used. Subjects with VCs of less than 2 L may require a smaller volume, just as with the washout volume. If only a very small sample is obtained, the gas may not accurately reflect the alveolar concentrations of CO and He, particularly in the presence of ventilation/perfusion abnormalities. Continuous analysis of the expirate using a mass spectrometer allows better identification of alveolar gas, but this method is not yet practical for clinical use. Newer, rapidly responding infrared analyzers that can simultaneously analyze multiple gases allow the entire breath to be analyzed. These instruments permit adjustment of the alveolar sampling window to allow a representative gas sample to be obtained.

Other procedural considerations related to the acceptability and reproducibility of the $D_{L_{CO}}SB$ are included in Chapter 11.

SELF-ASSESSMENT QUESTIONS

1. The pressure gradient for the diffusion of CO in the lung is:
   a. Equivalent to the partial pressure of inspired CO
   b. The difference between inspired and expired CO
   c. Equal to alveolar minus capillary partial pressure of CO
   d. Equal to the alveolar-arterial O_2 gradient

2. If the He and CO analyzers used for a $D_{L_{CO}}SB$ test are linear with respect to each other, the fractional concentration of CO at the beginning of the breath-hold ($F_{A_{CO_0}}$) is equal to:
   a. $F_{A_{He}}$
   b. $F_{A_{He}}/F_{I_{He}}$
   c. $F_{I_{CO}}$
   d. $Ln\ F_{I_{He}}$

3. Which of the following $D_{L_{CO}}$ methods is best suited to measuring diffusing capacity during exercise?
   a. $D_{L_{CO}}SB$
   b. $D_{L_{CO}}SS_1$
   c. $D_{L_{CO}}SS_2$
   d. $D_{L_{CO}}IB$

4. The membrane diffusion coefficient (resistance to diffusion by the alveolocapillary membrane) is estimated by:

a. The $D_{L_{CO}}SS_{He}$ method
b. Dividing the $D_{L_{CO}}$ by the Pa_{O_2}
c. Performing the $D_{L_{CO}}SB$ test at two different levels of alveolar oxygen tension
d. Subtracting $F_{A_{CO_{T_1}}}$ from $F_{A_{CO_{T_2}}}$ obtained from the $D_{L_{CO}}RB$

5. A subject has her $D_{L_{CO}}SB$ measured as 10.1 mL CO/min/mm Hg (STPD); her diffusing capacity measured by the $D_{L_{CO}}SS_1$ is 9.1 mL CO/min/mm Hg (STPD); these findings are consistent with:
a. Normal lung function
b. Normal difference in a subject with restriction
c. An improperly calibrated He analyzer
d. Inability to breath-hold near TLC

6. $D_{L_{CO}}$ is characteristically decreased by which of the following:
I. Radiation therapy of the lung
II. Emphysema
III. Pulmonary hemorrhage
IV. Exercise
a. I, II, III, IV
b. I, II, III
c. I, II only
d. III, IV only

7. In which of the following situations would the $D_{L_{CO}}$ be artificially increased:
a. Measurement is performed at 1500 meters above sea level
b. Subject smoked 1 hour prior to test
c. Measurement is made in the standing position
d. Subject has had right lung removed

8. A subject has the following measurements made:

	Measured Value
$D_{L_{CO}}SB$ (mL CO/min/mm Hg STPD)	10
pH	7.41
P_{CO_2} (mm Hg)	40
P_{O_2} (mm Hg)	89
Hb (g%)	9
O_2Hb (%)	88
COHb (%)	6

What $D_{L_{CO}}$ value should be reported:
a. 9.1 mL CO/min/mm Hg STPD
b. 10.6 mL CO/min/mm Hg STPD

   c. 12.6 mL CO/min/mm Hg STPD
   d. 13.3 mL CO/min/mm Hg STPD

9. A subject has a $D_{L_{CO}}SB$ of 8.3 mL CO/min/mm Hg (STPD), which is 38% of his predicted; his D_L/V_A ratio is calculated as 1.1. Which of the following is most consistent with these values:
   a. Pulmonary emphysema
   b. Pulmonary resection
   c. Pulmonary fibrosis
   d. Pulmonary edema

10. Differences in the calculation of $D_{L_{CO}}SB$ due to the timing of the breath-hold period may be minimized by:
    a. Having the subject practice breath-holding before testing
    b. Measuring breath-hold from the midpoint of inspiration
    c. Having the subject inspire and expire rapidly
    d. Limiting the breath-hold to less than 9 seconds

SELECTED BIBLIOGRAPHY

GENERAL REFERENCES

American Thoracic Society: Single breath carbon monoxide diffusing capacity (transfer factor): recommendations for a standard technique. *Am Rev Respir Dis* 136:1299, 1987.

Cotes JE: *Lung function assessment and application in medicine,* ed 4. Boston, 1979, Blackwell Scientific Publications.

Crapo RO, Forster RE: Carbon monoxide diffusing capacity. *Clin Chest Med* 10:187, 1989.

Ferris BG, editor: Epidemiology standardization project: recommended standardized procedure for pulmonary function testing. *Am Rev Respir Dis* 118(suppl 2:55):1, 1978.

Forster RE: Diffusion of gases across the alveolar membrane. In Farhi LE, Tenney SM, editors: *Handbook of physiology, volume 4: gas exchange, section 3: the respiratory system.* Bethesda, Md, 1987, American Physiologic Society.

Morris AH, Kanner RE, Crapo RO, et al: *Clinical pulmonary function testing,* ed 2. Salt Lake City, 1984, Intermountain Thoracic Society.

Symonds G, Renzetti AD Jr, Mitchell MM: The diffusing capacity in pulmonary emphysema. *Am Rev Respir Dis* 109:391, 1974.

West JB: *Pulmonary pathophysiology: the essentials,* ed 4. Baltimore, 1992, Williams and Wilkins.

Dᴸ**₍co₎SB**

Cotes JE, Dabbs JM, Elwood PC, et al: Iron-deficiency anaemia: its effects on transfer factor for the lung (diffusing capacity) and ventilation and cardiac frequency during submaximal exercise. *Clin Sci* 42:325, 1972.

Crapo RO, Morris AH: Standardized single breath normal values for carbon monoxide diffusing capacity. *Am Rev Respir Dis* 123:185, 1981.

Dinakara P, Blumenthal WS, Johnston RF, et al: The effect of anemia on pulmonary diffusing capacity with derivation of a correction equation. *Am Rev Respir Dis* 102:965, 1970.

Forster RE: The single-breath carbon monoxide transfer test 25 years on: a reappraisal. Physiologic considerations (editorial). *Thorax* 38:1, 1983.

Gaensler EA, Smith AA: Attachment for automated single breath diffusing capacity measurement. *Chest* 63:136, 1973.

Graham BL, Mink JT, Cotton DJ: Overestimation of the single breath carbon monoxide diffusing capacity in patients with air-flow obstruction. *Am Rev Respir Dis* 129:403, 1984.

Leech JA, Martz L, Liben A, et al: Diffusing capacity for carbon monoxide: the effects of different durations of breathhold time and alveolar volume and of carbon monoxide back pressure on calculated results. *Am Rev Respir Dis* 132:1127, 1985.

Kanner RE, Crapo RO: The relationship between alveolar oxygen tension and the single breath carbon monoxide diffusing capacity. *Am Rev Respir Dis* 133:676, 1986.

Mohsenifar Z, Tashkin DP: Effect of carboxyhemoglobin on the single breath diffusing capacity: derivation of an empirical correction factor. *Respiration* 37:185, 1979.

Ogilvie CM, Forster RE, Blakemore WS, et al: A standardized breathholding technique for the clinical measurement of the diffusing capacity of the lung for carbon monoxide. *J Clin Invest* 36:1, 1957.

Dᴸ**₍co₎SS**

Filey GF, Macintosh DJ, Wright GW: Carbon monoxide uptake and pulmonary diffusing capacity in normal subjects at rest and during exercise. *J Clin Invest* 33:530, 1954.

Davies NJH: Does the lung work? 4. What does the transfer of carbon monoxide mean? *Br J Dis Chest* 76:105, 1982.

Dᴸ**₍co₎IB**

Newth CJL, Cotton DJ, Nadel JA: Pulmonary diffusing capacity measured at multiple intervals during a single exhalation in man. *J Appl Physiol Respir Environ Physiol* 43:617, 1977.

6

Blood Gas Analysis, Capnography, and Related Tests

BLOOD PH

Description

The pH is the negative logarithm of the hydrogen ion (H^+) concentration in the blood, used as a positive number. The pH scale is unitless. The pH of water (7.00) is the center of the pH scale, while the physiologic range of blood pH encountered in clinical practice is from approximately 6.90 to 7.80.

Technique

Blood pH is measured by exposing the specimen to a glass electrode (see Fig. 9–13) under anaerobic conditions. Normally, pH measurements are made at 37° C. The pH of arterial blood is related to the Pa_{CO_2} by the Henderson-Hasselbalch equation:

$$pH = pK + \log \frac{[HCO_3^-]}{[CO_2]}$$

where:

pK = negative log of dissociation constant for carbonic acid (6.1)

$[HCO_3^-]$ = molar concentration of serum bicarbonate

$[CO_2]$ = molar concentration of CO_2

The Pa_{CO_2}, which is measured directly by the CO_2 electrode, may be multiplied by 0.03, the solubility coefficient for CO_2, to express the Pa_{CO_2} in mEq/L. The equation then may be written:

$$pH = 6.1 + \log \frac{[HCO_3^-]}{0.03(Pa_{CO_2})}$$

Because the pH and P_{CO_2} are measured by the blood gas analyzer, the bicarbonate can be easily calculated. Most blood gas analyzers perform this calculation along with others to derive values such as total CO_2 (dissolved CO_2 plus HCO_3^-) and standard bicarbonate (i.e., HCO_3^- corrected to a Pa_{CO_2} of 40 mm Hg). If the hemoglobin is measured or estimated, the base excess (BE) can be calculated. The BE is the difference between the actual buffering capacity of the blood and the normal buffer base at a pH of 7.40, approximately 48 mEq/L. The main buffers which affect the BE are the HCO_3^- and the Hb. Guidelines for quality control of blood gas analysis and for blood sampling are included in Chapter 11.

Significance and Pathophysiology

The pH of arterial blood in healthy adults averages 7.40 with a range of 7.35 to 7.45. Arterial pH below 7.35 constitutes acidemia. A pH above 7.45 constitutes alkalemia. A change of 0.3 pH units represents a two-fold change in H^+ concentration. When the pH falls from 7.40 to 7.10, with no change in P_{CO_2}, the concentration of hydrogen ions has doubled. Conversely, if the concentration of H^+ is halved, the pH rises from 7.40 to 7.70, assuming the P_{CO_2} remains at 40 mm Hg. Changes of this magnitude represent marked abnormalities in the acid-base status of the blood, and are almost always accompanied by clinical symptoms such as cardiac arrhythmias.

The pH may change depending on the body temperature of the subject. Alteration of body temperature affects the partial pressure of dissolved CO_2, which in turn influences pH as described in the previous equations (see Table 6–2). Although pH measurements are made at 37° C, the value reported is often corrected to the patient's temperature.

Acid-base disorders arising from respiratory origins are related to the P_{CO_2} and its transport in the form of carbonic acid (see P_{CO_2}, later in this chapter). If the pH is outside of its normal range, and the P_{CO_2} is not consistent with the observed disorder (i.e., acidemia or alkalemia), the condition is called nonrespiratory or metabolic (Table 6–1). The HCO_3^-, although it is normally a calculated blood gas value (as described above), is a useful indicator of the relationship between the pH and P_{CO_2}. In the presence of acidemia (i.e., pH less than 7.35) and a normal carbon dioxide tension (i.e., P_{CO_2} = 35 to 45 mm Hg), the HCO_3^- will be low and a nonrespiratory acidosis is present. If the P_{CO_2} is less

TABLE 6–1.

Acid-base Status

Status	pH	P_{CO_2}	HCO_3^-
Simple disorders			
Metabolic acidosis	Low	Normal	Low
Metabolic alkalosis	High	Normal	High
Respiratory acidosis	Low	High	Normal
Respiratory alkalosis	High	Low	Normal
Compensated disorders			
Compensated respiratory acidosis, or metabolic alkalosis	Normal*	High	High
Compensated metabolic acidosis, or respiratory alkalosis	Normal*	Low	Low
Combined disorders			
Metabolic/respiratory acidosis	Low	High	Low
Metabolic/respiratory alkalosis	High	Low	High

*Compensation cannot return values to within normal limits in severe acid-base disturbances. In addition, a normal pH may result in instances where there are respiratory and metabolic disturbances that occur together but are not compensatory.

than 35 mm Hg in the presence of acidosis, ventilatory compensation for the acidemia is likely occurring. The acid-base status would be considered partially compensated nonrespiratory (i.e., metabolic) acidosis. Complete compensation occurs if the pH returns to within the normal range when ventilation has reduced the P_{CO_2} to match the reduction in HCO_3^-.

In the presence of alkalemia (i.e., pH greater than 7.45) and a normal P_{CO_2} (i.e., 35 to 45 mm Hg), the calculated bicarbonate will be increased and a nonrespiratory (i.e., metabolic) alkalosis is present. If ventilatory compensation occurs, the P_{CO_2} will be slightly elevated. However, decreased ventilation is necessary to allow the CO_2 to rise, and may interfere with oxygenation. For this reason, the Pa_{CO_2} seldom rises above 50 to 55 mm Hg in compensation for a nonrespiratory (i.e., metabolic) alkalosis. Compensation may never be complete if the alkalosis is severe.

Combined respiratory and nonrespiratory acid-base disorders are characterized by abnormalities of both the P_{CO_2} and HCO_3^-. In combined acidosis, the P_{CO_2} is elevated (i.e., greater than 45 mm Hg) and the HCO_3^- is low (i.e., less than 22 mEq/L). In combined alkalosis, the HCO_3^- is high (i.e., greater than 26 mEq/L) and the P_{CO_2} is low (i.e., less than 35 mm Hg).

Technical problems encountered in the measurement of pH include contamination of the measuring electrode by protein or blood products and depletion of the potassium chloride (KCl) bridge between the measuring and reference electrodes (see Chapter 9). Excessive liquid heparin in the specimen does not alter the pH because of the buffering capacity of whole blood. However, changes in gas tensions resulting from dilution may occur. Arterial blood is normally used for pH determinations. Venous blood pH may be useful in detecting grossly abnormal acid-base disorders if an arterial sample cannot be obtained.

CARBON DIOXIDE TENSION (P_{CO_2})

Description

The P_{CO_2} is a measure of the partial pressure exerted by CO_2 in solution in the blood. The measurement is expressed in millimeters of mercury, (mm Hg or torr), or in kilopascals (kPa) used in the International System of Units (1 mm Hg = 0.133 kPa).

Technique

The P_{CO_2} is measured by submitting blood to a modified pH electrode (i.e., a Severinghaus electrode) that is contained in a jacket with a Teflon membrane at its tip (see Chapter 9). Inside the jacket is a bicarbonate buffer. As CO_2 diffuses through the membrane, it combines with water to form carbonic acid (H_2CO_3). The H_2CO_3 dissociates into H^+ and HCO_3^-, thereby changing the pH of the bicarbonate buffer. The change in pH is measured by the electrode and is proportional to the P_{CO_2}. The blood must be anticoagulated and kept in an anaerobic state in an ice-water bath until analysis. The P_{CO_2} also may be estimated using a transcutaneous electrode. Guidelines for quality control of blood gas analysis and for blood sampling are included in Chapter 11.

Significance and Pathophysiology

The arterial CO_2 tension (Pa_{CO_2}) of a healthy adult is approximately 40 mm Hg, and may range from 35 to 45 mm Hg. The P_{CO_2} of venous or mixed venous blood is seldom used clinically. Body temperature affects the Pa_{CO_2} as described in Table 6–2.

The Pa_{CO_2} is inversely proportional to the alveolar ventilation ($\dot{V}_A$) (see Chapter 2). When $\dot{V}_A$ decreases, CO_2 may be produced more rapidly than it is excreted by the lungs. This causes the Pa_{CO_2} to increase. The pH falls as the subject becomes acidotic, and the condition is called hypoventilation, or respiratory acidosis. Conversely, when CO_2 is removed by alveolar ventilation more rapidly than it is produced by the tissues, the Pa_{CO_2} falls. The pH rises as the subject becomes alkalotic, and the condition is called hyperventilation or respiratory alkalosis.

In the presence of increased dead space, high $\dot{V}_E$ may be required to provide adequate alveolar ventilation and keep the Pa_{CO_2} within normal limits.

TABLE 6-2.

Effects of Body Temperature on Blood Gas Values*

Temperature (C)	34°	37°	40°
pH	7.44	7.4	7.36
P_{CO_2}	35	40	46
P_{O_2}	79	95	114

*Temperature corrections based on algorithms from: *NCCLS: Definitions of Quantities and Conventions Related to blood pH and Gas Anaysis*, ed 2. [tentative standard]. (NCCLS Vol. 12, No. 11, 1991.)

Respiratory dead space occurs because some lung units are ventilated without being perfused by pulmonary capillary blood. Pulmonary embolization is an example of dead space–producing disease. Emboli may block pulmonary arterioles causing the ventilation of the affected lung units to be "wasted." In order to maintain a normal Pa_{CO_2}, total ventilation must be increased to compensate for the wasted ventilation.

The Pa_{CO_2} may be normal, or even reduced, in the presence of significant pulmonary disease. Subjects who have localized disorders such as lobar pneumonia may increase their $\dot{V}_E$ to produce more alveolar ventilation in functioning lung units. This mechanism compensates for lung units that do not participate in gas exchange. Hypoxemia is a common cause of hyperventilation (i.e., respiratory alkalosis). Hyperventilation may be seen in subjects with asthma, emphysema, and bronchitis, or foreign-body obstruction. Each of these disorders may cause hypoxemia and result in hyperventilation. Anxiety or central nervous system disorders may also cause hyperventilation.

Increased Pa_{CO_2} (i.e., hypercapnia) is commonly found in subjects who have advanced obstructive or restrictive disease. These individuals are characterized by markedly abnormal ventilation/perfusion ($\dot{V}/\dot{Q}$) patterns and the inability to maintain adequate alveolar ventilation. Not all subjects with advanced pulmonary disease retain CO_2. Those who become hypercapnic often have a low ventilatory response to CO_2 (see Chapter 2). Their response to the increased work of breathing imposed by the obstructive or restrictive disease is to allow the CO_2 to rise rather than to increase ventilation. The respiratory acidosis which results from the increased CO_2 tension is managed by renal compensation (see Table 6–1).

Elevated Pa_{CO_2} also may be seen in subjects who hypoventilate as a result of central nervous system or neuromuscular disorders. Whether CO_2 retention is the result of primary lung disease, central nervous system dysfunction, or neuromuscular disease, the pH is maintained close to normal. The kidneys retain and produce bicarbonate (HCO_3^-) to match the increased Pa_{CO_2}. This response may completely compensate for a mildly elevated Pa_{CO_2}, but can seldom produce a normal pH when the Pa_{CO_2} is greater than 65 mm Hg. When the disorder responsible for the increased Pa_{CO_2} is acute, such as foreign-body aspiration, little or no renal compensation may be observed.

Hypoxemia is always present in subjects who retain CO_2 while breathing air. As alveolar CO_2 increases, alveolar O_2 decreases. If the cause of the hypercapnia is primary lung disease, either obstructive or restrictive, the hypoxemia may be more severe because of ventilation/perfusion abnormalities. Oxygen therapy is commonly used in these subjects, and changes in the P_{CO_2} during breathing of supplementary O_2 must be carefully monitored. Some subjects with chronic hypoxemia have a decreased ventilatory response to CO_2, as noted above. Administering O_2 to these individuals may cause a reduction of the hypoxic stimulus to ventilation, resulting in a further elevation of the Pa_{CO_2}. Thus, O_2 therapy must be titrated to produce acceptable Pa_{O_2} values, usually 55 to 60 mm Hg, without hypercapnia and acidosis.

Technical problems related to the measurement of P_{CO_2} usually relate to the function of the P_{CO_2} electrode. If the electrode membrane is contaminated by protein or blood clots, the response time of the electrode may increase. Such contamination may affect both measurements and calibrations. Holes in the electrode membrane can also cause erroneous readings. Depletion of the bicarbonate electrolyte buffer within the electrode may also reduce accuracy and cause unacceptable drift. Measurement of end-tidal CO_2 ($P_{ET_{CO_2}}$) is sometimes used to track the Pa_{CO_2} (see Capnography section).

OXYGEN TENSION (P_{O_2})

Description

Oxygen tension, or P_{O_2}, is the measurement of the partial pressure exerted by O_2 dissolved in the blood. It is recorded in millimeters of mercury (mm Hg or torr), or in kilopascals (kPa), used in the International System of Units (1 mm Hg = 0.133 kPa).

Technique

The P_{O_2}, either arterial or mixed venous, is measured by exposing whole blood, obtained anaerobically, to a platinum electrode covered with a thin polypropylene membrane. This type of electrode is referred to as a polarographic electrode or a Clark electrode. Oxygen molecules are reduced at the platinum cathode after diffusing through the membrane (see Chapter 9). The P_{O_2} may also be measured using a transcutaneous electrode (see Chapter 9).

Arterial samples are usually obtained from either the radial or brachial artery. Before a radial artery puncture, the adequacy of collateral circulation to the hand via the ulnar artery should be established by means of the modified

Allen's test. The technologist performing the test occludes both the radial and ulnar arteries by pressing down over the wrist. The subject is instructed to make a fist, then open the hand and relax the fingers. The palm of the hand is blanched (i.e., pale and bloodless) because both of the arteries are occluded. The ulnar artery is released while the radial remains occluded. The hand should be reperfused rapidly (5 to 10 seconds) if the ulnar supply is adequate. If perfusion is inadequate, an alternate site should be used.

Mixed venous samples are drawn from a pulmonary artery (Swan-Ganz) catheter. Withdrawing a volume greater than the volume of the catheter assures that the sample is not diluted by the flush solution present in the catheter. Venous samples from peripheral veins are not useful for assessing oxygenation because venous blood reflects only the metabolism of the area drained by that particular vein.

The blood is usually collected in a heparinized syringe and sealed from the atmosphere immediately. Care must be taken that heparin solution does not dilute the sample. Heparin solution (sodium heparin) typically has a P_{O_2} of 150 mm Hg, and a P_{CO_2} near 0. If the volume of heparin solution is large in relation to the blood sample, the P_{O_2} and P_{CO_2} will be altered. The P_{O_2} will increase if it is less than 150 mm Hg, and the P_{CO_2} will decrease. Although liquid heparin is slightly acidic compared with blood, the pH is usually not directly affected. The large buffering capacity of whole blood prevents large changes in pH. In order to prevent dilution effects when a heparin solution is used, the following guidelines may be helpful:

1. Draw a small volume of sterile heparin into the syringe; typically, 0.25 mL of 1000μ/mL is sufficient for a 3-mL syringe.
2. Hold the syringe with the needle pointed up. Pull back the plunger so that the heparin solution coats the interior walls of the syringe.
3. Expel all of the heparin solution through the needle, leaving liquid only in the hub and lumen of the needle.
4. Obtain a blood sample volume of 2 to 3 mL, if possible.

Many blood gas kits available feature dry (lyophilized) heparin. Typically, dry heparin is applied to the lumen of the needle and the interior of the syringe. A small heparin pellet is often placed in the syringe to provide additional anticoagulation. After the syringe has been properly capped (see Infection Control and Safety, Chapter 11), the sample should be thoroughly mixed by rolling or gently shaking. Mixing helps prevent the blood sample from clotting, whether dry or liquid heparin is used.

Air contamination of arterial or mixed venous blood specimens can seriously alter blood gas values. Room air at sea level has a P_{O_2} of approximately 150 mm Hg and a P_{CO_2} near 0. If air bubbles are allowed to come into contact with a blood gas specimen, equilibration of gases between the sample and air begins to occur

TABLE 6–3.

Air Contamination of Blood Gas Samples

	In Vivo Values	Air Contamination*
pH	7.40	7.45
pco$_2$	40	30
Po$_2$	95	110

*Typical values that might occur when a blood gas specimen is exposed to air, either directly or by mixing with a solution that has been exposed to air (i.e., heparinized flush solution). The change in pH occurs because of the change in Pco$_2$.

(Table 6–3). Contamination happens commonly during sampling when air is left in the syringe before the sample is collected. Small bubbles also may be introduced if the needle does not connect tightly to the syringe. Other sources of air contamination include poorly fitting plungers and failure to properly cap the syringe.

Specimens may be collected in either glass or plastic syringes. Small changes in Po$_2$ may occur with the use of plastic syringes because of the partial pressure of oxygen dissolved in the plastic. Slower changes in the Po$_2$ may occur because of diffusion of gas through the walls or plunger tip of the plastic syringe. Glass syringes should have tightly fitting, matched plungers in order to avoid leakage of gas. Differences in Po$_2$ resulting from syringe material are usually not significant in most clinical situations, provided the specimen is handled properly. If the sample has a high Po$_2$ (i.e., greater than 150 mm Hg) or if precise Po$_2$ measurements are to be made as in a shunt determination, a glass syringe may be preferable.

The sample should be stored in an ice-water slush if analysis cannot be done immediately. Ice water reduces the metabolism of the red and white blood cells in the sample. Specimens with O$_2$ tensions in the normal physiologic range (i.e., 50 to 150 mm Hg) show minimal changes in Po$_2$ in 1 to 2 hours if kept in ice water. Changes in specimens held at room temperature are related to the metabolism of the cells in the blood, particularly white blood cells and platelets. Specimens with Po$_2$ values above 150 mm Hg are most susceptible to alterations resulting from gas leakage or cellular metabolism. When the Po$_2$ is 150 mm Hg or more, the Hb is almost completely bound with O$_2$. In such cases, a small change in oxygen content results in a large change in oxygen tension.

Capillary samples are useful in infants when arterial puncture is impractical. The area for collection (the heel is commonly chosen) should be heated by a warm compress, then lanced. Blood is then allowed to fill the required volume of heparinized glass capillary tubes. Squeezing the tissue should be avoided, as predominately venous blood will be obtained. The capillary tubes should be sealed carefully to avoid air bubbles. Guidelines for quality control of blood gas analyzers and for the safe handling of blood specimens are included in Chapter 11.

Significance and Pathophysiology

The Pa_{O_2} of a healthy young adult at sea level varies from 85 to 100 mm Hg, and decreases slightly with age. The Pa_{O_2} can be increased by a subject whose lung function is normal by hyperventilation to values as high as 120 mm Hg. Healthy persons breathing 100% O_2 may exhibit Pa_{O_2} values higher than 600 mm Hg. The alveolar P_{O_2} ($P_{A_{O_2}}$) for any particular inspired oxygen fraction can be calculated as described in the Shunt Calculation section. Decreased Pa_{O_2} can result from hypoventilation, diffusion defects, ventilation/blood flow imbalances, and inadequate atmospheric O_2 (high altitude).

Table 6–2 lists the changes that occur in Pa_{O_2} as a result of body temperatures above and below normal (37° C). The changes in oxygen tension as well as those in CO_2 tension are reflections of the solubility of the gas. Partial pressure of each gas is a measure of its activity. Hypothermia (low body temperature) is accompanied by decreased partial pressure. Hyperthermia (elevated body temperature) shows elevated gas tensions. It is noteworthy that modern blood gas analyzers perform their analyses at 37° C and allow "temperature corrections" to be made. Although the Pa_{O_2} varies with temperature, the clinical significance of correcting measurements is unclear. Blood gas values should be reported at 37° C. Extreme care should be taken to assure that blood gas analyzers are properly set to 37° C, as small variations can result in significantly altered measurements.

Because the P_{O_2} is the pressure of dissolved oxygen in blood, it is not influenced by the amount of Hb present or whether the Hb is capable of binding O_2. Hypoxemia (i.e., decreased oxygen content of the blood) may occur even though the Pa_{O_2} is normal or elevated, as occurs when O_2 is breathed. Hypoxemia commonly results from inadequate amounts or abnormal forms of Hb. Many automated blood gas analyzers provide a *calculation* of the oxygen saturation (Sa_{O_2}). Saturation is calculated from the Pa_{O_2} and pH, with the assumption that the normal oxygen-hemoglobin reaction occurs. The calculated saturation can be quite different from the actual saturation as measured by a spectrophotometer (see "Arterial and Mixed Venous Oxygen Saturation," this section). A common example is the subject with an elevated carboxyhemoglobin (COHb) from smoking or smoke inhalation. The subject's Pa_{O_2} may be within the normal range while the O_2 saturation is markedly decreased. Calculating saturation from P_{O_2} in this case could result in a dangerous overestimate of the oxygen content of the blood. Measured Sa_{O_2}, as described below, is preferred to the calculated value.

The ability of the Hb to bind O_2 at a particular pressure is quantified by the P_{50}, which specifies the partial pressure at which a specific hemoglobin is 50%

saturated. The P_{50} may be determined by tonometering (i.e., equilibrating) blood at several low oxygen tensions and then constructing an Hb-O_2 dissociation curve to estimate the partial pressure at which the Hb is 50% saturated. A second method allows estimation of the P_{50} by comparing the measured oxygen saturation using a spectrophotometer (see below) to the expected saturation based on a P_{50} of 26.7 mm Hg. Calculated saturations usually presume a value of 26 to 27 mm Hg as the P_{50}, although this may be quite different depending on the types of hemoglobins and interfering substances present.

The severity of impairment of arterial oxygenation is indicated by the Pa_{O_2} at rest. The Pa_{O_2} is a good index of the ability of the lungs to match pulmonary capillary blood flow with adequate ventilation. If ventilation matches perfusion, pulmonary capillary blood leaves the lungs with a P_{O_2} close to that of the alveoli. If ventilation is adequate and there is sufficient atmospheric O_2, pulmonary capillary blood is almost completely saturated. When either of these conditions is not met (i.e., poor ventilation or mismatching of gas and blood exists), pulmonary capillary blood has a reduced oxygen content. Arterial partial pressure of oxygen is reduced in proportion to the number of lung units contributing blood with low O_2 content. Well-ventilated and well-perfused lung units cannot compensate for their poorly functioning counterparts because pulmonary capillary blood leaving them is almost fully oxygenated already. Because of the shape of the oxygen-hemoglobin dissociation curve, O_2 binding to hemoglobin is almost complete when the Pa_{O_2} is greater than 60 mm Hg (i.e., 90% saturation). As the Pa_{O_2} falls from 60 to 40 mm Hg, saturation decreases from 90% to 75%, with increased symptoms of hypoxia (i.e., mental confusion, shortness of breath). The delivery of O_2 to the tissues, however, also depends on the Hb concentration and the cardiac output. Because most O_2 transported is bound to Hb, there must be an adequate supply (i.e., 12 to 15 g/dL) of functional hemoglobin. Adequate cardiac output (4 to 5 L/min) is necessary to deliver the oxygenated arterial blood to the tissues. Signs and symptoms of hypoxia may be present despite an adequate Pa_{O_2} because of severe anemia and/or reduced cardiac function.

The mixed venous oxygen tension ($P\bar{v}_{O_2}$) in healthy subjects at rest ranges from 37 to 43, with an average of 40 mm Hg. In healthy persons, the arterial O_2 content (Ca_{O_2}) averages 20 mL/dL, and the mixed venous O_2 content averages 15 mL/dL, resulting in a content difference of 5 mL/dL (or vol%). While arterial oxygen tension varies with the inspired O_2 fraction and the matching of ventilation and perfusion, the $P\bar{v}_{O_2}$ changes in response to alterations in cardiac output and oxygen consumption at the tissue level. If cardiac output increases while oxygen consumption ($\dot{V}_{O_2}$) remains constant, the difference in the O_2 contents of arterial and mixed venous blood [$C(a-\bar{v})_{O_2}$] decreases. Conversely, if cardiac output falls without a change in O_2 consumption, the $C(a-\bar{v})_{O_2}$ increases. Increased cardiac output sometimes occurs in response to pulmonary shunting, allowing mixed venous oxygen content to rise and reduce the deleterious effect of the shunt. Critically ill subjects often display low $P\bar{v}_{O_2}$ values and increased

$C(a-\bar{v})_{O_2}$ as a result of poor cardiovascular performance. Alterations in the $P\bar{v}_{O_2}$ often occur even though the Pao_2 may be within normal limits. A $P\bar{v}_{O_2}$ of less than 28 mm Hg in a critically ill patient, usually accompanied by an increased (i.e., greater than 6 vol%) $C(a-\bar{v})_{O_2}$, suggests a marked cardiovascular decompensation.

Resting subjects who have severe obstructive or restrictive diseases may show decreased arterial oxygen tension, occasionally as low as 40 mm Hg. Less advanced pulmonary disease may show little decrease in Pao_2 if hyperventilation is present or if the disease process affects both ventilation and perfusion in the same lung units. In subjects who have emphysema, the destruction of alveolar septa may eliminate pulmonary capillaries as well, resulting in poor ventilation and equally poor blood flow. These subjects may have severe airways obstruction but little or no decrease in Pao_2. Subjects who have chronic bronchitis or asthma, particularly during acute exacerbations, may have moderate or severe resting hypoxemia because of $\dot{V}/\dot{Q}$ abnormalities. Analysis of Pao_2 during exercise in subjects with obstructive disease often shows a decrease in Pao_2 commensurate with the extent of the disease process. The Pao_2 during exercise is correlated with the subject's $D_{L_{CO}}$ and FEV_1, but a wide range of variability exists. Subjects with markedly decreased $D_{L_{CO}}$ (i.e., less than about 50% of predicted) typically show low Pao_2 values both at rest and during exercise. The degree of arterial desaturation cannot be predicted from static pulmonary function measurements.

The Pao_2 may be decreased for nonpulmonary reasons such as anatomic shunts (intracardiac) or neuromuscular hypoventilation. Tissue hypoxia can occur because of inadequate or nonfunctional Hb, or because of poor cardiac output. The Pao_2 should be correlated with spirometry measurements (i.e., FEV_1, $FEF_{25\%-75\%}$), $D_{L_{CO}}$, ventilation (i.e., $\dot{V}_E$, V_T, V_D), and lung volume tests (i.e., VC, RV, TLC) to distinguish pulmonary from nonpulmonary causes of inadequate oxygenation.

OXYGEN SATURATION (Sao$_2$, S$\bar{v}_{O_2}$)

Description

Oxygen saturation measures the ratio of oxygenated Hb (O_2Hb) to either the total available Hb or to the functional Hb. Functional Hb is that portion of the total Hb which is capable of binding oxygen. This ratio of content to capacity is normally expressed as a percentage, but is sometime recorded as a simple fraction. The values may differ significantly depending on the method of calculation:

1. Oxyhemoglobin fraction of total Hb:

$$\frac{O_2Hb}{O_2Hb + RHb + COHb + MetHb}$$

2. Oxygen saturation of available Hb:

$$\frac{O_2Hb}{O_2Hb + RHb}$$

where:

$$RHb = \text{reduced hemoglobin concentration}$$

$$COHb = \text{carboxyhemoglobin concentration}$$

$$MetHb = \text{methemoglobin concentration}$$

Measurement of O_2 saturation using multiple wavelength spectrophotometers (i.e., co-oximeters) employs method 1 above while pulse oximeters normally use method 2.

Technique

Oxygen saturation of hemoglobin is commonly measured in one of several ways. In the first technique, O_2 content of arterial blood is measured volumetrically. Then the blood is exposed to the atmosphere so that the Hb may combine with O_2 under ambient conditions. The content is measured again and represents the oxygen binding capacity. Saturation is the original content divided by the capacity, determined after corrections for dissolved O_2 are made.

In the second technique, O_2 saturation is measured using a spectrophotometer (see Chapter 9). The spectrophotometer, or co-oximeter as it is sometimes described, uses method 1 as described above. The total Hb, O_2Hb, COHb, and MetHb are usually reported in conjunction with routine blood gas parameters.

In a third method, saturation is obtained noninvasively by means of a pulse oximeter (see Chapter 9). Pulse oximeters may use either the ear, finger, or another site for attachment of the probe. Pulse oximeters typically use only two wavelengths of light and employ method 2 as described above.

A fourth technique is used to measure mixed venous oxygen saturation. The $S\bar{v}_{O_2}$ may be measured by a reflective spectrophotometer in a pulmonary artery catheter (i.e., Swan-Ganz catheter). A special catheter that includes fiber-optic bundles is used to perform in vivo measurements. Descriptions of both the spectrophotometers and pulse oximeters are included in Chapter 9. Guidelines for quality control of blood gas analysis, as well as blood sampling, are included in Chapter 11.

Measurement of percent saturation allows calculation of the O_2 content of either arterial or mixed venous blood (Ca_{O_2} and $C\bar{v}_{O_2}$, respectively). The O_2 content is determined by the concentration of Hb, its saturation, and the partial pressure of dissolved O_2. This relationship is described by the equation (for arterial blood):

$$Cao_2 = (1.34 \times Hb \times Sao_2) + (0.0031 \times Pao_2)$$

where:

1.34 = the O_2 binding capacity of Hb in milliliters per gram (some clinicians prefer 1.39 mL/g)

Hb = hemoglobin concentration, in grams per deciliter

Sao_2 = oxygen saturation expressed as a fraction ($Sao_2/100$)

0.0031 = solubility coefficient for O_2 in mL/mm Hg

Pao_2 = partial pressure of O_2 in the specimen

The content derived by this calculation is expressed in milliliters of O_2 per 100 mL of blood (vol%). The first half of the equation (i.e., the terms in first parentheses) defines the volume of O_2 transported bound to Hb. The second half represents the O_2 transported in the dissolved form. The same calculation can be applied to a mixed venous sample by substituting the $S\bar{v}_{O_2}$ and $P\bar{v}_{O_2}$, respectively.

Significance and Pathophysiology

The Sao_2 for a healthy young adult with a Pao_2 of 95 mm Hg is approximately 97%. Because the O_2Hb dissociation curve is relatively flat when the Pao_2 is above 60 mm Hg (i.e., $Sao_2 \geq$ 90%), the saturation changes only slightly even when there is a marked change in Pao_2. The Pao_2, therefore, is a more sensitive indicator of oxygenation in lungs that do not have gross abnormalities. At a Pao_2 of approximately 150 mm Hg, the Hb becomes completely saturated (i.e., Sao_2 = 100%). At Pao_2 values above 150 mm Hg, all further increases in the O_2 content of the blood result from increased dissolved oxygen. Alterations in the $\dot{V}/\dot{Q}$ patterns in the lungs can be monitored by allowing the subject to breath 100% O_2 and measuring the changes in dissolved oxygen. In practice, this is accomplished using the clinical shunt equation (see Shunt Calculation, this section).

When the partial pressure of O_2 falls below 60 mm Hg, the Sao_2 decreases rapidly. Small decreases in Pao_2 result in large decreases in saturation. When the Sao_2 falls below 90%, the oxygen content of the blood decreases proportionately. At saturations less than 85% (i.e., Pao_2 <55 mm Hg), symptoms of hypoxemia increase and supplementary oxygen may be indicated.

Healthy persons have small amounts of hemoglobins that cannot carry oxygen. Carboxyhemoglobin (COHb) is present in blood resulting from metabolism and from environmental exposure to CO gas. Normal COHb, expressed as a percentage, is in the range of 0.5% to 2% of the total Hb. Sources of CO include smoking (cigarettes, cigars, and pipes), smoke inhalation, improperly vented furnaces, and automobile emissions. In smokers, the levels may be increased to between 3% and 15%, depending on the recent smoking history. Smoke inhalation or CO poisoning from other sources may also result in elevated COHb levels, sometimes as high as 50%. Because CO combines rapidly with Hb, even an exposure of short duration can cause a high level of COHb if high concentrations of CO are present. Because O_2Hb saturation falls as COHb rises, carboxyhemoglobin levels greater than 15% almost always result in hypoxemia. High levels of COHb can be rapidly fatal, because of the profound hypoxemia that occurs.

Carboxyhemoglobin absorbs light at wavelengths similar to O_2Hb. In the presence of high levels of COHb, arterial blood appears bright red. Cyanosis, which appears when there is an increased concentration of reduced Hb, is absent. In addition, the Pao_2 (i.e., the partial pressure of dissolved O_2) may be close to normal limits. Blood gas analysis that includes *calculated* saturation may be erroneously high. For this reason O_2Hb and COHb should be measured by blood oximetry whenever possible.

Carboxyhemoglobin interferes with oxygen transport in two ways: by binding competitively to the Hb, and by shifting the O_2Hb curve to the left. An increase in COHb results in a reduction of O_2Hb, with a decrease in O_2 content. The left shift of the dissociation curve causes the O_2 that is being carried to be bound more tightly to the Hb. The combination of these two effects can seriously alter O_2 delivery to the tissues. Concentrations of COHb in blood begin to decrease once the source of CO has been removed. Removal of CO from the blood depends on the minute ventilation and may require several hours to reduce even moderate levels to normal. Breathing 100% O_2 speeds the washout of CO and is indicated whenever dangerously high levels of COHb are encountered.

Methemoglobin (MetHb) results when the iron atoms of the hemoglobin molecule are oxidized from Fe^{++} to Fe^{+++}. The normal MetHb level is less than 1.5% of the total Hb. High levels of MetHb can result from ingestion of, or exposure to, strong oxidizing agents. Like COHb, MetHb reduces the oxygen carrying capacity of the blood by reducing the available hemoglobin and shifting the O_2Hb dissociation curve to the left.

The percent saturation of mixed venous blood ($S\bar{v}_{O_2}$) in healthy subjects is approximately 75%, when the $P\bar{v}_{O_2}$ is 40 mm Hg. Healthy subjects have a content difference, $C(a-\bar{v})_{O_2}$, of 5 vol%. Arterial blood typically carries about 20 vol% O_2, and mixed venous blood carries 15 vol% O_2. Pulmonary disease patterns that cause arterial hypoxemia may reduce the $S\bar{v}_{O_2}$ if the oxygen uptake and cardiac output remain constant. Normally, however, cardiac output increases to combat arterial hypoxemia resulting from intrapulmonary shunting. Increased cardiac output increases O_2 delivery to the tissues. This results in a reduced extraction of oxygen from the blood. The mixed venous blood then returns to the lungs with a normal or even increased oxygen saturation. When this blood is shunted, it has a higher oxygen content, thereby reducing the shunt effect. The $S\bar{v}_{O_2}$ may fall if the cardiac output is compromised, either with or without arterial hypoxemia.

$S\bar{v}_{O_2}$ is useful in monitoring cardiac performance in the critical care setting. Patients who have good cardiovascular reserves can maintain a mixed venous saturation in the range of 70% to 75%. Patients whose $S\bar{v}_{O_2}$ values are in the 60% to 70% range have a limited ability to deliver more oxygen to the tissues. $S\bar{v}_{O_2}$ values less than 60% usually indicate cardiovascular decompensation and tissue hypoxemia. The indwelling reflective spectrophotometer allows continuous monitoring of this important parameter. The $S\bar{v}_{O_2}$ also decreases during exercise. Despite increased cardiac output, O_2 extraction by the exercising muscles reduces the content of blood returning to the lungs.

Measurement of Sao_2 by most pulse oximeters is based on the relative absorption of light at two wavelengths. When only two wavelengths are analyzed, only two species of hemoglobin can be detected. Absorption in the red and near-infrared portions of the visible spectrum allows measurement of the oxyhemoglobin and reduced hemoglobin, providing an estimate of the oxygen saturation of *available* hemoglobin (see Description section). These measurements may be confounded by the presence of abnormal hemoglobins or other interfering substances that absorb light at similar wavelengths. Carboxyhemoglobin, which has a red color, absorbs light at a similar wavelength as O_2Hb. In the presence of increased amounts of COHb, the pulse oximeter "sees" the COHb as O_2Hb and will overestimate oxygen saturation. MetHb tends to force the O_2Hb saturation estimate toward 85%, but the effect is small unless large concentrations of MetHb are present. In the presence of dyes such as methylene blue or indocyanine green, which are sometimes injected for blood flow studies, the Sao_2 may be underestimated. The pulse oximeter will read lower than the true saturation.

Other technical problems in estimating Sao_2 by pulse oximetry include motion artifact, interference from external light sources, and altered perfusion at the sensor location. Movement of the probe causes the pulse oximeter to mistake the motion for arterial pulsation. If the motion is consistent and of long enough duration, as in the case of shivering, the Sao_2 tends to be forced toward 85% (see "Oximeters," Chapter 9). Decreased perfusion at the site of the oximeter sensor may also result in inaccurate estimates of Sao_2. Some potential causes of altered perfusion include hypotension, hypothermia, vasoconstrictor drugs, and redistribution of blood flow during exercise.

CAPNOGRAPHY

Description

Capnography includes continuous, noninvasive monitoring of expired CO_2, and analysis of the single-breath CO_2 waveform. Continuous monitoring of expired CO_2 allows trending of changes in alveolar and dead space ventilation. Analysis of a single breath of expired CO_2 measures the uniformity of both ventilation and pulmonary blood flow. P_{ETCO_2} is reported in mm Hg. The slope of the alveolar phase of the waveform is recorded as a percentage.

Technique

Continuous monitoring of expired CO_2 is performed by sampling gas from the subject's proximal airway. The gas is pumped to an infrared analyzer or to a mass spectrometer (see Chapter 9). The analyzer signal is then passed to either an oscilloscope, a recorder, or computerized data storage. The CO_2 waveforms may be displayed either individually (Fig. 6–1) or as a series of peaks to form a trend plot. The P_{ETCO_2} may be read from the peaks of the waveforms or obtained by a simple peak detector and displayed digitally. Continuous CO_2 monitoring is most commonly used in subjects with artificial airways in the critical care

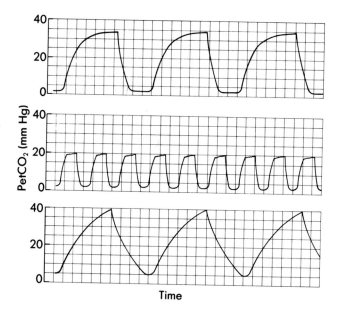

FIG 6–1.
Capnography tracings. Expired carbon dioxide (CO_2) is plotted vs. time in three subjects; in each example expiration is marked by the rapid increase in carbon dioxide to a peak (P_{ETCO_2}) followed by a return to baseline during inspiration. **Top,** a normal respiratory pattern with P_{ETCO_2} near 40 mm Hg and a relatively flat alveolar phase (see Fig. 6–2). **Middle,** a rapid respiratory rate and low end-tidal P_{CO_2} (20 mm Hg) such as might be found in a subject who is hyperventilating; the expiratory waveform has a normal configuration. **Bottom,** an abnormal expired CO_2 waveform consistent with $\dot{V}/\dot{Q}$ abnormalities; no alveolar plateau is present and the baseline does not return to close to zero.

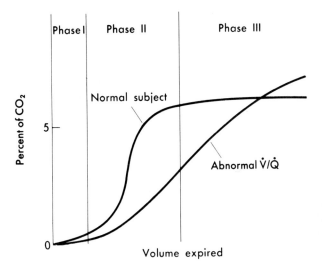

FIG 6–2.
Carbon dioxide (CO_2) elimination. A plot of expired CO_2 concentration against expired volume yields a curve distinctly similar to a single-breath nitrogen elimination (SBN_2) curve. Three phases can be defined: *Phase I* includes the expiration of upper airway dead space gas containing little CO_2. *Phase II* shows an abrupt rise in the percent of CO_2 as mixed bronchial and alveolar air is expired. *Phase III* shows the typical plateau as alveolar gas is monitored. Also illustrated is a waveform typical of abnormal ventilation/blood flow ratios. When different parts of the lungs have varying CO_2 concentrations and empty at dissimilar rates, the CO_2 elimination curve will show a constant rise during the entire expiration. The SBN_2 (see Chapter 4) test indicates abnormality of ventilation alone; the CO_2 waveform indicates abnormal matching of blood flow and ventilation, as only perfused alveoli contribute CO_2 to the expirate. If ventilation shifts to match uneven blood flow (or vice versa), the elimination curve will assure more of an S shape.

setting. The Pa_{CO_2} is often measured at intervals to establish the gradient with the PET_{CO_2}. Respiratory rate may be determined from the frequency of the CO_2 waveforms.

The change in CO_2 concentration of a single expiration may be recorded to obtain a washout curve (Fig. 6–2), as is done in the SBN_2 test. A rapid CO_2 analyzer is required. The washout curve is recorded by plotting expired CO_2 vs. volume or time. The slope of the alveolar plateau (i.e., Phase III of the curve) is recorded as a percent change in CO_2 per liter of volume. The PET_{CO_2} is also recorded from the maximal concentration at the end of the expiration.

Significance and Pathophysiology

In healthy individuals, the concentration of CO_2 in expired gas rises to a plateau as alveolar gas is expired and remains more or less constant (see Fig. 6–2). If all lung units empty CO_2 at exactly the same rate, the concentration of

CO_2 remains constant. However, even healthy lungs have ventilation and blood flow imbalances. Healthy lung units empty CO_2 at varying rates, and the CO_2 concentration rises slightly as the breath is expired. The end-tidal CO_2 theoretically should not exceed the $Paco_2$. In healthy subjects, the Pet_{CO_2} is usually quite close to the arterial value. When ventilation and perfusion become grossly mismatched as in many obstructive disease patterns, the CO_2 concentration at the end of the alveolar plateau may actually exceed the $Paco_2$. Because the $Paco_2$ reflects the gas exchange characteristics of the whole lung, the Pet_{CO_2} may differ significantly if some lung units are poorly ventilated.

Continuous CO_2 analysis provides several useful parameters for monitoring critically ill patients, particularly those requiring ventilatory support. End-tidal CO_2 measurements allow trending of changes in $Paco_2$ provided there is little or no change in the shape of the CO_2 waveform (i.e., indicating $\dot{V}/\dot{Q}$ abnormalities). Once a reference blood gas is obtained, Pet_{CO_2} can be utilized as a continuous and noninvasive monitor. Respiratory rate can be measured by analysis of the frequency of expired CO_2 waveforms. Marked changes such as hyperpnea or apnea can be quickly detected. Analysis of the individual CO_2 waveforms in conjunction with the $Paco_2$ may be helpful in identifying abrupt changes related to dead space–producing disorders such as pulmonary embolization or reduced cardiac output. Problems related to ventilatory support devices can be detected. Disconnection or leaks in breathing circuits can be recognized quickly by the loss of the CO_2 signal. Increased mechanical dead space (i.e., gas rebreathed in the ventilator circuit) can be identified by a baseline CO_2 concentration greater than zero. Irregularities in the shape of the waveform often signal that the patient is "out of phase" with the ventilator.

The shape of a single CO_2 expiration curve (see Fig. 6–2) is determined by the matching of ventilation to perfusion. Only those lung units which are both ventilated *and* perfused contribute CO_2 to the expirate. The CO_2 waveform in subjects without lung disease shows a flat initial segment of pure anatomic dead space gas containing little or no CO_2. This phase is followed by a rapid increase in CO_2 concentration reflecting a mixture of dead space and alveolar gas. Finally, an "alveolar" plateau occurs in which gas composition changes only slightly, because of different emptying rates of different lung units. The absolute concentration of CO_2 at the alveolar plateau depends on factors such as minute ventilation and CO_2 production. Dead space–producing disease, such as pulmonary embolization or a marked decrease in cardiac output, may show a profound decrease in the expired CO_2 concentration. In subjects having pulmonary disease, most notably airways abnormalities, the phases of the CO_2 washout curve may not be clearly delineated. The alveolar plateau may actually be a continuous slope throughout expiration, making measurement of even Pet_{CO_2} misleading.

Technical problems involved in capnography include the necessity of accurate calibration and management of the gas sampling system itself. Calibration using a known gas standard, preferably two-gas concentrations, is required if the system will be used to trend Pa_{CO_2}. Many systems use room air containing minimal CO_2 and a 5% CO_2 mixture for calibration (see Chapter 11, "Calibration and Quality Control of Gas Analyzers"). Condensation of water in the sampling tube or connectors can change the gas flow rate. Infrared analyzers (see Chapter 9) may be affected if the flow rate changes after calibration has been performed. Saturation of a water absorber column, if one is used, also can lead to inaccurate readings. Long sampling lines or low sampling flow rates can cause damping of the CO_2 waveform, making use of the shape for the estimation of $P_{ET_{CO_2}}$ inaccurate.

SHUNT CALCULATION ($\dot{Q}S/\dot{Q}T$)

Description

The shunt calculation measures that portion of the cardiac output which traverses the pulmonary system without participating in gas exchange. It is expressed as a ratio of shunted blood ($\dot{Q}s$) to total perfusion ($\dot{Q}t$). Shunt is recorded as a percent of the total cardiac output, or sometimes as a simple fraction.

Technique

There are two techniques for measuring the shunt fraction. The first uses the O_2 content differences, and is sometimes referred to as the physiologic shunt equation:

$$\frac{\dot{Q}s}{\dot{Q}t} = \frac{Cc_{O_2} - Ca_{O_2}}{Cc_{O_2} - C\bar{v}_{O_2}}$$

where:

Cc_{O_2} = O_2 content of end-capillary blood, normally estimated from
   the saturation associated with the calculated Pa_{O_2}

Ca_{O_2} = arterial O_2 content, measured from an arterial sample
   (see Oxygen Saturation section)

$C\bar{v}_{O_2}$ = mixed venous O_2 content, measured from a sample obtained
   from a pulmonary artery catheter

The denominator in this equation reflects potential arterialization of mixed venous blood, while the numerator reflects the actual arterialization.

In the second technique, the subject is allowed to breathe 100% O_2 for at least 20 minutes at atmospheric pressure. Oxygen breathing washes out all N_2 from the lungs, and the Hb becomes completely saturated. The percent of shunt is then calculated from the differences in dissolved O_2. This method is sometimes referred to as the clinical shunt equation:

$$\frac{\dot{Q}s}{\dot{Q}t} = \frac{(P_{AO_2} - Pa_{O_2}) \times 0.0031}{C(a - \bar{v})_{O_2} + [(P_{AO_2} - Pa_{O_2}) \times 0.0031]}$$

where:

P_{AO_2} = alveolar O_2 tension

Pa_{O_2} = arterial O_2 tension

$C(a\text{-}\bar{v})_{O_2}$ = arteriovenous O_2 content difference

0.0031 = conversion factor to volume percent for O_2

P_{AO_2}, when the subject is breathing 100% O_2, can be estimated as follows:

$$P_{AO_2} = P_B - P_{AH_2O} - Pa_{CO_2}/0.8$$

where:

P_B = barometric pressure

P_{AH_2O} = partial pressure of water vapor at body temperature (47 mm Hg)

Pa_{CO_2} = arterial CO_2 tension (measured from an arterial blood gas sample)

0.8 = respiratory exchange ratio

When using either method, the shunt fraction or ratio may be multiplied by 100 and the result reported as a percentage (i.e., 0.20 ratio $\times$ 100 equals a 20% shunt).

The second method of calculating the shunt is accurate only when the hemoglobin is completely saturated. This normally requires a Pa_{O_2} of greater than 150 mm Hg. A Sa_{O_2} of 100% is usually easily achieved by breathing pure O_2. See the Appendix for a more detailed description of the technique. In situations where breathing 100% O_2 does not raise the Pa_{O_2} high enough to completely saturate the Hb, the content difference method (first method above) should be used.

Significance and Pathophysiology

In healthy subjects, less than 5% of the cardiac output is shunted through the pulmonary system. An increased shunt fraction indicates that some lung units have low ventilation in relation to their blood flow. These patterns may be found in both obstructive and restrictive disease patterns. However, even in severe obstructive or restrictive diseases, blood flow may be decreased to the areas of poor ventilation by the lesions themselves. In emphysema, destruction of the alveolar septa obliterates pulmonary capillaries. As the terminal airways loose their support, they also have reduced blood flow. In lung units that are poorly ventilated, pulmonary arteriole vasoconstriction redirects blood flow away from the affected area. In these cases, there may be a minimal amount of shunting, even though severe ventilatory impairment exists.

Perhaps most common is increased shunting caused by acute disease patterns such as atelectasis or aspiration of a foreign body. Diseases such as pneumonia or the adult respiratory distress syndrome (ARDS) usually result in a shunt-like effect resulting from the reduction of ventilation in relation to blood flow in a large number of lung units. Foreign-body aspiration may cause shunting by blocking the airway and depriving all distal lung units of ventilation.

The accuracy of the shunt measurement using the dissolved O_2 differences depends on the accuracy of the Po_2 determinations. In small shunts, the Hb still becomes 100% saturated, and the difference between alveolar and arterial Po_2 values results simply from the amount of O_2 dissolved. The difference in the actual content of dissolved oxygen vs. the amount that could potentially dissolve is the basis for the calculation. The actual value for percent of shunt is also largely dependent on the value of the O_2 content difference between arterial and mixed venous blood [$C(a-\bar{v})_{O_2}$] used in the denominator of the equation. Because the $a-\bar{v}$ content difference is determined not only by the lungs but also by the cardiac output and perfusion status, the value used in the equation ideally should be measured rather than estimated. Arterial content can be measured or calculated easily from a sample taken from a peripheral artery. However, mixed venous content can only be measured accurately from a sample taken from the pulmonary artery. In subjects who do not have the right heart catheterized, an estimated value must be used. $C(a-\bar{v})_{O_2}$ values from 4.5 to 5.0 vol% are reasonable $a-\bar{v}$ content differences in subjects who have good cardiac outputs and perfusion states. Values of 3.5 vol% are probably more realistic in patients who are critically ill.

In instances when the $a-\bar{v}$ content difference cannot be reliably estimated or when the Hb cannot be maximally saturated by breathing 100% O_2, the alveolar-arterial oxygen gradient ($A-aD_{O_2}$) may be used as an index for matching of ventilation to blood flow. The $\dot{Q}s/\dot{Q}t$ does not directly provide absolute values for $\dot{Q}s$, but if the cardiac output ($\dot{Q}t$) is known, $\dot{Q}s$ can be determined easily.

Several technical considerations should be noted regarding the shunt measurement. The first method (O_2 content differences) requires placement of a pulmonary artery catheter to obtain mixed venous O_2 content. The second method (dissolved O_2 differences) should also use measured $C(a-\bar{v})_{O_2}$. In addition, this method requires inhalation of pure O_2 for 20 minutes, which may be contraindicated in subjects whose main respiratory drive is hypoxemia.

Breathing 100% O_2 washes N_2 out of the lungs completely. In subjects who have poorly ventilated lung units, the washout of N_2 plus the removal of O_2 by the perfusing blood flow may reduce the size of alveoli to their critical limit and cause alveolar collapse. The net effect of this "nitrogen shunting" may be clinical shunt values that are falsely high, as a certain amount of shunting is induced by the testing procedure.

Measurement of the shunt fraction is often performed in conjunction with the determination of the V_D/V_T ratio (see Chapter 2) to assess both types of gas exchange abnormalities together.

SELF-ASSESSMENT QUESTIONS

1. When the pH falls from 7.40 to 7.10, with no change in the P_{CO_2}, the concentration of H^+ has:
   a. Decreased by half
   b. Increased twofold
   c. Changed by 0.3 mEq/L
   d. Decreased to 45 mEq/L

2. A subject who displays the signs and symptoms of severe hypoxemia has the following blood gases:
   pH = 7.44
   P_{CO_2} mm Hg = 36
   P_{O_2} mm Hg = 83
   Sa_{O_2} % = 94
   COHb % = 1.7
   Hb g/dL = 7.3
   Which of the following best describes these findings:
   a. The subject has nonrespiratory alkalosis
   b. The subject has a decreased Ca_{O_2}
   c. The P_{O_2} measurement is erroneous
   d. The dissolved O_2 content is extremely low

3. What is the $C(a-\bar{v})_{O_2}$ in a patient with the following arterial and mixed venous blood gases:

	Arterial	Mixed Venous
Hb g/dL	15.1	15.1
Saturation (%)	92	70
P_{O_2} mm Hg	73	39

   a. 3.01 vol%
   b. 3.92 vol%

    c. 4.55 vol%
    d. 5.11 vol%

4. Which of the following statements are true concerning hyperventilation:
    I. The Pa_{O_2} is greater than 100 mm Hg
    II. The pH is greater than 7.45
    III. The respiratory rate is greater than 25 breaths per minute
    IV. The tidal volume is greater than 500 mL
    a. I, II, III, IV
    b. I, III, IV
    c. III, IV only
    d. II only

5. Carbon monoxide interferes with O_2 transport by:
    a. Oxidizing the iron atoms in the Hb molecule
    b. Shifting the O_2Hb dissociation curve to the right
    c. Competing for O_2 binding sites on the Hb molecule
    d. Reducing the solubility of O_2 in the plasma

6. The following serial blood gases are obtained from the same patient breathing room air:

Time	9:10 A.M.	9:20 A.M.
pH	7.39	7.38
P_{CO_2} mm Hg	41	26
P_{O_2} mm Hg	92	109
Hb g/dl	14.4	11.5

Which of the following best explain these results:
    a. The subject began hyperventilating
    b. The subject was started on supplementary O_2
    c. The second sample was contaminated with heparin solution
    d. The first sample contained air bubbles

7. A subject has the following arterial blood gases:
    pH = 7.38
    Pa_{CO_2} = 42
    Pa_{O_2} = 65
    HCO_3^- = 24
    These are best described as:
    a. Normal acid-base status, mild hypoxemia
    b. Compensated metabolic alkalosis, moderate hypoxemia
    c. Uncompensated respiratory acidosis with mild hypoxemia
    d. Compensated respiratory acidosis, moderate hypoxemia

8. Which of the following can cause a profound decrease in the concentration of expired CO_2?
   I. Pulmonary embolization
   II. Pulmonary shunting
   III. Decreased minute ventilation
   IV. Decreased cardiac output
   a. I, III only
   b. II, III only
   c. I, IV only
   d. II, IV only

9. Measurement of oxygen saturation by pulse oximetry may produce an erroneous reading in the presence of:
   a. Decreased concentration of Hb
   b. Shivering
   c. Metabolic acidosis
   d. Respiratory alkalosis

10. A patient with a pulmonary artery catheter in place has the following blood gas measurements while breathing 100% O_2 at a barometric pressure of 750 mm Hg:

	Arterial	Mixed Venous
Po_2 (mm Hg)	377	44
Pco_2 (mm Hg)	40	46
Saturation (%)	100	76
Hb (vol%)	14.2	14.2

What is this subject's approximate percent of shunt?
   a. 6%
   b. 8%
   c. 13%
   d. 16%

SELECTED BIBLIOGRAPHY

GENERAL REFERENCES

Morris AH, Kanner RE, Crapo RO, et al: *Clinical pulmonary function testing*, ed 2. Salt Lake City, 1984, Intermountain Thoracic Society.

Shapiro BA, Harrison RA, Cane RD, et al: *Clinical application of blood gases*, ed 4. Chicago Yearbook Medical Publishers, 1989.

Shapiro BA, Cane RD: Blood gas monitoring: yesterday, today, and tomorrow. *Crit Care Med* 17:573, 1989.

West JB: *Pulmonary pathophysiology: the essentials,* ed 4. Baltimore, 1992, Williams and Wilkins.

West JB: *Respiratory physiology: the essentials,* ed. 4. Baltimore, 1991, Williams and Wilkins.

BLOOD GASES

Definitions of quantities and conventions related to blood pH and gas analysis, ed 2. (tentative standard). National Committee for Clinical Laboratory Standards, Publication C12-T2, 1991.

Blood gas preanalytical considerations: specimen collection, calibration, and controls (tentative guideline). National Committee for Clinical Laboratory Standards, Publication C27-T, 1989.

Bageant RA: Variations in arterial blood gas measurements due to sampling techniques. *Respir Care* 20:565, 1975.

Barker SJ, Tremper KK: Pulse oximetry: applications and limitations. In Tremper KK, Barker SJ, editors: *International Anesthesiology Clinics.* Boston, 1987, Little, Brown and Co.

Hansen JE: Arterial blood gases. *Clin Chest Med* 10:227, 1989.

Raffin TA: Indications for arterial blood gas analysis. *Ann Intern Med* 105:390, 1986.

Severinghaus JW: Blood gas calculator. *J Appl Physiol* 21:1108, 1966.

Siggard-Anderson O: Acid-base and blood gas parameters: arterial or capillary blood. *Scand J Clin Lab Invest* 21:289, 1968.

SHUNT AND CAPNOGRAPHY

Cane RD, Shapiro BA, Harrison RA, et al: Minimizing errors in intrapulmonary shunt calculations. *Crit Care Med* 8:294, 1980.

Carlon GC, Ray C, Miodownik S, et al: Capnography in mechanically ventilated patients. *Crit Care Med* 16:550, 1988.

Cheng EY, Renschler MF, Mihm FG, et al: Noninvasive respiratory monitoring of patients during weaning from mechanical respiratory support. *Anesth Analg* 65:S29, 1986.

Harrison RA, Davison R, Shapiro BA, et al: Reassessment of the assumed a-v oxygen content difference in the shunt calculation. *Anesth Analg* 54:198, 1975.

Wiedemann HP, McCarthy K: Noninvasive monitoring of oxygen and carbon dioxide. *Clin Chest Med* 10:239, 1989.

7

Exercise Testing

The efficiency of the cardiopulmonary system may be quite different during periods of increased metabolic demands than at rest. Therefore, tests designed to assess ventilation, gas exchange, and cardiovascular function during exercise can provide information not obtainable with tests of cardiopulmonary function performed at rest. Exercise testing allows evaluation of the heart and lungs under conditions of increased metabolic demand. Limitations to work are not entirely predictable from any single resting measurement of pulmonary function. Exercise capacity may be estimated from the FEV_1 or $D_{L_{CO}}$, but cannot be accurately predicted. To define work limitations, an exercise test is necessary. In all forms of exercise testing, measured parameters of cardiopulmonary function are assessed in relation to the work load (i.e., the level of exercise).

The primary indication for performing an exercise test is dyspnea on exertion. Other indications include exercise-induced bronchospasm and arterial desaturation. Exercise testing can detect:

1. The presence and nature of ventilatory limitations to work.
2. The presence and nature of cardiovascular limitations to work.
3. The extent of conditioning or deconditioning.
4. The maximum tolerable work load and safe levels of daily exercise.
5. The extent of disability for rehabilitation purposes.
6. O_2 desaturation and appropriate levels of supplemental O_2 therapy.

Exercise testing may be indicated in apparently healthy individuals, particularly in adults older than 40 years. Exercise testing is indicated to assess fitness prior to engaging in vigorous physical activities, such as running. Cardiopulmonary exercise testing may be useful in assessing risk of postoperative complications, particularly in subjects undergoing thoracotomy. Chapter 12 includes examples of exercise studies (see Cases 7, 8, and 9).

WORK-LOAD DETERMINATION AND EXERCISE PROTOCOLS

Exercise tests can be divided into two general categories depending on the protocols used to perform the test: progressive multistage tests and steady-state tests. Progressive multistage exercise tests examine the effects of increasing work loads on various cardiopulmonary parameters, without necessarily allowing a steady state to be achieved. These protocols are often used to determine the work load at which the subject reaches a maximum oxygen uptake ($\dot{V}_{O_{2_{max}}}$). Multistage protocols also can determine maximal ventilation or maximal heart rate. Progressive multistage protocol allows trending of various exercise parameters.

In a typical progressive multistage test, the work load of the exercising subject is increased at predetermined intervals (Table 7-1). Measurements of cardiopulmonary parameters are performed continuously. The work load may be increased at intervals of 1 to 6 minutes. If measurements are made using a manual system (see Fig. 7–3), data is usually collected during last 30 to 60 seconds of each interval. Complex measurements, such as blood sampling or measurement of cardiac output, may require longer intervals. Computerized measurements (see Fig. 7–4) generally permit shorter intervals to be used. The combination of intervals and work increments chosen should allow the subject to reach exhaustion or limitation by symptoms within a reasonable period. A progressive test lasting 8 to 10 minutes after a warm-up is ideal. If a cycle ergometer (see Fig. 7–2) is used, a "ramp" (i.e., a continuously increasing work load) test may be performed.

During multistage tests using short intervals (i.e., 1 to 3 minutes or a ramp protocol), a steady state of gas exchange, ventilation, and cardiovascular response may not be attained. Healthy subjects may reach a steady state in 2 to 3 minutes at low and moderate work loads. Attainment of a steady state, however, is not necessary if the primary objective of the evaluation is to determine the maximum values (oxygen uptake, heart rate, or ventilation). Short exercise intervals also lessen muscle fatigue that may occur with prolonged tests. Short-interval or ramp protocols may allow better delineation of gas exchange ($\dot{V}_{O_2}$, $\dot{V}_{CO_2}$) kinetics. If a progressive multistage test using intervals of 4 to 6 minutes is used, a steady state (i.e., relatively constant gas exchange, ventilation, and cardiovascular response) may result. This phenomenon should not be confused with steady-state tests as discussed in the next paragraph.

Steady-state tests are designed to assess cardiopulmonary function under conditions of constant metabolic demand. Steady-state conditions are usually defined in terms of heart rate, oxygen consumption ($\dot{V}_{O_2}$), or ventilation ($\dot{V}_E$). If the heart rate remains unchanged for 1 minute at a given work load, a steady state may be assumed. Steady-state tests are useful for assessing responses to a known work load. Steady-state protocols may be used to evaluate the effectiveness of various therapies or pharmacologic agents on exercise ability. For example, a progressive multistage test may be performed initially to

TABLE 7–1.

Exercise Protocols

Treadmill	Speed (MPH)/Grade (%)	Interval	Comment
Bruce	1.7 / 10 2.5 / 12 3.4 / 14 4.2 / 16 5.0 / 18 5.5 / 20 6.0 / 22	3 minutes	Large work-load increments; 1.7/0 and 1.7/5 may be used as preliminary stages for de-conditioned subjects
Balke	3.3–3.4 / 0 increasing grade by 2.5% to exhaustion	1 minute	Small work-load increments; may use 3 MPH and 2-minute intervals for deconditioned subjects, or reduce slope changes to 1%
Jones	1.0 / 0 2.0 / 0 2–3.5 / 2.5 increasing grade by 2.5% to exhaustion	1 minute	Small work-load increments and low starting work load

Cycle Ergometer	Work load	Interval	Comment
Astrand	50 W (300 kpm) to ex-haustion	4 minutes	Large work-load increments and long intervals; 33 W (200 kpm) may be used for females
"Ramp"	10 W/min to exhaustion	contin-uous	Requires electronically braked ergometer; different work rates may be used to alter ramp slope
Jones	16 W/min (100 kpm) to exhaustion	1 minute	Smaller increments (50 kpm) may be used for decon-ditioned subjects

Other	Description	Interval	Comment
Master step test	Either constant or variable step height combined with increasing step rates	variable	Simple to perform; work load may be difficult to quantify
12-minute walk	Distance covered in 12 minutes	12 minutes	Simple; useful in subjects with limited reserves or following rehabilitation

determine a subject's maximum tolerable work load. Then a steady-state test is used to evaluate specific parameters at a submaximal level, such as at 50% and 75% of the highest $\dot{V}o_2$ achieved. The subject exercises for 5 to 8 minutes at a predetermined level to allow a steady state to develop. Measurements are performed during the last 1 or 2 minutes of the period. Successive steady-state determinations at higher power outputs may be made continuously or spaced with short periods of light exercise or rest. A similar protocol may be used for evaluation of exercise induced bronchospasm (see Chapter 8).

Two methods of varying exercise work load are commonly employed: the treadmill and the cycle ergometer (Figs. 7–1 and 7–2). The work load on the treadmill is adjusted by changing the speed or slope of the walking surface, or both. The speed of the treadmill may be calibrated in either miles per hour or in kilometers per hour. Treadmill slope is registered as "percent grade" on most devices. Percent grade refers to the relationship between the length of the walking surface and the elevation of one end above level. A treadmill with a 6-foot surface, and one end elevated 1 foot above level, would have an elevation of $\frac{1}{6} \times 100$, or approximately 17%. The primary advantages of the treadmill are that it elicits walking, jogging, or running, which are familiar forms of exercise. An additional advantage is that maximal levels of exercise can be easily attained, even in conditioned healthy subjects. However, the actual work performed

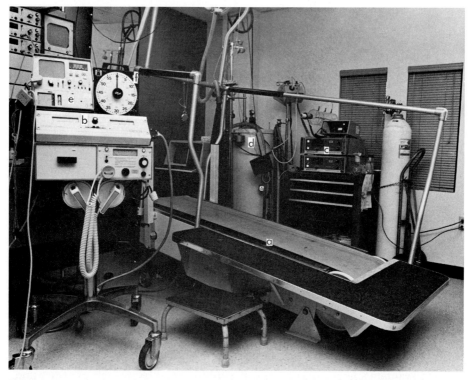

FIG 7–1.
Typical exercise laboratory setup. **A,** motor-driven treadmill with adjustable slope and speed, side rails, and platform. **B,** treadmill controls with speed and slope indicators. **C,** gas analyzers (O_2 and CO_2). **D,** Tissot spirometer for ventilation measurements. **E,** cardiac monitor/recorder. **F,** electric timer.

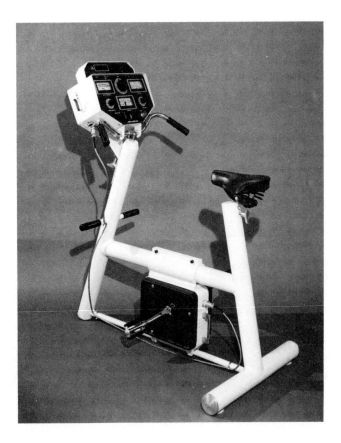

FIG 7–2.
Electronically braked cycle ergometer. A typical cycle ergometer with continuous adjustable electronic braking. Included are controls for adjusting the pedaling resistance, a timer, and analog meters for pedaling frequency (rpm) and external work load (watts). (Courtesy of Warren E. Collins, Inc., Braintree, MA.)

during treadmill walking is a function of the weight of the subject. Subjects who have different weights walking at the same speed and slope perform different work loads. Different walking patterns or stride length also may affect the actual amount of work being done. Subjects who grip the handrails of the treadmill may use their arms to reduce the amount of work being performed. For these reasons, estimating $\dot{V}_{O_2}$ from a subject's weight and the speed and slope of the treadmill may produce erroneous results.

The cycle ergometer allows the work load to be varied by adjustment of the resistance to pedaling and by the pedaling frequency, usually specified in revolutions per minute (rpm). The flywheel of a mechanical ergometer turns against a belt or strap, both ends of which are connected to a weighted physical balance. The diameter of the wheel is known and the resistance can be easily measured. When the pedaling speed (usually 50 to 90 rpm) is determined, the amount of work performed can be accurately calculated. One of the chief advantages of the cycle ergometer is that the work load is independent of the weight of the subject. Unlike the treadmill, $\dot{V}_{O_2}$ can be reasonably estimated if the pedaling speed and resistance are carefully measured. In addition, the work load can be changed rapidly by adjusting the tension on the flywheel. Other advantages include smaller size and better stability of the subject for gas collection, blood sampling, and blood pressure monitoring. Electronically braked cycle ergometers (see Fig. 7–2) provide a smooth, rapid, and more reproducible means of changing exercise work load than mechanical ergometers. Electronically braked ergometers allow continuous adjustment of the work load independent of pedaling speed. This feature permits the exercise level to be ramped (i.e., the work load increases continuously rather than in increments). The ramp test allows the subject to advance from low to high work loads quickly, and provides all the information normally sought during a progressive maximal exercise test. A ramp protocol typically requires computerization for adjustment of the work load and rapid collection of physiologic data.

There are some differences in the maximal workload attainable between the treadmill and the cycle ergometer. These differences are attributed primarily to the muscle groups used. In most subjects, cycling does not produce as high a maximum O_2 consumption as walking on the treadmill (i.e., approximately 7% less). Ventilation and lactate production may be slightly greater on the cycle ergometer because of the different muscle groups used. These differences between the treadmill and cycle ergometer are not significant in most clinical situations. The choice of device may be dictated by the subject's clinical condition and the types of measurements to be made.

Work load may be expressed quantitatively in several ways:

1. *Work* is normally expressed in kilopond-meters (kpm). One kpm equals the work of moving a 1 kg mass a vertical distance of 1 m against the force of gravity.

2. *Power* is expressed in kilopond-meters per minute (i.e., work per unit of time) or in watts. One watt equals 6.12 kpm/min (100 watts $\cong$ 600 kpm/min).

3. *Energy* is expressed by oxygen consumption ($\dot{V}_{O_2}$), in liters or milliliters per minute (STPD), or in terms of multiples of the resting O_2 uptake (METs). Resting or baseline $\dot{V}_{O_2}$ can be measured as described in the following paragraphs or estimated. For purposes of standardization, 1 MET is often considered to be 3.5 mL O_2/min/kg.

For purposes of exercise evaluation, it is particularly useful to relate the ventilatory, blood gas, and hemodynamic measurements to the $\dot{V}_{O_2}$ as the independent variable. This requires measurement of ventilation and analysis of expired gas during exercise.

VENTILATION DURING EXERCISE

Collection and analysis of expired gas during graded exercise testing provides a noninvasive means of obtaining the following parameters:

- Minute ventilation ($\dot{V}_E$)
- Tidal volume (V_T)
- Frequency of breathing; respiratory rate (f_b)
- Oxygen consumption; oxygen uptake ($\dot{V}_{O_2}$)
- Carbon dioxide production ($\dot{V}_{CO_2}$)
- Respiratory exchange ratio (RER)
- Ventilatory equivalent for oxygen ($\dot{V}_E/\dot{V}_{O_2}$)
- Ventilatory equivalent for CO_2 ($\dot{V}_E/\dot{V}_{CO_2}$)

Exhaled gas may be collected by using a one-way breathing circuit and a collection system, usually a bag or balloon (Fig. 7–3). A second method includes a flow transducer (Fig. 7–4) with a mixing chamber. The third and most sophisticated method employs a computerized breath-by-breath system (Fig. 7–5). The volume measuring device in any system should be routinely calibrated before each procedure (see Chapter 11). Tissot or other large volume spirometers are typically used in systems in which gas is collected in a bag. Volume-based spirometers usually remain accurate for extended periods if leaks are not present in tubing or valves. Pneumotachometers derive volumes by integration of expiratory flow (see Chapter 9). Pneumotachometers are used in both mixing-chamber and breath-by-breath systems. Flow-based spirometers (i.e., pneumotachometers) should be checked by applying a known volume and/or flow signal. They also may be calibrated by being connected in series with a volume-based spirometer of known accuracy.

Gas analyzers should be calibrated and checked before each test procedure. Some laboratories perform calibrations before and after testing in order to detect instrument drift. Two-point calibrations using gases that approximate the physiologic range to be tested provide the best means of maintaining the accuracy of the analyzers. Three-point calibration is necessary to check the linearity of the analyzers. For tests conducted without supplementary O_2, room air (i.e., 20.93% O_2 and 0.03% CO_2) and a gas mixture containing 12% to 16% O_2 with 5% to 7% CO_2 provide suitable gases for a two-point calibration. If tests are to be conducted with the subject breathing supplementary O_2, the oxygen analyzer should be calibrated with a gas that approximates the $F_{I_{O_2}}$.

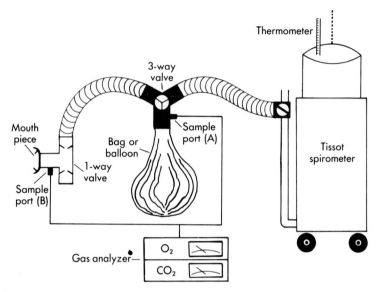

FIG 7–3.
System for collection and analysis of expired gas. The subject inspires from a one-way valve and expires through large-bore tubing into a Douglas bag, a meteorologic balloon, or directly into a counterweighted Tissot spirometer. A three-way valve controls the breathing circuit. A sample may be collected over a timed interval into the bag or balloon. $F_{E_{O_2}}$ and $F_{E_{CO_2}}$ are determined by extracting a sample from *port A*. The volume in the bag/balloon may then be emptied into the Tissot spirometer for a volume measurement. Temperature of the gas in the spirometer is measured for conversion of gas volumes to BTPS and STPD. Alternatively, the volume may be collected directly into the Tissot spirometer, with a small sample collected in the bag/balloon for gas analysis; gas in the bag/balloon is then returned to the spirometer for the volume determination. Measurements may be obtained by sampling gas at *port B,* allowing for determination of end-tidal CO_2 and O_2, as well as respiratory rate. A valve or solenoid may be used to sample alternatively between ports A and B, so that individual breaths and mixed expired gas can be analyzed.

The one-way valve of the breathing circuit should have a low resistance (i.e., 1 to 2 cm H_2O at 100 L/min) and a small dead space. In healthy subjects, a valve dead space of 100 mL is acceptable. In subjects who have dead space–producing disease or very small tidal volumes, a valve with reduced dead space may be required. Some breath-by-breath systems allow the user to reject small breaths. If this feature is employed, the volume of the rejected breath should be matched to the valve dead space. Only breaths that do not clear the valve dead space should be discarded. If a large number of breaths are rejected, the valve dead space may be too large for the subject.

If a gas collection system (either a bag/balloon or mixing chamber) is being used, the subject should be allowed to breathe through the circuit with a noseclip in place long enough to wash out room air with expired gas. The exact washout volume, or time, depends on the volume of the collection system. A bag or balloon should be filled and emptied at least once before collecting gas. Circuits employing a mixing chamber and pneumotachometer can usually be washed out quickly. Breath-by-breath systems (see Fig. 7–5) normally require minimal washout, as fractional gas concentrations are sampled directly at the mouthpiece. If supplementary O_2 is breathed, the inspiratory portion of the breathing circuit as well as the subject's lungs should be in equilibrium before gas sampling is begun.

Depending on the protocol and equipment used, gas collection and analysis are performed over a specified interval during each exercise level. For steady-state protocols, gas collection is usually performed after 4 to 6 minutes at a constant work load. In progressive multistage protocols, the appropriate sampling may be performed during the last minute of each stage. In breath-by-breath systems, sampling is normally done continuously, with data

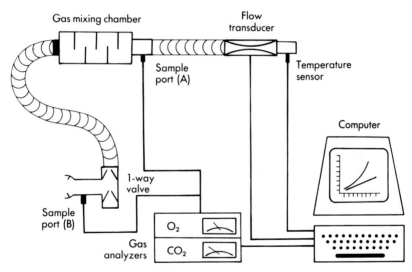

FIG 7–4.
Mixing-chamber type system for analysis of expired gas. The subject inspires room air through a one-way valve and expires through large-bore tubing into a mixing chamber that has a volume of about 5 L. Baffles in the chamber cause the gas to be thoroughly mixed so that it is representative of mixed expired gas. A small volume is extracted at *sample port A* and directed to the O_2 and CO_2 analyzers for determination of the $F_{E_{O_2}}$ and $F_{E_{CO_2}}$. The expired gas then passes through a flow-sensing (i.e., pneumotachometer) device from which volumes can be derived by integration. A temperature probe at the flow transducer provides data for conversion of the gas volume from ambient temperature to BTPS and STPD. Signals from the gas analyzers, flow transducer, and temperature sensor may be recorded directly on an analog recorder or converted to digital signals for processing by computer. Analysis of individual breaths of expired gas can be obtained by sampling at *port B*. This technique allows end-tidal CO_2 and O_2 concentrations, as well as respiratory rate, to be conveniently determined. A valve or solenoid can be used to sample alternatively between ports A and B, so that breath-by-breath and mixed expired samples can be analyzed.

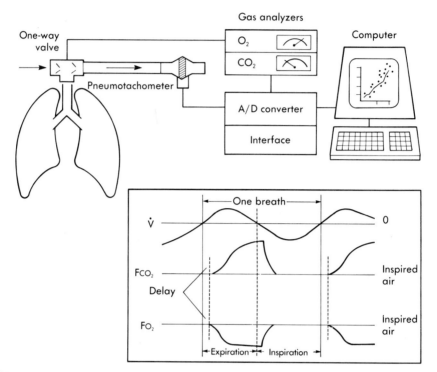

FIG 7–5.
Breath-by-breath system for determination of $\dot{V}_{O_2}$, $\dot{V}_{CO_2}$, and ventilation. The subject inspires room air through a one-way valve and expires through a pneumotachometer or similar flow-sensing device. Gas is continuously sampled at the subject's mouth for O_2 and CO_2. The flow signal and the signals from the gas analyzers are all integrated to derive volume, $F_{E_{O_2}}$, and $F_{E_{CO_2}}$, and to calculate $\dot{V}_E$, $\dot{V}_{O_2}$, $\dot{V}_{CO_2}$, rate, and V_T. In order to perform the necessary calculations and corrections, computerization is required. The *insert* shows the simultaneous recording of flow $(\dot{V})$ and fractional concentrations of O_2 and CO_2. During expiration, F_{CO_2} rises and F_{O_2} falls. Because of the lag time required to transport gas from the mouthpiece to the analyzers and because of the response time of the analyzers themselves, gas concentrations and flow are out of phase. By storing appropriate delay corrections (determined from calibrations) in the computer, the necessary signals can be aligned. Ventilatory and gas exchange parameters can be monitored and displayed on a breath-by-breath basis. In many applications, the breath-by-breath data are averaged over a short interval (10 to 60 seconds).

being displayed for each breath. Breath-by-breath data also may be averaged over several breaths. In gas collection or mixing-chamber systems, six raw data parameters are measured for each sample collected:

1. *Volume* expired, in liters.
2. *Temperature* of the gas at the measuring device, in degrees Celsius.
3. *Time* of the collection, in seconds or minutes.

4. *Respiratory rate* during the collection interval.
5. Fraction of mixed expired O_2 ($F_{E_{O_2}}$)
6. Fraction of mixed expired CO_2 ($F_{E_{CO_2}}$)

These data can be recorded manually or by a multichannel recorder with appropriate analog signals. Similarly, the data may be entered into a computer either manually, or *on-line,* by means of an analog-to-digital (A/D) converter (see Chapter 10). On-line data reduction offers the advantage of immediate feedback of all measurements, as well as greater flexibility for using different exercise protocols (see Table 7–1). Breath-by-breath analysis requires that signals from the flow-sensing or volume-measuring transducer be integrated with the gas analyzer signals for $F_{E_{O_2}}$ and $F_{E_{CO_2}}$. The lag time, or phase delay, between the volume and gas analyzer signals is corrected (see Fig. 7–5). This can be done by computer if the appropriate delay times are measured during calibration.

Minute Ventilation ($\dot{V}E$)

The $\dot{V}E$ is the total volume of gas expired per minute by the exercising subject, expressed in liters, BTPS. The normal adult at rest respires 5 to 10 L/min. During exercise, this value may increase to more than 200 L/min in trained subjects and commonly exceeds 100 L/min in healthy individuals (Figs. 7–6 and 7–7). The tremendous increase in ventilation provides adequate removal of CO_2, the primary product of exercising muscles, even at high work loads. The $\dot{V}E$ may be calculated according to the following equation:

$$\dot{V}E = \frac{\text{volume expired} \times 60}{\text{collection time, in seconds}} \times \text{BTPS factor}$$

Sample calculations and BTPS factors are contained in the Appendix. Ventilation increases linearly with an increasing work load (i.e., $\dot{V}_{O_2}$) at low and moderate levels of exercise. In healthy subjects, this increase in ventilation during exercise follows the rise in $\dot{V}_{CO_2}$. As higher levels of work are achieved (i.e., greater than about 60% of the $\dot{V}_{O_{2_{max}}}$), metabolic demand exceeds the capacity for energy production solely by aerobic pathways. In order to meet the increasing energy demands, anaerobic glycolysis assumes an increasing role. The main product of these reactions is lactate. As the blood lactate level rises, buffering occurs via the carbonic acid (H_2CO_3) pathway, and the result is an increase in the total $\dot{V}_{CO_2}$. In healthy subjects, ventilation increases with increasing CO_2 production facilitating its removal.

Relating the $\dot{V}_{E_{max}}$ achieved to resting measures of ventilatory function may provide indexes of the role of ventilatory limitations to exercise. The dyspnea index is an example of quantifying ventilation during exercise with a routine pulmonary function measurement, the MVV (see Chapter 3). This index relates

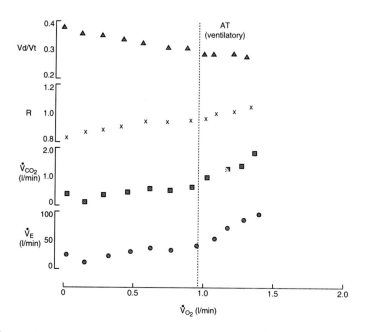

FIG 7–6.

Normal ventilation/gas exchange responses during exercise. Four parameters are plotted against $\dot{V}_{O_2}$ as a measure of work rate as they might appear in a healthy young adult. The *dotted vertical line* represents the anaerobic threshold *(AT)*. Because the threshold is determined from expired gas analysis, it is called the ventilatory threshold. $\dot{V}_E$ increases linearly with work rate at low and moderate work loads up to the AT, as does $\dot{V}_{CO_2}$. At higher levels, both $\dot{V}_E$ and $\dot{V}_{CO_2}$ increase at a faster rate, as anaerobic metabolism (lactic acidosis) is buffered by HCO_3^- and CO_2 is produced. The ratio of $\dot{V}_{CO_2}$ to $\dot{V}_{O_2}$ (RER) follows a similar pattern as RER approaches, then exceeds 1.00. V_D/V_T initially decreases rapidly as the V_T increases; it then continues to fall but at a slower rate (see text).

the $\dot{V}_E$ achieved during a submaximal exercise level, usually 6 minutes at 0% grade and 2 mph, to the MVV, and is calculated by this equation:

$$\text{dyspnea index} = \frac{\dot{V}_E \text{ during the last minute}}{\text{MVV}} \times 100$$

Values greater than 50% for this calculation are consistent with severe dyspnea. A valid MVV maneuver is essential or the dyspnea index may be overestimated.

The MVV can be similarly related to the $\dot{V}_E$ achieved at the highest work load attained ($\dot{V}_{E_{max}}$). The $\dot{V}_{E_{max}}$ may approach the MVV if there is a primary ventilatory limitation to exercise, particularly if the MVV is reduced. The $\dot{V}_{E_{max}}$ also may be compared with the FEV_1 multiplied by 35, because of the correlation between the MVV and the $FEV_1 \times 35$. The $FEV_1 \times 35$ provides a satisfactory estimate of the ventilation that can be maintained for 1 to 4 minutes both in healthy subjects and in those with moderate ventilatory impairment. In healthy subjects, maximal exercise will produce a $\dot{V}_E$ that may range from 20% to 50% of the MVV. The difference between $\dot{V}_{E_{max}}$ and MVV is often referred to as the "ventilatory reserve." The ventilatory reserve is calculated:

$$\text{ventilatory reserve} = [1 - (\dot{V}_{E_{max}}/\text{MVV})] \times 100$$

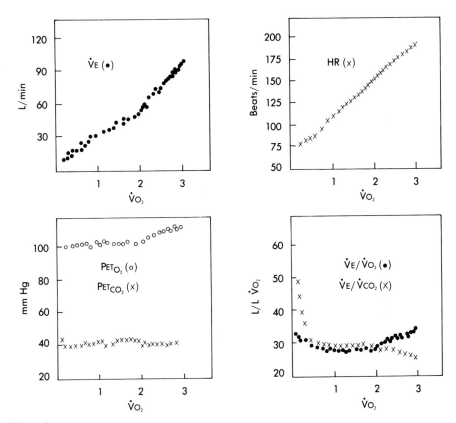

FIG 7–7.
Breath-by-breath exercise data. Four plots of data obtained using a breath-by-breath technique, as in Figure 7–5. Although data are recorded for each breath, the plots represent 30 second averages. All parameters are plotted against $\dot{V}_{O_2}$ as the measure of work being performed. $\dot{V}_E$ increases linearly up to about 2 L/min $\dot{V}_{O_2}$; heart rate *(HR)* increases linearly throughout the test. $P_{ET_{O_2}}$ and $P_{ET_{CO_2}}$ (end-tidal partial pressures of O_2 and CO_2, respectively) remain relatively constant up to approximately 2 L/min $\dot{V}_{O_2}$. At this point, end-tidal O_2 begins to increase and the end-tidal CO_2 begins to fall. A similar pattern is seen on the plot of ventilatory equivalents for O_2 and CO_2 ($\dot{V}_E/\dot{V}_{O_2}$ and $\dot{V}_E/\dot{V}_{CO_2}$, respectively). A primary advantage of breath-by-breath analysis is that these plots may be viewed in "real time" as they occur, thus allowing modification of the testing protocol as required. The data in this example indicate the occurrence of the ventilatory threshold (AT) at approximately 2 L/min of $\dot{V}_{O_2}$.

TABLE 7–2.

Exercise Variables and Dyspnea

	Cardiac	Ventilatory	Deconditioned	Poor Effort
$\dot{V}_{O_2max}$	Less than 80% of predicted	Less than 80% of predicted	Less than 80% of predicted	Less than 80% of predicted
$\dot{V}_{E_{max}}$	Less than 50% of MVV	Greater than 70% of MVV	Less than 50% of MVV	Variable
Anerobic threshold	Achieved at low $\dot{V}_{O_2}$	Usually not achieved	Achieved at low $\dot{V}_{O_2}$	Not achieved
Heart rate	Greater than 85% of predicted	Less than 85% of predicted	Greater than 85% of predicted	Less than 85% of predicted
ECG/signs of ische-mia	S-T changes, arrhythmias, chest pain	Usually normal	Normal	Normal
Sa_{O_2}	Greater than 90%	Often less than 90%, hypoxemia	Greater than 90%	Greater than 90%

*This table compares the usual findings for the exercise variables listed in subjects with dyspnea caused by cardiac disease, pulmonary disease, or deconditioning. Some subjects may have dyspnea because of a combination of causes. Poor effort during exercise may result from improper instruction, lack of understanding by the subject, or lack of motivation by the subject.

where:

$$\dot{V}_{E_{max}} = \text{ventilation at the highest exercise level reached}$$

$$\text{MVV} = \text{maximal voluntary ventilation in liters per minute}$$

The ventilatory reserve is usually expressed as a percentage. The $FEV_1 \times 35$ is often used in place of the MVV. In healthy subjects, the ventilatory reserve seldom exceeds 50%. In subjects with pulmonary disease, it typically exceeds 70% (Table 7–2). Subjects who have airways obstruction may actually achieve a $\dot{V}_E$ during exercise that equals the MVV. Because their MVV is less than predicted, exercise is limited by their inability to further increase ventilation.

At high levels of ventilation in healthy subjects (i.e., greater than 120 L/min), increases in O_2 uptake gained by increased ventilation serve mainly to supply O_2 to the respiratory muscles. The same phenomenon may occur at much lower levels of ventilation in subjects with abnormal lung parenchyma or airways from increased work of breathing. Because of the enormous ventilatory reserve in the healthy subject, exercise is seldom limited by ventilation. Maximal exercise is normally limited by inability to further increase cardiac output or inability to extract more O_2 at the tissue level in the exercising muscles. Some highly trained athletes may achieve ventilatory limitation. Aerobic training can improve cardiovascular function so that ventilation, not cardiac output, limits maximal work.

Tidal Volume (V$_T$) and Respiratory Rate (f, or f$_b$)

Tidal volume (V$_T$) during exercise is usually calculated by dividing the $\dot{V}_E$ by the respiratory rate (f$_b$). Breath-by-breath systems may accumulate individual breaths and then report the average V$_T$ over a short interval, or after a fixed number of breaths have been analyzed. In healthy subjects, V$_T$ increases at low and moderate work loads. Increased V$_T$ accounts for the rise in ventilation, with only a small initial increase in f$_b$. This pattern continues until the V$_T$ approaches approximately 60% of VC. Further increases in total ventilation are accomplished by increasing the rate of breathing.

Subjects who have airway obstruction may be able to increase their $\dot{V}_E$, but cannot attain predicted values. If the VC is markedly reduced by the obstructive process, there may be little reserve to accommodate an increased V$_T$. Obstructed subjects, who have a relatively normal VC but increased resistance to flow, may increase their V$_T$ at a low f$_b$ during exercise in an effort to minimize the work of breathing. This pattern continues until the V$_T$ reaches a plateau, as described above. Then the respiratory rate must be augmented to further increase $\dot{V}_E$. Because of flow limitations, particularly during the expiratory phase, increases in respiratory rate must be accomplished by shortening the inspiratory portion of each breath. Reduction of the inspiratory time in relation to the total breath time (i.e., T_i/T_{tot}) requires the inspiratory muscles to generate increasingly greater flows. The increased load placed on the muscles of inspiration typically results in dyspnea.

Unlike the pattern in obstruction, V$_T$ may remain relatively fixed in restrictive disease states, with increases in $\dot{V}_E$ during exercise accomplished primarily by rapid respiratory rates. It is mechanically more efficient for subjects who have "stiff" lungs to move small tidal volumes at fast rates to increase ventilation. Flow limitation may be close to normal while the work of distending the lung is increased in restrictive patterns. The mechanism of increasing ventilation primarily by increasing flow places a load on the respiratory muscles. In combination with hypoxemia, this increased load often results in extreme shortness of breath.

OXYGEN CONSUMPTION ($\dot{V}_{O_2}$), CO_2 PRODUCTION ($\dot{V}_{CO_2}$), AND RESPIRATORY EXCHANGE RATIO (RER) IN EXERCISE

$\dot{V}_{O_2}$

$\dot{V}_{O_2}$ is the volume of O_2 taken up by the exercising (or resting) subject in liters or milliliters per minute, STPD. Oxygen consumption is also commonly reported in milliliters per kilogram of body weight (i.e., mL/kg). $\dot{V}_{O_2}$ is a result of the ventilation per minute and the rate of extraction from the gas breathed (i.e., the difference between the $F_{I_{O_2}}$ and the $F_{E_{O_2}}$, see the following paragraph). Healthy subjects at rest have a $\dot{V}_{O_2}$ of approximately 0.25 L/min (STPD), or about 3.5 mL

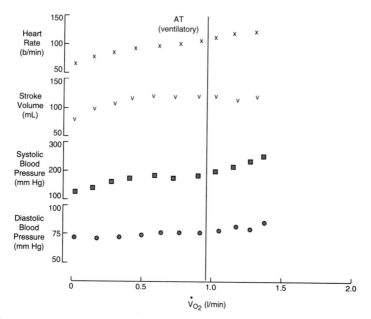

FIG 7–8.

Normal cardiovascular responses during exercise. Four cardiovascular parameters are plotted against $\dot{V}_{O_2}$ as a measure of work rate, as they might appear in a normal healthy adult. Heart rate (HR) increases linearly with work, with the maximum value attained determined by the age of the subject. Stroke volume (SV) increases initially at low to moderate work loads, but then becomes relatively constant. Cardiac output, which equals HR × SV, increases at low and moderate work loads because of increases in both HR and SV. At higher levels of work, increases in HR are responsible for increasing cardiac output. Systolic blood pressure increases by about 100 mm Hg (torr) in a linear fashion, while diastolic pressure increases only slightly.

O_2/min/kg. During exercise, $\dot{V}_{O_2}$ may increase to over 4 L/min (STPD) in trained subjects. The $\dot{V}_{O_2}$ serves as the best single measure of the work load being performed. Exercise limitation caused by gas exchange abnormalities or inappropriate cardiovascular responses may be quantified by relating specific parameters to the $\dot{V}_{O_2}$. Figures 7–6, 7–7, and 7–8 provide examples of ventilatory and cardiovascular measurements as they relate to the $\dot{V}_{O_2}$ in healthy subjects. By analyzing these parameters as the $\dot{V}_{O_2}$ increases in the exercising subject, the causes of work limitations may be defined. Exercise limitation may be a result of pulmonary disease, cardiac disease, deconditioning, or a combination of these factors.

To calculate $\dot{V}_{O_2}$ and $\dot{V}_{CO_2}$, the fractional concentrations of O_2 and CO_2 in expired gas must be analyzed. Exhaled gas is sampled from a collection device (see Fig. 7–3), a mixing chamber (see Fig. 7–4), or a breath-by-breath system (see Fig. 7–5). In systems that accumulate a volume of gas (i.e., a bag, balloon, Tissot spirometer, or mixing chamber), a sample pump is typically used to draw gas through the O_2 and CO_2 analyzers. Water vapor is removed from the mixed expired sample by drawing the gas through a calcium chloride drying tube. If the gas sample is removed before the volume is measured, the $\dot{V}_E$ should be corrected for the volume withdrawn. If exhaled gas is sampled continuously, the output of the sample pump may be returned to the volume measuring device.

In breath-by-breath systems, fractional gas concentrations are sampled at the mouth using rapid gas analyzers. The signals from the gas analyzers are integrated with the expiratory flow signal to provide the volumes of O_2 and CO_2 exchanged for each breath (see Fig. 7–5).

The $\dot{V}_{O_2}$ is calculated from an accumulated gas volume using this equation:

$$\dot{V}_{O_2} = \left(\left[\left(\frac{1 - F_{E_{O_2}} - F_{E_{CO_2}}}{1 - F_{I_{O_2}}} \right) \times F_{I_{O_2}} \right] - F_{E_{O_2}} \right) \times \dot{V}_E(\text{STPD})$$

where:

$$F_{E_{O_2}} = \text{fraction of } O_2 \text{ in the expired sample}$$

$$F_{E_{CO_2}} = \text{fraction of } CO_2 \text{ in the expired sample}$$

$$F_{I_{O_2}} = \text{fraction of } O_2 \text{ in inspired gas (room air} = 0.2093)$$

and ventilation is corrected to STPD by:

$$\dot{V}_E(\text{STPD}) = \dot{V}_E(\text{BTPS}) \times \left(\frac{P_B - 47}{760} \right) \times 0.881$$

The term

$$\left(\frac{1 - F_{E_{O_2}} - F_{E_{CO_2}}}{1 - F_{I_{O_2}}} \right)$$

is a factor to correct for the small differences between inspired and expired volumes.

Oxygen consumption at the highest level of work attainable by normal subjects is termed the $\dot{V}_{O_{2\text{max}}}$. The $\dot{V}_{O_{2\text{max}}}$ is characterized by a plateau of the oxygen uptake despite increasing external work loads. The $\dot{V}_{O_{2\text{max}}}$ is useful for comparing exercise capacity between subjects. The $\dot{V}_{O_{2\text{max}}}$ also may be used to compare a subject to his or her age-related predicted value of $\dot{V}_{O_{2\text{max}}}$. Equations for deriving predicted $\dot{V}_{O_{2\text{max}}}$ are included in the Appendix. One measure of impairment is the percentage of expected $\dot{V}_{O_{2\text{max}}}$ attained by the exercising subject. Stature, gender, age, and fitness level all affect the "normal" maximal oxygen consumption. Because of these factors, most prediction equations show a large variability (i.e., $\pm 20\%$). Subjects who have reductions in $\dot{V}_{O_{2\text{max}}}$ of 20% to 40% may be considered to have mild to moderate impairment. Those who have $\dot{V}_{O_{2\text{max}}}$ values less than 60% of their predicted may have severe exercise impairment.

Several studies have attempted to estimate $\dot{V}_{O_2}$ based on the height and weight of the subject and the speed and slope of a treadmill, or length of time spent walking. For the most part, O_2 uptake values estimated from treadmill walking are sufficiently variable, so their use is limited. Power output from a well-calibrated cycle ergometer may be used to estimate $\dot{V}O_2$ more accurately than from treadmill exercise. The values obtained are typically less influenced by weight or stride, but the actual $\dot{V}O_2$ may differ significantly from the estimate.

$\dot{V}CO_2$

The $\dot{V}CO_2$ is a direct reflection of the state of metabolism and is expressed in liters or milliliters per minute, STPD. Pulmonary ventilation, consisting of alveolar ventilation ($\dot{V}A$) and dead space ventilation ($\dot{V}D$), may be related in terms of the $\dot{V}CO_2$. The fraction of alveolar carbon dioxide (F_{ACO_2}) is directly proportional to $\dot{V}CO_2$ and inversely proportional to the $\dot{V}A$. The concentration of CO_2 in the lung is determined by CO_2 production and the rate of removal from the lung by ventilation. This relationship may be expressed:

$$F_{ACO_2} = \frac{\dot{V}CO_2}{\dot{V}A}$$

The $\dot{V}CO_2$ in a healthy person at rest is about 0.20 L/min (STPD). It may increase to more than 4 L/min (STPD) during maximal exercise in trained individuals. The adequacy of $\dot{V}A$ in response to the increase in $\dot{V}CO_2$ is indicated by the maintenance of the $Paco_2$. Alveolar ventilation keeps $Paco_2$ in equilibrium with alveolar gas at low and moderate work loads. At high work loads, $\dot{V}A$ increases dramatically to actually reduce $Paco_2$ (see $\dot{V}CO_2$ in the next paragraph).

The $\dot{V}CO_2$ may be calculated using this equation:

$$\dot{V}CO_2 = (F_{ECO_2} - 0.0003) \times \dot{V}E$$

where:

F_{ECO_2} = fraction of CO_2 in expired gas

0.0003 = fraction of CO_2 in room air (may vary)

$\dot{V}E$ (STPD) = calculated as in the equation for $\dot{V}O_2$

Respiratory Exchange Ratio (RER)

The RER is defined as the ratio of $\dot{V}CO_2$ to $\dot{V}O_2$ at the mouth. It is calculated by dividing the $\dot{V}CO_2$ by the $\dot{V}O_2$, and is expressed as a fraction. In some circumstances RER is assumed to be equal to 0.8, but for exercise evaluation or for metabolic studies, the actual value is calculated. The RER normally varies between 0.70 and 1.00 in resting subjects, depending on the nutritional substrate being metabolized (see Metabolic Measurements, Chapter 8). The RER only reflects the respiratory quotient (RQ) at the cellular level when the subject is in a true steady state. The RER may differ significantly from RQ depending on the subject's ventilation. The RER typically increases from a resting level of between 0.75 and 0.85 as work increases. When anaerobic metabolism (see the next paragraph) begins to produce CO_2 from the buffering of lactate, the $\dot{V}CO_2$ approaches the $\dot{V}O_2$. As exercise continues, the $\dot{V}CO_2$ exceeds $\dot{V}O_2$ and the RER becomes greater than 1.00. The RER is frequently increased at rest, as most subjects hyperventilate while breathing into the gas collection apparatus. In exercise tests in which a steady state is allowed to develop (i.e., 4 to 6 minutes at a constant work load), RER may approach or equal the RQ, and reflects the ratio of $\dot{V}CO_2/\dot{V}O_2$ at the cellular level. Under steady-state conditions, the $\dot{V}CO_2$ reflects the CO_2 produced metabolically at the cellular level.

Anaerobic Threshold (AT)

Measurement of $\dot{V}E$ and analysis of exhaled gases during exercise allows a noninvasive estimate of the anaerobic threshold, or AT. The AT occurs when the energy demands of the exercising muscles exceed the body's ability to produce energy by aerobic metabolism. The AT is an index of fitness in healthy subjects. The AT is also used to assess cardiac performance in subjects with known or suspected heart disease. Historically, anaerobic metabolism has been assessed by noting an increase in the blood lactate level of an exercising subject. Analysis of $\dot{V}E$ and $\dot{V}CO_2$ in relation to work load ($\dot{V}O_2$) can be used to detect the onset of anaerobic metabolism without drawing blood. This threshold is commonly referred to as the ventilatory AT.

At low and moderate work loads, $\dot{V}E$ increases linearly with increases in $\dot{V}CO_2$. When the body's energy demands exceed the capacity of aerobic pathways, further increases in energy are produced anaerobically. The primary product of anaerobic metabolism is lactate. The increased lactic acid (from lactate) is buffered by HCO_3^- resulting in an increase in CO_2 in the blood. $\dot{V}CO_2$ measured from exhaled gas increases because CO_2 is being produced by both the exercising muscles and by the buffering of lactate. In order to maintain the pH near normal levels, $\dot{V}E$ increases to match the increase in $\dot{V}CO_2$. This pattern of increasing ventilation and CO_2 production can be detected when these parameters are plotted against $\dot{V}O_2$ (see Fig. 7–6). Determination of the ventilatory AT may be accomplished by visual inspection of an appropriate plot. Numerical analysis also can be used to determine the inflection point as displayed by the graph (Fig. 7–9). Several different algorithms have been used to determine the ventilatory AT. One of the most common techniques uses regression analysis to determine the "breakpoint" at which $\dot{V}E$ and $\dot{V}CO_2$ change abruptly (Beaver method). Noninvasive AT determination may be useful in assessing cardiac and pulmonary diseases. In healthy subjects, the AT occurs between approximately 60% and 70% of the $\dot{V}O_{2max}$. Patients who have cardiac disease typically display an AT at lower work loads ($\dot{V}O_2$). Occurrence of the anaerobic threshold at less than 40% of the $\dot{V}O_{2max}$ is considered abnormally low. Patients who have a ventilatory

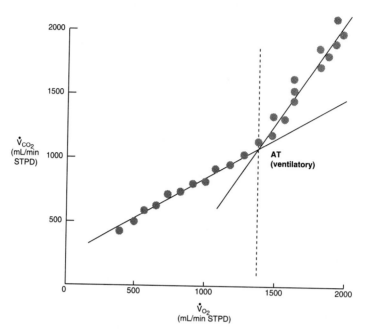

FIG 7–9.

V-slope determination of the ventilatory threshold *(AT)*. By plotting $\dot{V}_{CO_2}$ against $\dot{V}_{O_2}$, an inflection point can typically be identified, indicating an abrupt increase in CO_2 production. A more precise method is to fit two regression lines to the data gathered. One line is a best-fit line through the low and moderate work-load portion of the data, the second a best-fit line through the high work-load points. These lines are recalculated repeatedly until the best statistical "fit" is obtained. The point at which the two lines intersect is representative of the onset of lactate production, the anaerobic threshold.

limitation to exercise (i.e., pulmonary disease) may be unable to exercise at a high enough work load to reach their anaerobic threshold. In subjects who have pulmonary disease, O_2 delivery may be limited by the lungs rather than by cardiac output or extraction by the exercising muscle.

Aerobic training improves cardiac performance and O_2 delivery to the tissues, resulting in a delay in the AT until higher work loads are reached. Measurement of the AT is often used to select a training level. Maximum training effects seem to occur when the subject exercises at a work load slightly below the AT. In subjects who are sedentary, deconditioning may occur. Deconditioning may be present when the AT occurs at a lower than expected work load, and there is no evidence of cardiac or pulmonary disease.

The AT also may be determined by inspecting graphs of the ventilatory equivalents for O_2 and CO_2 (see the next section) plotted against $\dot{V}_{O_2}$. When the $\dot{V}_E/\dot{V}_{O_2}$ increases without an increase in $\dot{V}_E/\dot{V}_{CO_2}$, the AT has been reached. A similar pattern can be seen when the end-tidal O_2 and CO_2 gas tensions are plotted (see Fig. 7–7).

Sample calculations of $\dot{V}E$, $\dot{V}O_2$, $\dot{V}CO_2$, and RER, as used with one of the gas accumulation methods, are included in the Appendix.

VENTILATORY EQUIVALENTS FOR O_2 AND CO_2, AND O_2 PULSE IN EXERCISE

$\dot{V}E/\dot{V}O_2$

The minute ventilation during exercise may be related to the amount of work being performed (expressed as the $\dot{V}O_2$). This ratio is called the ventilatory equivalent for O_2, or $\dot{V}E/\dot{V}O_2$. It is calculated by dividing the $\dot{V}E$ (BTPS) by the $\dot{V}O_2$ (STPD) and expressing the ratio in liters of ventilation per liter of O_2 consumed per minute. The $\dot{V}E/\dot{V}O_2$ is a measure of the efficiency of the ventilatory pump at various work loads.

Ventilation at low and moderate work loads increases linearly with increasing $\dot{V}O_2$ and $\dot{V}CO_2$. The absolute level of ventilation depends on the response to CO_2, on the adequacy of $\dot{V}A$, and on the V_D/V_T ratio. In healthy subjects, the ratio remains in the range of 20 to 30 L/L $\dot{V}O_2$ until higher levels of work are reached. At work loads above 60% to 75% of the $\dot{V}O_{2max}$, $\dot{V}E$ is more closely related to $\dot{V}CO_2$. As ventilation increases to match the $\dot{V}CO_2$ above the AT, the ventilatory equivalent for O_2 also increases.

Ventilation helps determine the volume of O_2 that can be transported per minute. Therefore, it is often useful to evaluate the level of total ventilation required for a particular work load to assess the role of the lungs in exercise limitations. In some pulmonary disease patterns, the $\dot{V}E/\dot{V}O_2$ may be close to normal at rest, but increases with exercise out of proportion to increases in either $\dot{V}O_2$ or $\dot{V}CO_2$. This usually occurs in individuals who have severe $\dot{V}/\dot{Q}$ abnormalities that worsen with increasing cardiac output during exercise. Some subjects who have pulmonary disease may have an elevated $\dot{V}E/\dot{V}O_2$ at rest (i.e., greater than 40 L/L $\dot{V}O_2$) that falls during exercise but does not return to the normal range. Many subjects hyperventilate during the resting phase at the beginning of an exercise evaluation. The result is an increased $\dot{V}E/\dot{V}O_2$ that usually returns to the normal range during exercise. This pretest hyperventilation is also usually denoted by an RER of greater than 1.0 that returns to a normal level once the subject begins exercise.

$\dot{V}E/\dot{V}CO_2$

The ventilatory equivalent for CO_2 ($\dot{V}E/\dot{V}CO_2$) is calculated in a manner similar to that used for the $\dot{V}E/\dot{V}O_2$. Carbon dioxide production (STPD) is divided by minute ventilation (BTPS). The normal level is in the range of 25 to 35 L/L $\dot{V}_{CO_2}$. The $\dot{V}_E$ tends to match $\dot{V}_{CO_2}$ from low up to high work loads. Hence the $\dot{V}_E/\dot{V}_{CO_2}$ remains constant in healthy subjects until the highest work loads are reached. The $\dot{V}_E/\dot{V}_{CO_2}$ may be useful for estimating the maximum tolerable work load in subjects who have moderate or severe ventilatory limitations. The ventilatory equivalents for O_2 and CO_2, measured using a breath-by-breath technique, may be useful in identifying the onset of the AT. Anaerobic metabolism is usually accompanied by a steady increase in the $\dot{V}_E/\dot{V}_{O_2}$ while the $\dot{V}_E/\dot{V}_{CO_2}$ remains constant or falls slightly. This same pattern may also be seen on a breath-by-breath display of $P_{ET_{O_2}}$ and $P_{ET_{CO_2}}$ (see Fig. 7–7). A markedly elevated $\dot{V}_E/\dot{V}_{CO_2}$ (i.e., greater than 50 L/L $\dot{V}_{CO_2}$) also may be observed in pulmonary hypertensive disease.

O_2 Pulse

The efficiency of the circulatory pump may be related to the work load, expressed as the $\dot{V}_{O_2}$, during exercise by the O_2 pulse. The O_2 pulse is defined as the volume of O_2 consumed per heartbeat. The heart rate (HR) may be read manually from a standard ECG or from an accurate analog signal. The $\dot{V}_{O_2}$ in milliliters per minute (STPD) is divided by the HR per minute. The quotient is expressed as milliliters of $\dot{V}_{O_2}$ per heartbeat. In healthy subjects, the O_2 pulse varies between 2.5 and 4.0 mL O_2/beat at rest. The O_2 pulse increases to 10 to 15 mL O_2/beat during strenuous exercise.

In patients with cardiac disease, the O_2 pulse may be normal or even low at rest, but does not rise to expected levels during exercise. This pattern is consistent with an inappropriately high HR for a particular level of work. The cardiac output is the product of the HR and stroke volume (SV). Cardiac output normally increases linearly with increasing exercise (see Fig. 7–8). A low O_2 pulse is generally consistent with an inability to increase the SV. The O_2 pulse may even fall in subjects with poor left ventricular function. The pattern of low O_2 pulse with increasing work rate may be seen in subjects with coronary artery disease or valvular insufficiency, but is most pronounced in the cardiomyopathies. Tachycardia or tachyarrhythmias tend to lower the O_2 pulse because of the abnormally elevated HR. Conversely, beta-blocking agents, which tend to reduce HR, may falsely elevate the O_2 pulse. The O_2 pulse is often considered an index of fitness. At similar power outputs, a fit subject will have a higher O_2 pulse than one who is deconditioned. Fitness is generally accompanied by a lower HR, both at rest and at maximal work loads. Conditioning exercises (i.e., aerobic training) tend to increase SV. As a result, the heart beats less frequently to produce the same cardiac output. Trained subjects can thus achieve higher work rates before reaching their limiting cardiac frequency.

GAS EXCHANGE AND EXERCISE BLOOD GASES

Blood gas sampling during exercise testing, although invasive, is often indicated in subjects with primary pulmonary disorders. An indwelling arterial catheter permits analysis of blood gas tensions (i.e., Pa_{O_2}, Pa_{CO_2}), saturation (Sa_{O_2}), O_2 content (Ca_{O_2}), pH, and lactate levels at various work loads. The indwelling catheter, in conjunction with a suitable pressure transducer (Fig. 7–10), allows continuous monitoring of systemic blood pressure as well. Arterial catheterization, at either the radial or brachial sites, has been demonstrated to be relatively safe. An arterial catheter is indicated if multiple blood specimens are required. Subjects who have resting blood gas abnormalities may be candidates for arterial catheterization for exercise evaluation. An arterial line may be helpful in titrating supplementary O_2 in subjects who desaturate during exercise. See Chapter 11, Infection Control and Safety, for precautions concerning insertion of arterial catheters.

An alternative technique is to obtain a specimen by a simple arterial puncture at peak exercise. Use of a cycle ergometer for testing allows better stabilization of the radial or brachial artery sites. The sample should be obtained within 15 seconds of peak exercise because gas tensions, particularly Pa_{O_2}, may change rapidly. A potential disadvantage of the single puncture is that if the specimen cannot be obtained within 15 seconds, the procedure must be repeated.

Oxygen saturation during exercise may be monitored using a pulse oximeter on either the ear or finger sites (see Chapter 9). Oxygen saturation measured by pulse oximetry is sometimes referred to as the Sp_{O_2}. Whether the pulse oximeter is attached at the finger or ear site, the probe should be adequately secured. Motion artifact is a common problem, particularly with treadmill exercise.

An advantage of pulse oximetry is that it provides continuous measurements of saturation, in distinction to the discrete measurements of arterial sampling. Such in vivo measurements are extremely valuable in evaluating subjects who have pulmonary disease. These subjects frequently display rapid changes in Pa_{O_2} and Sa_{O_2} during exercise. Pulse oximetry may overestimate the true saturation if a significant concentration of COHb is present. Inadequate perfusion of the ear or finger also may confound oximetry during exercise testing. Motion artifact, light scattering within the tissue at the probe site, and dark skin pigmentation all may cause discrepancies between the Sp_{O_2} and the actual Sa_{O_2} (see Sa_{O_2}, Chapter 6). A single arterial sample, preferably at peak exercise, may be used to correlate the Sp_{O_2} reading with true saturation if the specimen is analyzed with a multiwavelength blood oximeter (see Chapter 9). Once adequate correlation between Sa_{O_2} and Sp_{O_2} during exercise is established, further blood sampling may be unnecessary.

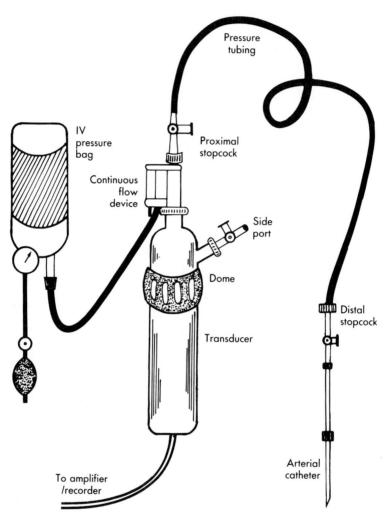

FIG 7–10.
Pressure transducer setup for continuous arterial monitoring. The components for continuous monitoring of systemic blood pressure via an arterial catheter. The catheter is normally inserted into the radial or brachial artery. Pressure tubing connects the catheter to a continuous flow device that maintains a constant pressure (and a small flow of solution) against the arterial line to prevent back flow of blood into the system. The continuous flow device also allows flushing of the system. Connected in line with the tubing is a pressure transducer assembly. Pressure changes in the system are transmitted via a thin membrane at the base of the dome to a pressure transducer. Blood samples may be drawn by inserting a heparinized syringe at the distal stopcock, closing the proximal stopcock to block the continuous flow device, and withdrawing (the blood pressure signal is temporarily lost during sampling). A similar assembly can be used for connection to a Swan-Ganz catheter for pulmonary artery monitoring during exercise.

In healthy subjects, the Pa_{O_2} tends to remain constant, even up to relatively high work loads. The alveolar P_{O_2} increases at maximal exercise as a result of the increased ventilation accompanying the rise in $\dot{V}_{CO_2}$. The alveolar-arterial (A-a) gradient, normally about 10 mm Hg, widens as a result of the increase in alveolar oxygen tension. The A-a gradient also increases somewhat because of a lower mixed venous oxygen content. The $P(A-a)_{O_2}$ may increase to 20 to 30 mm Hg in healthy subjects during heavy exercise because of these mechanisms.

A fall in the Pa_{O_2} with increasing exercise can result from increased right to left shunting. Similarly, inequality of $\dot{V}_A$ in relation to pulmonary capillary perfusion may result in a reduced Pa_{O_2}. Diffusion limitation at the alveolocapillary interface also can affect Pa_{O_2}. Because exercise reduces the mixed venous oxygen tension ($P\bar{v}_{O_2}$), the presence of a shunt or $\dot{V}/\dot{Q}$ inequality may result in a decrease in the Pa_{O_2}, or a widening of the $A\text{-}a_{O_2}$ gradient. This change in Pa_{O_2} may occur without an absolute change in the magnitude of the shunt. Mixed venous blood with a lowered O_2 content (resulting from extraction by the exercising muscles) passes through abnormal lung units and then mixes with normally arterialized blood.

In some subjects who have decreased Pa_{O_2} and increased $P(A-a)_{O_2}$ at rest, oxygenation may improve with exercise. Increased cardiac output or redistribution of ventilation during exercise may actually cause an increase in the Pa_{O_2}. This improvement in the Pa_{O_2} may occur as a result of an increased PA_{O_2} caused by a reduction of PA_{CO_2} at moderate to high work rates. Improved $\dot{V}/\dot{Q}$ relationships resulting directly from the changes in ventilation and/or cardiac output also may improve the Pa_{O_2}. Because the Pa_{O_2} may either increase or decrease during exercise, measuring Pa_{O_2} during exercise may be particularly valuable in subjects with known or suspected pulmonary disorders.

A Pa_{O_2} falling to less than 55 mm Hg or an Sa_{O_2} decreasing to less than 85% is sufficient reason for terminating the exercise evaluation. Subjects with hypoxemia at rest or at very low work rates should be tested with supplementary O_2 via a controlled delivery system (e.g., a nasal cannula) in order to determine an appropriate exercise O_2 prescription. Different levels of supplementary oxygen may be required for rest and for various activities of daily living. Correlation of Pa_{O_2} using supplementary oxygen to different exercise work loads allows relatively precise titration of therapy to the patient's needs.

In healthy subjects, the Pa_{CO_2} remains relatively constant at low and moderate work rates. The $\dot{V}_A$ increases to match the increase in $\dot{V}_{CO_2}$. The end-tidal CO_2 increases at submaximal work loads, indicating that less ventilation is "wasted" (V_D/V_T decreases). At work loads in excess of 50% to 60% of the $\dot{V}_{O_2 max}$, the metabolic acidosis resulting from anaerobic metabolism stimulates $\dot{V}_E$ to increase. This occurs in response to the augmented $\dot{V}_{CO_2}$ from the buffering of lactic acid. Ventilation thus increases in excess of that required to keep the Pa_{CO_2} constant. A progressive decrease in Pa_{CO_2} ensues, resulting in respiratory compensation for the acidosis associated with anaerobic metabolism (see Figs. 7–6 and 7–7). The $P_{ET_{CO_2}}$ decreases along with the Pa_{CO_2} at high work rates.

Some individuals who have airways obstruction may be able to increase their $\dot{V}_A$ to maintain a normal Pa_{CO_2} at low work loads. At higher work loads, however, they may be unable to reduce the Pa_{CO_2} to compensate for the metabolic acidosis. In many subjects who have airways obstruction, the level of maximal exercise is limited by the lack of ventilatory reserve. These individuals typically do not reach the AT. They are unable to attain a work load sufficient to induce anaerobic metabolism. In subjects with severe airflow obstruction, $\dot{V}_A$ may not be able to match the increase in $\dot{V}_{CO_2}$, resulting in hypercapnia and respiratory acidosis. Increased work of breathing and reduced sensitivity to CO_2 combined with the increased $\dot{V}_{CO_2}$ of exercise allow the Pa_{CO_2} to rise.

The pH, like Pa_{CO_2}, is regulated by the $\dot{V}_A$ at low work rates. The $\dot{V}_A$ increases in proportion to the $\dot{V}_{CO_2}$ up to the AT. At work rates above the AT, proportional increases in ventilation maintain the pH at near-normal levels. Most of the buffering of lactic acid is provided by HCO_3^- and a decrease in the Pa_{CO_2}. At the highest work rates (i.e., above 80% of the $\dot{V}_{O_{2max}}$), the pH decreases despite hyperventilation, as the compensation for lactic acidosis becomes incomplete. In the presence of airways obstruction, ventilatory limitations may prevent compensation above the AT, with the development of significant respiratory acidosis. However, subjects who have moderate or severe obstruction generally cannot exercise up to a level that elicits anaerobic metabolism. Acidosis observed in these subjects may result primarily from increased Pa_{CO_2}.

Arterial blood gases drawn during exercise allow several other parameters of gas exchange to be determined. These include physiologic dead space, alveolar ventilation, and the V_D/V_T ratio.

The V_D (see Chapter 2), comprised of anatomic and alveolar dead space, makes up that part of the $\dot{V}_E$ that does not participate in gas exchange. The V_D/V_T ratio expresses the relationship between "wasted" and tidal ventilation for the average breath. The healthy adult subject at rest has a $\dot{V}_A$ of 4 to 7 L/min (BTPS), and a V_D/V_T ratio of approximately 0.25 to 0.35. The volume of dead space normally increases during exercise in conjunction with increased $\dot{V}_E$. Because of increases in V_T and increased perfusion of well-ventilated lung units (i.e., the apices), the V_D/V_T ratio falls. This pattern is expected in healthy subjects (see Fig. 7–6). The V_D/V_T may fall in mild or moderate pulmonary disease states. In severe airways obstruction or in pulmonary vascular disease, the V_D/V_T typically remains fixed or even increases. An increase in the V_D/V_T is indicative of increased ventilation in relation to perfusion, and is often associated with pulmonary hypertension. The $\dot{V}_A$ during exercise normally increases proportionately more than the $\dot{V}_E$ because the V_D/V_T falls. In subjects whose V_D/V_T ratio remains fixed or rises, the adequacy of $\dot{V}_A$ must be assessed in terms of the Pa_{CO_2} and not simply by the magnitude of the $\dot{V}_E$.

Calculation of V_D, $\dot{V}_A$, and V_D/V_T requires measurement of the $Paco_2$. The V_D may be calculated using the following equation:

$$V_D = \left(V_T \times \left[1 - \frac{FE_{CO_2} \times (P_B - 47)}{Paco_2} \right] \right) - V_{D_{sys}}$$

where:

V_T = tidal volume, in liters (BTPS)

FE_{co_2} = fraction of expired CO_2

$P_B - 47$ = dry barometric pressure

$Paco_2$ = arterial CO_2 tension

$V_{D_{sys}}$ = dead space of the one-way breathing valve, in liters

Once the V_D is determined, $\dot{V}_A$ (BTPS) can be calculated using this equation:

$$\dot{V}_A = \dot{V}_E - (f_b \times V_D)$$

where:

$\dot{V}_E$ = minute ventilation (BTPS)

f_b = respiratory rate

V_D = respiratory dead space (BTPS)

The V_D/V_T ratio may be calculated as the quotient of the V_D (as determined above) and the V_T, averaged from the $\dot{V}_E$ and f_b. Alternately, the V_D/V_T may be derived simply from the difference between arterial and mixed expired CO_2 at each exercise level:

$$V_D/V_T = \frac{(Paco_2 - Peco_2)}{Paco_2}$$

where:

PE_{co_2} = partial pressure of CO_2 in expired gas

CARDIOVASCULAR MONITORS DURING EXERCISE

Continuous monitoring of HR and ECG during exercise are essential for safe performance of the test. Intermittent or continuous monitoring of blood pressure (BP) is equally important in assuring that exercise testing is safe. Recording of HR, ECG, and BP allows work limitations caused by cardiac or vascular disease to be identified and quantified. The level of fitness or conditioning can be gauged from the HR response in relation to the maximal work rate achieved during exercise.

Shortness of breath brought on by exertion is perhaps the most widespread indication for cardiopulmonary exercise evaluation. The combination of cardiovascular parameters (i.e., HR, SV) and data obtained from analysis of exhaled gas (i.e., $\dot{V}o_2$, AT) permits assessment of dyspnea on exertion. Table 7–2 generalizes some of the basic relationships between cardiovascular and pulmonary exercise responses. These relationships help delineate whether exertional dyspnea is a result of cardiac or pulmonary disease, or whether the subject is simply deconditioned. In some instances, poor effort may mimic exertional dyspnea. Comparison of data from cardiovascular and exhaled gas monitors can elucidate inadequate subject effort.

Heart Rate and Electrocardiogram

Heart rate and rhythm may be monitored continuously using one or more modified chest leads. Standard precordial chest-lead configurations (V_1–V_6) allow comparison with resting 12-lead tracings. Twelve-lead monitoring during exercise is practical with devices that incorporate adequate filters (digital or analog). Electrocardiographic instruments designed for exercise testing eliminate movement artifact and may provide sensitive ST segment monitoring. Limb leads normally must be moved to the torso for ergometer or treadmill testing (modified leads). Resting ECGs should be performed to record differences between the standard and modified leads. Single-lead monitoring allows only for gross arrhythmia detection and rate determination. It may not be adequate for testing subjects with known or suspected cardiac disease.

The ECG monitoring device should be able to provide tracings sufficiently free of motion artifact to allow assessment of intervals and segments up to the subject's maximum HR (HR_{max}). Computerized arrhythmia recording, or manual "freeze-frame" storage may be of value for careful evaluation of conduction abnormalities, while allowing the testing protocol to continue. Some digital ECG systems generate computerized "median" complexes averaged from a series of beats. These may be helpful in analyzing ST segment depression. The "raw" or nondigitized ECG should also be available. Heart rate should ideally be analyzed by visual inspection of a tracing with manual measurement of the rate, rather than by an automatic sensor. Most HR meters average the R-R intervals over several beats. Inaccurate HRs may occur with variable rhythms, such as nodal or ventricular arrhythmias, or because of motion artifact. Tall P or T waves may be falsely identified as R waves and cause automatic calculation of HR to be incorrect. Accurate measurement of HR is necessary to determine the subject's maximum rate in comparison with their age-related predicted maximum. Significant S-T segment changes should be easily identifiable from the tracing up to the predicted HR_{max}.

Motion artifact is the most common cause of unacceptable recordings during exercise. Allowing the subject to practice the exercise (ergometer or treadmill) not only familiarizes the subject, but permits the adequacy of the ECG signal to be checked. Carefully applied electrodes, proper skin preparation, and secured lead wires greatly minimize movement artifact. Electrodes specifically designed for exercise testing are helpful. Most of these use extra adhesive to assure electrical contact, even when the subject begins perspiring. The skin sites should be carefully prepared. Removal of surface skin cells by gentle abrasion is recommended. Subjects with excessive body hair may require shaving of the electrode site to insure good electrical contact. Lead wires must be securely attached to the electrodes. Devices which limit the movement of the lead wires can greatly reduce motion artifact. Spare electrodes and lead wires should be available to avoid test interruption in the event of an electrode failure.

The HR normally increases linearly with increasing work load, up to an age-related maximum. Several formulas are available for predicting HR_{max}. For most predicted HR_{max} values, a variability of ± 10 to 15 beats/min exists in healthy adult subjects. Two commonly used equations for predicting HR_{max} are:

$$1.\ HR_{max} = 220 - Age_{years}$$
$$2.\ HR_{max} = 210 - (0.65 \times Age_{years})$$

Equation 1 yields slightly higher predicted values in young adults, while equation 2 produces higher values in older adults. Other methods of predicting HR_{max} vary depending on the type of exercise protocol utilized in deriving the regression data. Specific criteria for terminating an exercise test should include factors based on symptom limitation as well as HR and blood pressure changes (see Safety section).

Heart rate increases almost linearly with increasing $\dot{V}o_2$, and is the main factor affecting the increase in cardiac output. Increases in SV account for a smaller portion of the increase in cardiac output, primarily at low and moderate work loads (see Fig. 7–8). While the HR changes from approximately 70 beats/min up to 200 beats/min, the SV increases from 80 mL to approximately 110 mL in healthy upright subjects. Reduced HR response may occur in subjects who have ischemic heart disease or complete heart block. Low HR also is common in subjects who have been treated with drugs that block the effects of the sympathetic nervous system (beta blockers). The HR response also may be reduced if the autonomic nervous system is impaired or if the heart is denervated, as occurs in cardiac transplantation.

Except in trained subjects, low HR contributes to low cardiac output. Inability to increase the cardiac output almost always results in a reduced $\dot{V}_{O_{2_{max}}}$. Reductions in SV are usually related to the preload or afterload of the left ventricle. Increased HR response, in relation to the work load, implies that the SV is compromised. When the SV is fixed, increased cardiac output is accomplished primarily by increased frequency.

In subjects who have heart disease (i.e., coronary artery disease, cardiomyopathies), increased HR is typically accompanied by ECG changes such as arrhythmias and/or ST segment depression. Deconditioned subjects without heart disease show a high HR at lower than maximal work loads, but usually without ECG abnormalities. Depression of the ST segment greater than 1 mm for a duration of 0.08 seconds is usually considered evidence of ischemia. ST depression at low work loads that increases with HR and continues into the postexercise period is usually indicative of multivessel coronary artery disease. ST depression accompanied by exertional hypotension or marked increase in diastolic pressure is usually associated with significant coronary disease. The predictive value of ST segment changes during exercise must be related to the subject's clinical history and risk factors for heart disease.

The most common arrhythmia occurring during exercise testing is the ventricular premature contraction (VPC). VPCs are associated with an increased incidence of myocardial ischemia and are considered dangerous because they may precede more serious lethal arrhythmias. Exercise-induced VPCs occurring at a rate of more than 10 per minute are often found in ischemic heart disease. Increased VPCs during exercise also may be seen in mitral valve prolapse. Coupled VPCs (couplets) often precede ventricular tachycardia or ventricular fibrillation. Occurrence of couplets or frequent VPCs may be indications for terminating the exercise evaluation. Some subjects with VPCs at rest or at low work loads may have these ectopic beats suppressed as the exercise intensity increases. The most serious ventricular ectopic beats are sometimes seen in the immediate postexercise phase.

Blood Pressure (BP)

Systemic BP may be monitored intermittently using the standard cuff method. Continuous monitoring of BP may be accomplished by connection of a pressure transducer to an indwelling arterial catheter (see Fig. 7–10). An indwelling line allows continuous display and recording of systolic, diastolic, and mean arterial pressures. In addition, the catheter provides ready access for arterial blood sampling when multiple specimens are required. Arterial catheterization normally can be easily accomplished using either the radial or brachial site. The catheter must be adequately secured to prevent loss of patency during vigorous exercise. Insertion of arterial catheters presents some risk of blood splashing. Adequate protection for the individual inserting the catheter, as well as for those withdrawing specimens, is essential. See Chapter 11, Infection Control and Safety, for specifics regarding arterial sampling via catheters.

Automated blood pressure monitors using a self-inflating cuff also may be used during exercise testing. These devices, as well as manual cuffs, may not be able to detect the usual blood pressure sounds during vigorous exercise, particularly with treadmill walking.

Systolic BP increases in healthy subjects during exercise from 120 mm Hg to approximately 200 to 250 mm Hg. Diastolic pressure normally rises only slightly (10 to 15 mm Hg) or not at all. The mean arterial pressure rises from approximately 90 mm Hg to about 110 mm Hg, depending on the changes in systolic and diastolic pressures. The increase in systolic pressure is caused almost completely by increased cardiac output, particularly the SV. Although the cardiac output may increase five-fold (i.e., from 5 to 25 L/min), the systolic pressure only increases two-fold. The systolic pressure only doubles because of the tremendous decrease in peripheral vascular resistance. Most of this decrease in resistance results from vasodilatation in exercising muscles. Increases in the systolic pressure to greater than 250 to 300 mm Hg should be considered an indication for terminating the exercise evaluation (see Table 7–4). Similarly, if the systolic pressure fails to rise with an increasing work load, or if the diastolic pressure falls markedly, the cardiac output is not increasing appropriately. The exercise test should be terminated and the subject's condition stabilized. Variations in blood pressures during exercise often result from the subject's respiratory efforts. Phasic changes with respiration are particularly common in subjects who develop large transpulmonary pressures because of lung disease. Differences of as much as 30 mm Hg between inspiration and expiration may be seen during continuous monitoring of arterial pressure.

In maximal tests in which the subject is taken to HR_{max}, it may be impossible to obtain a reliable BP at peak exercise. Even with an arterial catheter, motion artifact may prevent recording of a usable tracing. The systolic pressure may transiently drop, and the diastolic may fall to zero at the termination of exercise. In order to minimize the degree of hypotension resulting from the abrupt cessation of heavy exercise, the subject should "cool down." This is easily accomplished by having the subject continue exercising at a low work rate until BP and HR have stabilized at or slightly above baseline levels.

Safety

Safe and effective exercise testing for cardiopulmonary disorders requires careful pretest evaluation to identify contraindications to the test procedure (Table 7–3). A preliminary workup should include a complete history and physical examination by either the referring physician or the physician performing the stress test. Preliminary laboratory tests should include a 12-lead ECG, a chest x-ray film, baseline pulmonary function studies before and after

TABLE 7–3.

Contraindications to Exercise Testing

Pa_{O_2} less than 40 mm Hg on room air
Pa_{CO_2} greater than 70 mm Hg
FEV_1 less than 30% of predicted
Recent (within 4 weeks) myocardial infarction
Unstable angina pectoris
Second- or third-degree heart block
Rapid ventricular/atrial arrhythmias
Orthopedic impairment
Severe aortic stenosis
Congestive heart failure
Uncontrolled hypertension
Limiting neurologic disorders
Dissecting/ventricular aneurysms
Severe pulmonary hypertension
Thrombophlebitis or intracardiac thrombi
Recent systemic or pulmonary embolus
Acute pericarditis

bronchodilators, and routine laboratory examinations such as complete blood count and serum electrolytes. Subjects on methylxanthine bronchodilators should have a recent theophylline level measurement, particularly if the primary indication for exercise testing is ventilatory limitation.

The risks and benefits of the entire exercise procedure should be explained or demonstrated to the subject. Appropriate informed consent should be obtained. A physician experienced in exercise testing should supervise the test. Submaximal tests on subjects younger than 40 years old with no known risk factors may be performed by qualified technologists or nurses, provided a physician is immediately available. Criteria for terminating the exercise evaluation before the specified end point or symptom limitation occurs are listed in Table 7–4.

Following termination of the exercise evaluation for whatever reason, the subject should be monitored until HR, BP, and ECG return to pretest levels. Electrocardiographic monitoring should continue for at least 15 minutes, with tracings made at frequent intervals immediately postexercise.

Personnel conducting exercise tests should be trained in handling cardiovascular emergencies and should be certified in cardiopulmonary resuscitation. The laboratory should have available resuscitation equipment, including:

1. Standard intravenous medications (epinephrine, atropine, lidocaine, isoproterenol, propanolol, procainamide, sodium bicarbonate, and calcium gluconate).
2. Syringes, needles, intravenous infusion apparatus.

3. Portable O_2 and suction equipment.
4. Airway equipment, endotracheal tubes, and laryngoscope.
5. DC defibrillator and appropriate monitor.

TABLE 7–4.
Indications for Terminating Exercise Tests

Monitoring system failure
2-mm horizontal or down-sloping ST depression or elevation
T wave inversion or Q waves
Sustained supraventricular tachycardia
Ventricular tachycardia
Multifocal premature ventricular beats
Development of second- or third-degree heart block
Exercise-induced left or right bundle branch block
Progressive chest pain (angina)
Sweating and pallor
Systolic pressure greater than 250 mm Hg
Diastolic pressure greater than 120 mm Hg
Failure of systolic pressure to increase, or a drop of 10 mm Hg
   with increasing work load
Lightheadedness, mental confusion, or headache
Cyanosis
Nausea or vomiting
Muscle cramping

CARDIAC OUTPUT (FICK METHOD)

Cardiac output is commonly measured by thermal or dye dilution, or by the direct or indirect Fick method. The Fick methods require exhaled gas analysis and are often used in conjunction with exercise testing.

Direct Fick Method

The direct Fick method is as follows:

$$\dot{Q}_T = \frac{\dot{V}_{O_2}}{C(a\text{-}\bar{v})_{O_2}} \times 100$$

where:

$\dot{Q}_T$ = cardiac output, in liters per minute

$\dot{V}_{O_2}$ = oxygen consumption, in liters per minute

$C(a\text{-}\bar{v})_{O_2}$ = arterial–mixed venous O_2 content difference, in vol%

   100 = factor to correct $C(a\text{-}\bar{v})_{O_2}$ to liters (content differences are normally reported in vol% or milliliters per deciliter)

The $\dot{V}_{O_2}$ is measured as described previously. The $C(a\text{-}\bar{v})_{O_2}$ is obtained by measuring or calculating the oxygen content in both the arterial and mixed venous samples (see Chapter 6).

Indirect Fick Method

The indirect Fick method uses the CO_2 content differences and the $\dot{V}_{CO_2}$. This method is also called the CO_2 rebreathing technique:

$$\dot{Q}_T = \frac{\dot{V}_{CO_2}}{C(\bar{v}\text{-}a)_{CO_2}} \times 100$$

where:

$\dot{Q}_T$ = cardiac output, in liters per minute

$\dot{V}_{CO_2}$ = CO_2 production, in liters per minute

$C(\bar{v}\text{-}a)_{CO_2}$ = mixed venous–arterial CO_2 content difference, in vol%

   100 = factor to correct $C(\bar{v}\text{-}a)_{CO_2}$ to liters (content differences are normally reported in vol% or milliliters per deciliter)

The $\dot{V}_{CO_2}$ is measured as described previously. The content difference for CO_2 can be obtained completely noninvasively or in conjunction with arterial blood gas analysis. In order to calculate the mixed venous CO_2 content, the $P\bar{v}_{CO_2}$ must be measured using a rebreathing technique. This measurement is accomplished while the subject is connected to the typical circuit used for exhaled gas analysis during exercise. The subject, either at rest or during exercise, is switched to a rebreathing bag. This bag contains a mixture of CO_2 in air that is slightly higher than the $P_{A_{CO_2}}$, and has a volume of 1 to 2 times the V_T. In general, the concentration of CO_2 in the bag must be adjusted between 7% and 15%, and the volume between 1 and 3 L. The bag CO_2 during rebreathing is usually estimated from the subject's end-tidal CO_2 (Fig. 7–11). If the volume and CO_2 concentration in the bag are appropriate, a rapid equilibrium between the bag and mixed venous blood is quickly achieved. The subject rebreathes rapidly from the bag until an equilibrium between the CO_2 in the bag and in the alveoli occurs. Equilibrium may not be accomplished if there is too much or too little CO_2 in the bag. In this case, a different concentration is prepared and the maneuver repeated. Because no CO_2 is removed from the lungs during rebreathing (due to the slightly higher CO_2 concentration in the bag), the fractional concentration

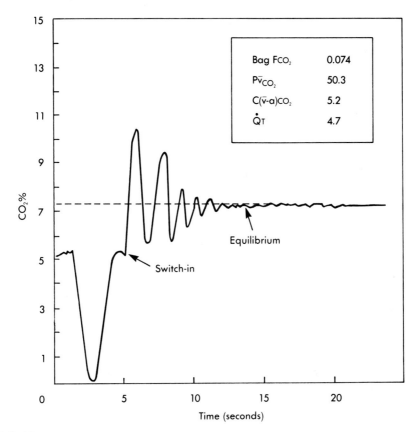

Bag F_{CO_2} — 0.074

$P\bar{v}_{CO_2}$ — 50.3

$C(\bar{v}-a)_{CO_2}$ — 5.2

$\dot{Q}_T$ — 4.7

FIG 7–11.
Cardiac output determination by CO_2 rebreathing. Expired CO_2 is sampled at the mouth with a breath-by-breath system. The $\%CO_2$ is plotted against time as the subject is switched from breathing room air to rebreathing from a bag containing 7% to 15% CO_2. After switch-in, the subject takes several fast deep breaths until an equilibrium is established, as identified by a flat CO_2 tracing. In order for the maneuver to work correctly, the CO_2 concentration in the bag must be slightly higher than the subject's alveolar CO_2. The fractional concentration of CO_2 in the bag *(bag F_{CO_2})* is then used to estimate the mixed venous CO_2. A modified form of the Fick equation, using CO_2 contents in arterial and mixed venous blood, is then used along with the $\dot{V}_{CO_2}$ to determine the cardiac output.

at equilibrium closely resembles that in the pulmonary capillaries. The partial pressure can be determined from the fractional concentration of CO_2. The content can be estimated from the partial pressure of CO_2.

A similar method of rebreathing does not require a special mixture of CO_2, but simply monitors the rise in concentration of CO_2 in the bag during rebreathing. From the exponential increase in CO_2, an equilibrium value can be estimated. The most accurate application of the exponential method requires computerized curve fitting. Once the mixed venous tension of CO_2 is known, the CO_2 content may be calculated or read from a standard nomogram. (The reader is referred to the excellent text by Jones et al. in the Selected Bibliography at the end of this chapter).

The CO_2 content of arterial blood can be estimated similarly using either a measured Pa_{CO_2}, or an estimated value derived from the end-tidal and mixed-expired CO_2 values, V_T, and respiratory rate:

$$Pa_{CO_2} = P_{ET_{CO_2}} + 4.4 - 0.0023V_T + 0.03f_b - 0.09P_{E_{CO_2}}$$

where:

$$P_{ET_{CO_2}} = \text{partial pressure of end-tidal } CO_2$$

$$V_T = \text{tidal volume}$$

$$f_b = \text{frequency of breathing (respiratory rate)}$$

$$P_{E_{CO_2}} = \text{partial pressure of mixed expired } CO_2$$

Or, Pa_{CO_2} can be estimated:

$$Pa_{CO_2} = P_{E_{CO_2}} \div \left(1 - \frac{V_D + V_{D_{sys}}}{V_T}\right)$$

where:

$$P_{E_{CO_2}} = \text{partial pressure of mixed expired } CO_2$$

$$V_D = \text{subject's respiratory dead space (estimated)}$$

$$V_{D_{sys}} = \text{dead space of the breathing circuit}$$

Either of these methods of estimating Pa_{CO_2} presumes normal lung function. Completely noninvasive cardiac output may not be practical if the subject has lung disease by static measures of pulmonary function.

After the CO_2 contents of mixed venous and arterial blood are calculated, the difference is divided into the $\dot{V}_{CO_2}$, measured immediately before the rebreathing maneuver. These calculations may be performed manually or, because of their complexity, by computer. Corrections to the calculated CO_2 contents must be made if the subject's Hb is less than 15 g%, or if the Sa_{O_2} is much less than 95%. Both Hb concentration and O_2 saturation affect the CO_2 dissociation curve. A correction for slight differences between the alveolar and arterial CO_2, which occurs primarily during exercise, may be necessary so that the bag P_{CO_2} accurately reflects $P\bar{v}_{CO_2}$.

Equilibrium must be achieved quickly before recirculation occurs. As with all breath-by-breath measurements, a rapid-responding CO_2 analyzer is necessary. Attainment of equilibrium can be complicated by having a CO_2 concentration in the rebreathing bag that is either too high or too low. Similarly, an inadequate volume in the bag to match the subject's tidal breathing can prevent equilibrium from being reached. In order to rapidly adjust the gas concentrations and bag volume during exercise, an automated (i.e., computerized) gas mixing system may be helpful.

Thermodilution Method

Most modern pulmonary artery (Swan-Ganz) catheters incorporate circuitry for measurement of cardiac output by thermodilution. A sensitive thermistor is placed near the tip of the catheter. This thermistor is connected to a small, dedicated computer. A cool (usually 10 to 20° C) saline solution is injected at the level of the right atrium. The thermistor senses the change in temperature as the solution is pumped through the right ventricle and into the pulmonary artery. The computer then integrates the change in temperature and the time required for the change to occur. From these inputs, the flow per unit of time or cardiac output can be calculated. Thermodilution cardiac output determination is the most common technique used in critical care settings. The method is also practical for exercise testing.

Cardiac output in healthy subjects is approximately 4 to 6 L/min at rest. It may rise during exercise to as high as 25 to 35 L/min. Cardiac output is the product of HR and SV:

$$\dot{Q}_T = HR \times SV$$

where:

$$HR = \text{heart rate in beats per minute}$$

$$SV = \text{stroke volume in liters or milliliters}$$

In healthy upright subjects, the SV is approximately 70 to 100 mL at rest. The SV increases to 100 to 140 mL with low or moderate exercise. The HR increases almost linearly with increasing work rate as described above, so that at low work loads the increase in cardiac output results from a combination of HR and SV. At moderate and high work loads, further increases in $\dot{Q}_T$ result mainly from increases in the HR. The SV increases very little during exercise in the supine position, but is slightly higher at rest than in the upright subject. Derivation of the SV from $\dot{Q}_T$ and HR is useful in quantifying poor cardiac performance in subjects with coronary artery disease, cardiomyopathy, or other diseases which affect myocardial contractility.

Subjects who reach their predicted $\dot{V}_{O_{2max}}$ and their predicted HR_{max} typically have a normal cardiac output and SV. A subject who has a reduced $\dot{V}_{O_{2max}}$, but achieves a maximal predicted HR, often has a low cardiac output because of a low SV. Limited cardiac output in the face of increasing exercise work load is often accompanied by an early onset of anaerobic metabolism. Reduced cardiac output is typical in both atrial and ventricular arrhythmias, in valvular insufficiency, and in cardiomyopathies.

In subjects who are fit, the SV may be increased both at rest and during exercise. Endurance (aerobic) training normally results in increased SV. Other benefits of aerobic training include reductions in systolic BP and ventilation. Fit subjects typically have lower resting HRs than their sedentary counterparts. Because HR (i.e., cardiac output) is the limiting factor to exercise in most individuals, fit subjects are able to reach a higher $\dot{V}_{O_{2max}}$. Depending on the frequency, intensity, and duration of training, fit individuals are able to maintain a higher level of work for longer periods because of improved cardiac performance.

The main disadvantage of the direct Fick method is that placement of a pulmonary artery catheter is required to obtain a mixed venous sample. The indirect Fick method (CO_2 rebreathing) is somewhat complicated, and requires careful attention to the correct CO_2 concentration in the rebreathing bag. Additionally, if arterial P_{CO_2} is estimated rather than measured, the content differences may be erroneous. In subjects with obstructive pulmonary disease, this may be a serious limitation. The CO_2 rebreathing technique appears to work well despite uneven distribution of ventilation.

The thermodilution method also requires placement of a pulmonary artery catheter—a highly invasive procedure. Thermodilution cardiac output measurements may be erroneous in the presence of significant valvular disease, particularly if regurgitation of blood through the valve occurs.

SELF-ASSESSMENT QUESTIONS

1. Which of the following exercise protocols best can be described as a "ramp" test:
   a. Treadmill, 2 mph, grade increase of 5% every 3 minutes
   b. Treadmill, 10% grade, speed increase of 2.5 mph every 3 minutes
   c. Cycle ergometer, 10 watts per minute continuous increase
   d. Cycle ergometer, increasing resistance 50 watts every 2 minutes

2. Which of the following affect the amount of work performed during treadmill exercise?

    I. Stride length of the subject
    II. Speed of the treadmill belt
    III. Slope of the treadmill belt
    IV. Body weight of the subject
    a. I, II, III, IV
    b. II, III, IV
    c. II, III only
    d. I, IV only

3. A patient has the following values measured by exhaled gas analysis at maximal exercise:

$F_{I_{O_2}} = 0.21$

$F_{E_{O_2}} = 0.16$

$F_{E_{CO_2}} = 0.04$

$\dot{V}_E$ liters (STPD) $= 33.0$

What is this subject's $\dot{V}_{O_2}$ in liters per minute (STPD)?
    a. 1.32
    b. 1.65
    c. 1.73
    d. 5.28

4. Which of the following gas mixtures would be most appropriate for calibrating the analyzers used for exhaled gas analysis during exercise:
    a. 100% O_2, room air
    b. 40% O_2, 5% CO_2
    c. room air, 24% O_2, 7% CO_2
    d. room air, 12% O_2, 5% CO_2

5. A subject whose FEV_1 is 1.1 L has the following results of an exercise test (values in parentheses are percents of predicted):

$\dot{V}_{O_{2max}}$ L/min (STPD) $= 1.77$ (51%)

HR_{max} beats/min $= 117$ (73%)

$\dot{V}_{E_{max}}$ L/min (BTPS) $= 37$

Which statement best describes these results:
    a. Mild exercise impairment, poor effort
    b. Moderate exercise impairment, probably deconditioning
    c. Severe exercise impairment, with cardiovascular limitation
    d. Severe exercise impairment, with ventilatory limitation

6. In order to perform breath-by-breath exhaled gas analysis to determine $\dot{V}_{O_2}$, which of the following is necessary:
    a. Phase delay of the gas analyzers must be determined
    b. Expiratory circuit must be thoroughly washed out

c. Volume of the mixing chamber must be accurately measured

d. A small volume (less than 1 L) collection bag is needed

7. The anaerobic threshold (AT) may be identified by which of the following:

I. Increase in blood lactate

II. Increase in blood pH

III. A change in the rate of $\dot{V}co_2$ in relation to $\dot{V}o_2$

IV. A plateau in the $\dot{V}o_2$

a. I, II, III

b. I, III only

c. II, IV only

d. I, IV only

8. A subject has a $\dot{V}E/\dot{V}o_2$ of 44 L/L O_2 at rest before beginning an exercise test; which of the following best explains this value:

a. Anxiety hyperventilation

b. Systemic hypertension

c. Normal resting value

d. Erroneous measurement of $\dot{V}E$

9. A subject has the following results of an exercise test:

	Maximal Exercise	Predicted
HR (beats/min)	167	171
ST change (mm)	−3	<1
$\dot{V}o_2$ (mL/min/kg)	22	36
$\dot{V}E$ (L/min)	43	97
Sao_2 (%)	92	>90

Which of the following best describes these findings:

a. Coronary artery disease

b. Chronic obstructive pulmonary disease

c. Mild deconditioning

d. Poor subject effort

10. Which of the following are normal findings at maximal exercise in healthy subjects:

I. Vd/Vt less than 0.3

II. $\dot{V}o_{2max}$ equal to 10 mL/min/kg

III. $\dot{V}E/\dot{V}co_2$ greater than 50 L/L CO_2

IV. O_2 pulse greater than 10 mL/beat

a. I, II, III

b. II, III, IV

    c. II, III only

    d. I, IV only

11. Which of the following are contraindications for performing an exercise test:

    a. Pao_2 less than 40 mm Hg on room air

    b. FEV_1 less than 70% of predicted

    c. Sinus tachycardia

    d. Dyspnea of unknown origin

12. At high work loads, increasing cardiac output is achieved by:

    a. Increasing stroke volume (SV)

    b. Increasing vascular resistance

    c. Increasing heart rate (HR)

    d. Decreasing dead space to tidal volume ratio (V_D/V_T)

SELECTED BIBLIOGRAPHY

GENERAL REFERENCES

American College of Sports Medicine: *Guidelines for graded exercise testing and exercise prescription*, ed 3. 1986, Lea and Febiger.

Hansen JE: Exercise instruments, schemes, and protocols for evaluating the dyspneic patient. *Am Rev Respir Dis* 129(suppl):S25, 1984.

Hansen JE, Sue DY, Wasserman K: Predicted values for clinical exercise testing. *Am Rev Respir Dis* 129(suppl):S49, 1984.

Hellerstein HK, Brock LL, Bruce RA: *Exercise testing and training of apparently healthy individuals: a handbook for physicians.* New York, 1972, Committee on Exercise American Heart Association.

Jones NL: *Clinical Exercise Testing*, ed 3. Philadelphia, 1988, WB Saunders.

McKelvie RS, Jones NL: Cardiopulmonary exercise testing. *Clin Chest Med* 10:277, 1989.

Wasserman K, Hansen J, Sue D, et al: *Principles of exercise testing and interpretation.* Philadelphia, 1986, Lea and Febiger.

Wasserman K, Whipp BJ: Exercise physiology in health and disease. *Am Rev Respir Dis* 112:219, 1975.

Weber KT, Janicki JS: *Cardiopulmonary exercise testing: physiologic principles and clinical applications.* Philadelphia, 1986, WB Saunders.

VENTILATION, GAS EXCHANGE, AND BLOOD GASES

Beaver WL, Wasserman K, Whipp BJ: A new method for detection of anaerobic threshold by gas exchange. *J Appl Physiol* 60:2020, 1986.

Eschenbacher WL, Mannina A: An algorithm for the interpretation of cardiopulmonary exercise tests. *Chest* 97:263, 1990.

Jones NL: Normal values for pulmonary gas exchange during exercise. *Am Rev Respir Dis* 129(suppl):S44, 1984.

Jones NL: Exercise testing in pulmonary evaluation: rationale, methods and the normal respiratory response to exercise, Parts I and II. *New Engl J Med* 293:541, 1975.

Neuberg GW, Friedman SH, Weiss MB, et al: Cardiopulmonary exercise testing: the clinical value of gas exchange data. *Arch Intern Med* 148:2221, 1988.

Sue DY, Hansen JE, Blais M, et al: Measurement and analysis of gas exchange during exercise using a programmable calculator. *J Appl Physiol* 49:456, 1980.

Wasserman K: The anaerobic threshold measurement in exercise testing. *Clin Chest Med* 5:77, 1984.

Weber KT, Janicki JS, McElroy PA, et al: Concepts and applications of cardiopulmonary exercise testing. *Chest* 93:843, 1988.

Whipp BJ, Ward SA, Wasserman K: Ventilatory responses to exercise and their control in man. *Am Rev Respir Dis* 129(suppl):S17, 1984.

CARDIOVASCULAR MONITORING DURING EXERCISE

Bruce RA: Value and limitations of the electrocardiogram in progressive exercise testing. *Am Rev Respir Dis* 129(suppl):S28, 1984.

Ellestad MH, Allen WA, Wan MCK, et al: Maximal treadmill stress testing for cardiovascular evaluation. *Circulation* 39:517, 1969.

Pollack ML, Bohannon RL, Cooper KH, et al: A comparative analysis of four protocols for maximal stress testing. *Am Heart J* 92:39, 1976.

Stone HL, Liang IYS: Cardiovascular response and control during exercise. *Am Rev Respir Dis* 129(suppl):S13, 1984.

8

Specialized Test Regimens

The diagnosis of specific pulmonary disorders requires that an appropriate battery of tests be performed. It is often unnecessary to perform all of the various tests available. In many instances, simple spirometry and/or blood gas analysis provides sufficient information to delineate a disease process or recommend a course of therapy. Lung volume determination and diffusing capacity may be necessary to quantify changes to the pulmonary parenchyma, or to assess the overall gas exchange. Specialized test regimens, such as those described in this chapter, often consist of standard tests performed under special conditions. The FEV_1, for example, may be analyzed before and after bronchodilator administration, inhalation challenge, or exercise to quantify airway reactivity. The subject's pulmonary history and clinical condition at the time of testing often aid in the selection of appropriate tests and assist in the interpretation of the results.

PULMONARY HISTORY AND RESULTS REPORTING

Accurate interpretation of pulmonary function studies—from simple screening spirometry to the complete cardiopulmonary evaluation—requires clinical information pertinent to possible pulmonary disorders. An ordered array of questions that can be easily answered by the subject provides the most useful type of history. The interpreter of pulmonary function studies may have little clinical information concerning the subject other than that obtained at the time of testing. An appropriate history should be taken as a routine part of pulmonary function testing, and should include the following:

1. Age, sex, standing height, weight, race, current diagnosis
2. Family history: Did anyone in your immediate family (mother, father, brother, or sisters) ever have:
   Tuberculosis
   Emphysema

Chronic bronchitis
Asthma
Hay fever or allergies
Cancer
Other lung disorders

3. Personal history: Have you ever had, or been told that you had:
Tuberculosis
Emphysema
Chronic bronchitis
Asthma
Recurrent lung infections
Colds
Pneumonia or pleurisy
Allergies or hay fever
Chest injury
Chest surgery

4. Occupation: Have you ever worked:
In a mine, quarry, or foundry
Near gases or fumes (if so, what kind?)
In a dusty place (if so, what kind?)

5. Smoking habits: Have you ever smoked:
Cigarettes (_____/day)
Cigars (_____/day)
Pipe (_____/day)
How long? (_____years)
Do you still smoke?   Y   N
Do you live with a smoker?   Y   N

6. Cough: Do you ever cough:
In the morning   Y   N
At night   Y   N
At a particular time of the year_____
Blood (when _____)
Phlegm (when _____)
(color _____)
(volume _____)

7. Dyspnea: Do you get short of breath:
At rest   Y   N
On exertion (when _____)
At night   Y   N

8. Subject disposition at the time of test
Dyspneic   Y   N
Wheezing   Y   N
Coughing Y   N

Cyanotic Y   N
Apprehensive   Y   N
Cooperative   Y   N
9. Current medications (for Heart, Lung, or Blood Pressure)
_____ (Last taken:)
_____ (Last taken:)

Most of these types of questions can be answered by "Yes," "No," or circling an appropriate response. In addition, space may be provided for comments either by the subject or history taker. An outline history of this type provides a basis for evaluation of the various tests. In instances in which the physician performs the test, such history may be redundant if a medical history is available.

Interpretation of pulmonary function tests is best made if the clinical question asked of the test is considered. The clinician requesting the test should indicate the reason for the test. Examples of clinical questions asked of pulmonary function studies include: "Does the patient have airway obstruction?" or "Does the patient have hyperreactive airways?" The clinical information, including the reason for the test, should be used in the decision as to what is normal or abnormal. Clinical information as provided by the history is especially important when the subject displays values that are borderline. For example, an FEV_1 that is 80% of the expected value would be interpreted differently in a healthy young subject tested as part of a routine physical than it would be in a smoker who complained of increasing dyspnea.

Standardized reporting helps simplify test interpretation. A common method of recording test results follows a format such as that outlined in Figure 8–1. Test results are usually reported in conjunction with the appropriate reference values (i.e., predicted normal values). The corresponding percent of predicted normal values is calculated by dividing the measured value by the reference value and multiplying by 100. Many studies providing reference values are available for the more common pulmonary function tests. The reference values chosen for a particular laboratory should represent the methodology used as well as the patient population being tested. For example, a laboratory using a water-sealed spirometer at or near sea level might select reference values obtained using similar equipment. Because trying to match methodologies may not always be practical, reference values representing a large and diverse population are usually most appropriate. (See the Appendix for a more detailed discussion of selecting normal values.)

In addition to the reference value itself, the standard deviation (SD) or standard error of estimate (SEE) for any normal reference value should be considered in the final interpretation of lung function. The SD and SEE are measures of the *variability* in the sample population tested to generate the reference values. Using a statistical approach (i.e., SD or SEE) to define the difference between the subject's measured value and the reference value is

Name: _____ Sex: M   F   Age: _____ Height: _____ Weight: _____

Date: _____ P_B: _____ Temp: _____ Technologist: _____

Test	Prebronchodilator			Postbronchodilator		
	Pred	Pre-	%Pred	Post-	%Pred	%Chg
Spirometry						
FVC (L)						
FEV_1 (L)						
$FEV_{1\%}$						
$FEF_{25\%-75\%}$ (L/sec)						
PEF (L/sec)						
$FEF_{25\%}$ (L/sec)						
$FEF_{50\%}$ (L/sec)						
$FEF_{75\%}$ (L/sec)						
$FEF_{50\%}/FIF_{50\%}$						
MVV (L/min)						
Lung Volumes						
VC (L)						
IC (L)						
ERV (L)						
FRC (L)						
RV (L)						
TLC (L)						
RV/TLC%						
Diffusing Capacity						
$DL_{CO}SB$ (ml/min/mm Hg)						
DL_{CO} - corrected						
DL/V_A						
Blood Gases						
pH						
PCO_2 (mm Hg)						
PO_2 (mm Hg)						
HCO_3^- (mEq/L)						
SaO_2 (%)						
Hb (gm/dl)						

Interpretation:

Interpreted by: _____

FIG 8–1.

Typical pulmonary function report form. Categories of tests (i.e., spirometry, lung volumes, DL_{CO}, blood gases) are listed at the left. The first column contains the reference or predicted value for each parameter. The actual values before and after bronchodilator are listed in their respective columns, as are the percents of predicted. The far right column contains the calculated percent change from before to after bronchodilator. Some report formats include the standard deviation (SD) or standard error of estimate (SEE) in a separate column. Calibration factors (for the spirometer) as well as a notation regarding the reference values used are often included in the final report.

usually more sound than using simple percentages. Perhaps the best method to estimate the extent of abnormality is to calculate the *confidence interval* (CI) for each reference value. The CI is defined as follows:

$$CI = 1.65 \times SD$$

where:

SD = the standard deviation for a particular parameter

1.65 = the number of SDs below the mean that includes 95% of the normal population

This method accounts for the variability associated with each individual pulmonary function parameter. For tests in which the subject could be considered abnormal if the measured value is either higher or lower than the reference, such as residual volume, the CI is calculated using 1.96 SDs. There are problems in reporting the relation between measured and reference values using confidence intervals. Some parameters, such as the $FEF_{25\%-75\%}$, are so variable in the normal population that 1 CI may include extremely low or even negative values. Considering how variable a specific parameter is in the normal population is important when using that parameter to diagnose pulmonary abnormalities (see "Selecting and Using Reference Values" in the Appendix).

In addition to comparison with reference values, the reported pulmonary function results should be referenced to any previous studies of the subject. Comments on serial tests should include whether there has been a significant change in function, and if so, to what extent. Some pulmonary function software allows calculation of percent of change for serial tests in a manner similar to that used for before- and after-bronchodilator studies (see next section). Reporting of serial test results is important in longitudinal studies designed to assess the rate of decline of a specific pulmonary function parameter (i.e., FEV_1, FVC, etc.).

Reporting of results should include any other information that is pertinent to the interpretation of the test. Some laboratories "adjust" reference values for certain ethnic groups in order to more accurately reflect the expected values. If reference values are race corrected or standardized in some other way, that fact should be included in the final report. If multiple reference sets are used to accommodate subjects of different ethnic origins or to provide a complete set of normals, the source of the reference equations should be reported. When a computer-assisted interpretation is generated, it should be clearly marked as such. Some test parameters are corrected before reporting, such as correcting the $D_{L_{CO}}$ for Hb, COHb, or altitude. If corrections to the measured value are made, both the uncorrected and corrected data should be available so that the interpreter can evaluate the effect of the correction on the measurement. In general, questionable test results should not be reported. In many instances, it may not be possible to differentiate between an abnormal finding and an erroneous one. In such instances, the questionable values should be noted as such. Including predefined criteria for acceptability in the interpretation of each test may be helpful in explaining questionable results (see Chapter 11 for Criteria for Acceptability).

BEFORE- AND AFTER-BRONCHODILATOR STUDIES

One of the most practical applications of pulmonary function testing is the determination of a course of therapy in the management of airway obstructive disease. Pulmonary function tests, particularly spirometry, can be performed before and after bronchodilator administration to determine the reversibility of airways obstruction. An $FEV_{1\%}$ less than 70% (slightly lower in older adults) is a good indication for performing bronchodilator studies. Some subjects whose FEV_1 and FVC are "within normal limits" may display a low $FEV_{1\%}$ if the FVC is greater than 100% of predicted while the FEV_1 is slightly reduced. Although any pulmonary function parameter may be measured before and after bronchodilator therapy, the FEV_1 and/or specific airway conductance (SGaw) are usually evaluated.

The subject may be given a normal array of tests, including spirometry, lung volume measurements, and diffusing capacity. Functional residual capacity determinations done by He dilution or the open-circuit nitrogen method should be performed prior to bronchodilator administration. This provides a baseline for comparison of changes in lung volume compartments that may result from bronchodilatation. Even though indices of flow, such as the FEV_1, $FEF_{25\%-75\%}$, and SGaw, usually show the greatest change, lung volumes and D_{LCO} also may respond to bronchodilator therapy.

In subjects referred for bronchodilator testing, routine bronchodilator therapy should be withheld before the procedure. Beta agonists should be withheld for 8 hours. Sustained action beta adrenergics and methylxanthines should be withheld for 12 hours. Slow-release theophylline preparations (i.e., those designed for once per day dosing) may need to be withdrawn 24 hours prior to testing. Cromolyn sodium also should be withheld for 24 hours. Prednisone and other corticosteroids may be continued before testing at a stable dosage. Atropine-like drugs (i.e., parasympatholytics) should be withheld for 8 hours. Some subjects may be unable to manage their symptoms with prolonged withdrawal of bronchodilators. In these instances, it is important to note how long before testing the medication was last used. Some subjects who have used bronchodilators shortly before testing (i.e., within 4 hours) still show significant improvement following a repeated dose.

The bronchodilator, usually a beta-adrenergic agent, can be administered by an aerosol generator, intermittent positive-pressure breathing (IPPB), or a metered-dosage device. A metered-dose inhaler (MDI) typically provides a more reproducible administration of bronchodilator. The MDI mouthpiece should be held slightly away from the subject's open mouth. As the subject inspires from FRC, the MDI is activated. The subject should inspire slowly to TLC, hold the breath for 3 to 5 seconds, and then exhale slowly. A second inhalation may be given after a few minutes. For subjects who are unable to coordinate the activation of the metered dose device with a slow, deep inspiration, the use of an aerosol reservoir, or spacer, may provide a more consistent delivery of medication. A small-volume, jet-powered nebulizer may be used to administer a larger volume of bronchodilator over a longer interval.

Depending on the type of bronchodilator used and the means of administration, the therapy should last long enough to achieve the maximum effects. With MDIs, two or more "puffs" spaced over several minutes may result in greater bronchodilatation. The first inhalation promotes bronchodilatation. The aerosol inspired with the subsequent inhalation may then penetrate deeper into the airways. Most aerosolized bronchodilators begin taking effect on inhalation and continue for an indefinite period, usually at least an hour. Some beta-adrenergic preparations have a slower onset, and peak response may not occur for 10 to 15 minutes following inhalation of the drug. Evaluation of atropine-like drugs may require a delay of 45 to 60 minutes or longer following inhalation.

Reversibility of airways obstruction and improvement in flow rates is considered significant for increases of greater than 12% and 200 mL for either the FEV_1 or FVC. If the SGaw is assessed, an increase of 30% to 40% is usually considered significant. The percent of change is calculated as follows:

$$\% \text{ change} = \frac{\text{postdrug} - \text{predrug}}{\text{predrug}} \times 100$$

where:

postdrug = the test parameter after administration

predrug = the test parameter before administration

Any pulmonary function parameter that worsens following bronchodilator administration will produce a negative value using this scheme. In addition, parameters that have small absolute values (for example, an $FEF_{25\%-75\%}$ less than 0.5 L/sec) may show large percent changes even though the actual improvement in flow is minimal. The FEV_1 is the most commonly assessed parameter for quantifying bronchodilator effects. If the $FEF_{25\%-75\%}$ or $\dot{V}_{max50\%}$ are used, they should be considered secondarily. Increases in the FVC also usually indicate that instantaneous flow rates (i.e., $\dot{V}_{max50\%}$, etc.) should be volume adjusted (see Chapter 3). If the FVC increases more than the FEV_1 following bronchodilator administration, the $FEV_{1\%}$ may actually decrease. The $FEV_{1\%}$ should not be used to judge bronchodilator response. Total expiratory time must be considered in obstructed subjects who show a large increase in FVC. Typically, the FVC may increase just because the subject expired longer than in a predrug trial. Spirometry software that allows superimposition of flow-volume loops (at TLC) provides graphic analysis of the extent of improvement in flows at all lung volumes.

Disease patterns involving the bronchial (and bronchiolar) musculature show the most pronounced change from "before" to "after." Improvements of greater than 50% in parameters such as the FEV_1 and $FEF_{25\%-75\%}$ may occur in uncomplicated asthma. Moderate or severe chronic obstructive diseases may fail to show any improvement and may sometimes yield poorer results for the "after" tests because of the exertion of performing the forced expiratory tests several times. A common cause of little or no bronchodilator response is inadequate deposition of the inhaled drug resulting from a poor inspiratory maneuver. Some subjects show a "paradoxical" response to bronchodilator therapy. In these individuals, flows may actually decrease following the bronchodilator. Some subjects may have a significant response to one drug, but little or no response to another.

Most clinicians require a 12% to 15% increase in FEV_1 from the predrug baseline to define a significant response. Changes of less than 8%, or of less than 150 mL, are within the variability of the usual measurement of FEV_1. Such small changes may occur with testing and are unlikely to be significant. Because bronchodilators effect the greatest change in flows, repetition of the lung volume tests and $D_{L_{CO}}$ are usually unnecessary. If the VC increases, it is normally at the expense of the previously increased RV. However, if symptomatic improvement occurs with bronchodilator in the absence of increased flows, it may be a result of changes in the lung volume compartments. Changes in $D_{L_{CO}}$ or in the matching of ventilation to perfusion also may occur. A common change is that in which the VC increases only slightly, but the FEV_1 shows a significant increase. This may be caused by the opening of previously obstructed airways without a notable increase in the actual volume of air moved by a forced expiratory maneuver. Failure of the FEV_1 to increase by more than 12% to 15% does not preclude the use of bronchodilator therapy, particularly if symptomatic improvement or increased exercise tolerance is demonstrated. Many subjects with obstructive lung disease may show minimal response to inhaled bronchodilator on initial testing, but significant improvement on subsequent tests. Repeat testing may be indicated in subjects with clinical signs of obstruction who would benefit from bronchodilator therapy.

A paradoxical fall in Pa_{O_2} may occur in some subjects following administration of inhaled bronchodilator. This hypoxemia is thought to result from alterations in the matching of ventilation and blood flow in the lungs following bronchodilator administration. The beta-adrenergic drug enters the circulatory system via the lungs and is then distributed to poorly ventilated lung regions during recirculation. An increased blood flow to poorly ventilated lung units results in an increased venous admixture, with a fall in Pao_2. Blood gas analysis before and after bronchodilators may be required to document the paradoxical hypoxemia, particularly if flows improve but symptoms of hypoxemia worsen. Other complications of inhaled beta-adrenergic drugs usually center on aggravation of cardiac arrhythmias or hypertension. Careful monitoring of HR and blood pressure in susceptible subjects before and after bronchodilator administration should be part of the testing regimen. Subjects who develop tachycardia, sweating, or other signs of adverse cardiovascular response should have testing terminated and be immediately evaluated by a physician.

BRONCHIAL CHALLENGE TESTING

Bronchial challenge testing is used to determine the extent of airway hyperreactivity. Challenge tests are typically performed in subjects with symptoms of bronchospasm who have normal pulmonary function studies or uncertain results of bronchodilator studies. There are several commonly used provocative agents that can be used to assess airway hyperreactivity. These include:

- Methacholine challenge
- Histamine challenge
- Eucapnic hyperventilation (using either cold or room-temperature gas)
- Exercise

Each of these agents may trigger bronchospasm, but in slightly different ways. Methacholine is a chemical stimulus that increases parasympathetic tone in bronchial smooth muscle. Histamine triggers a similar response producing bronchoconstriction. Hyperventilation, either at rest or during exercise, results in heat and water loss from the airway. This provokes bronchospasm in susceptible subjects. With each of these agents, the subject's FEV_1 (or other measures of air flow) is assessed before and after exposure.

Methacholine Challenge

Bronchial challenge by inhalation of methacholine is performed by having the subject inhale increasing doses of the drug. Spirometry, and sometimes airway conductance (i.e., SGaw), is measured after each dose. Most clinicians consider the test result positive when inhalation of methacholine precipitates a 20% decrease in the FEV_1. The methacholine concentration at which this 20% decrease occurs is referred to as the provocative dose or $PD_{20\%}$. In the doses usually employed (Table 8–1), normal subjects do not display decreases greater than 20% in the FEV_1. Therefore the methacholine challenge test is highly specific for airway hyperreactivity. Some subjects who have hyperreactive airways may display decreases in FEV_1 less than 20%, even at the highest dose of methacholine.

Subjects to be tested should be asymptomatic, with no coughing or obvious wheezing. Their baseline FEV_1 should be greater than 80% of their expected value. For subjects with known obstruction or restriction, the FEV_1 should exceed 80% of their highest previously observed value. If the subject is taking bronchodilators, they should be withheld according to the schedule presented in Table 8–2.

Baseline spirometry is performed to establish that the subject's FEV_1 is greater than 80% of predicted or the previously observed best value. Subjects who demonstrate obstruction based on reduced $FEV_{1\%}$ or other flows do not require challenge testing to document airway hyperreactivity. Obstructed subjects may be tested, however, to establish the degree of hyperreactivity. Subjects who have a restrictive process (i.e., reduced FEV_1 and FVC) also may be tested for hyperreactive airways. The FEV_1 measured before inhalation of the aerosolized drug is referred to as the "baseline."

A small-volume, gas-powered nebulizer may be used to generate the methacholine aerosol. The nebulizer should generate an aerosol with a particle size in the range of 2 to 5 µm (mass median diameter). This particle range promotes deposition in the medium and small airways. A dosimeter may provide a true "quantitative" challenge test by delivering a consistent volume of drug. The dosimeter (or nebulizer) should be activated during inspiration, either automatically by a flow sensor or manually by the subject. A driving pressure of 20 psi is typically used for most dosimeters. An activation time of 0.5 to 0.6 seconds allows a fixed volume of aerosol to be generated with each breath. By limiting the period of aerosol production, the last part of the inhalation carries

TABLE 8–1.

Units for Methacholine Challenge*

Methacholine Concentration (mg/mL)	Cumulative No. of Breaths	Cumulative Units/ Five Breaths	Cumulative No. of Minutes
0.075	5	0.375	3
0.15	10	1.125	6
0.31	15	2.68	9
0.62	20	5.78	12
1.25	25	12.00	15
2.50	30	24.50	18
5.00	35	49.50	21
10.00	40	99.50	24
25.00	45	225.00	27

*One methacholine unit is arbitrarily defined as one inhalation of 1 mg/mL of methacholine in diluent. The quantity of drug required to provoke a 20% decrease in FEV_1 is expressed in X units/X minutes, for example, 12 methacholine units/15 minutes.

TABLE 8–2.
Withholding Bronchodilators Before Bronchial Challenge

1. Beta-adrenergic agents (oral or inhaled) should be withheld for 12 hours.
2. Anticholinergic aerosols should be withheld for 12 hours.
3. Short- and intermediate-action theophylline preparations should be withheld for 18 to 24 hours.
4. Sustained-action theophylline preparations should be withheld for 48 hours.
5. Cromolyn sodium should be withheld for 48 hours.
6. Antihistamines should be withheld for 48 hours.
7. Subjects receiving corticosteroids should be challenged while taking a stable dosage.
8. Caffeine-containing drinks (cola, coffee) should be withheld for 6 hours.
9. Beta-blocking agents may increase the response.

the aerosol into the lung. Ideally, the dosimeter or nebulizer should have an output sufficiently high so that 1 mL of solution can be aerosolized during the course of the inhalations at each level. If multiple nebulizers are used for the increasing dilutions, their outputs should be similar. Continuous low- or high-flow nebulization schemes also may be used. Aerosol output and flow rates should be kept as constant as possible to ensure reproducibility.

The subject begins by inhaling five breaths of nebulized diluent, usually normal saline. The breaths should be slow and deep. The subject should inspire from FRC to TLC, with a short breath-hold (2 to 5 seconds) at TLC to maximize aerosol deposition. After 3 minutes, spirometry is performed. The highest FEV_1 following inhalation of the diluent value then becomes the "control." If the FEV_1 is not reduced 10% from the baseline, inhalation of methacholine is begun. Some subjects, usually those who have highly reactive airways, may have a positive response (i.e., a 10% decrease in FEV_1) to the diluent alone. As with routine spirometry, three acceptable FVC maneuvers should be obtained. The two best FEV_1 and FVC values should be within 5%. If the FEV_1 values are not reproducible (i.e., within 5%), the validity of further testing may be questionable. Because the objective of the test is to detect a fall in the FEV_1, results that cannot be reproduced may lead to a false-positive interpretation.

Two dosage protocols with slightly different methacholine dilutions are commonly used:

Methacholine Dosing Schedules

0.025 mg/mL	0.075 mg/mL
0.250 mg/mL	0.150 mg/mL
2.50 mg/mL	0.310 mg/mL
5.00 mg/mL	0.620 mg/mL
10.0 mg/mL	1.25 mg/mL
25.0 mg/mL	2.50 mg/mL
	5.00 mg/mL
	10.0 mg/mL
	25.0 mg/mL

The six-dilution set allows the test to be completed more quickly. The nine-dilution protocol employs smaller differences between concentrations at the lower levels. Each of these dilutions may be prepared from a 25 mg/mL stock solution. The stock solution is prepared by dissolving the powdered drug in an aqueous diluent containing 0.5% NaCl, 0.275% $NaHCO_3$, and 0.4% phenol. This diluent has a pH of 7.0 and helps to sterilize the solution. Methacholine is fairly stable after mixing and usually may be kept for up to 4 months if refrigerated at 4°C. The lowest dosage (0.025 mg/mL) is the least stable and may need to be prepared immediately before testing.

One-milliliter volumes are suitable for five inhalations in commonly used nebulizers. Other dilutions may be used but should be arranged in such a way that the dosages range from approximately 0.1 mg/mL to 25 mg/mL. An adequate number of intermediate concentrations should be used (usually 5) so that a 20% decrease in FEV_1 can be detected without inducing a more severe response. A bolus technique also may be used. In this protocol, the subject inhales multiple breaths of a fixed concentration, with spirometry performed after each 5 breaths.

The subject inhales five breaths (as described for the diluent above) from the nebulizer beginning with the lowest concentration. Spirometry is repeated at 3 minutes, with the "best" test selected from duplicate or triplicate efforts. The percent of decrease is calculated as follows:

$$\% \text{ decrease} = \frac{X - Y}{X} \times 100$$

where:

$$X = \text{control (following diluent) } FEV_1$$

$$Y = \text{current } FEV_1 \text{ following methacholine inhalation}$$

A 20% or greater decrease in the FEV_1 is considered a positive test. The decrease should be sustained. Additional spirometry efforts may be necessary to distinguish an actual decrease from variability in the maneuvers. If the test is negative, then five breaths of the next higher dilution are administered and the measurements repeated. If the test is borderline positive (i.e., a fall of 15% to 20%), less than five inhalations of the next dilution may be given.

At each concentration, the subject should be observed and questioned for the perception of symptoms such as chest tightness or wheezing. Auscultation may be helpful in detecting the beginning of bronchospasm. As soon as a 20% fall in the FEV_1 is observed, administration of the methacholine is terminated. The bronchospasm may be reversed by means of an appropriate bronchodilator, usually by inhalation. Spirometry should be performed following reversal to document the efficacy of the bronchodilator in reversing the effects of the methacholine (Fig. 8–2).

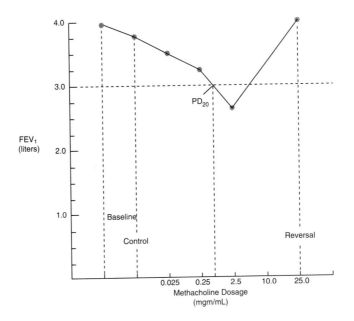

FIG 8–2.
Methacholine challenge test. Results of data gathered during an inhalation challenge test are shown. The dosage of the challenge agent (methacholine in this case) is plotted on a logarithmic scale on the X axis. The flow parameter measured is plotted on the Y axis. In this plot, the first point represents the baseline FEV_1 of approximately 4 L. The control (i.e., the FEV_1 after inhalation of the diluent) is plotted next. The FEV_1 after each successive dose of methacholine is plotted until a 20% decrease occurs. In this plot, the FEV_1 fell by more than 20% with a dosage of 2.5 mg/mL. A vertical line drawn from the point at which the dose response curve crosses the 20% line defines the PD_{20}. The subject was then given an inhaled bronchodilator to reverse the effect of the provocative agent, and this response is plotted.

Several methods of quantifying the results of the procedure are commonly used. The dilution that produced the 20% decrease in FEV_1 is most often reported as the PD_{20}. A more precise method totals the amount of methacholine inhaled to produce the requisite decrease by multiplying the number of breaths by the dilution. This method requires a dosimeter or metered-dosage type of nebulizer, so that a known quantity of drug is given with each inhalation. Table 8–1 lists the cumulative amounts of methacholine delivered using the five-breath routine and the nine-dilution dosage schedule listed above.

Methacholine challenge testing presents some risk to the subject, so a physician familiar with the procedure should be immediately available. Technologists administering bronchial challenge tests should be thoroughly familiar with the procedure, and with the signs and symptoms of bronchospasm. Medication for reversal of the bronchospasm (i.e., epinephrine), as well as for resuscitation, should be immediately available in the event of an adverse reaction.

The spirometer used should meet the minimal standards set by the American Thoracic Society (see Chapter 11) and should provide spirometric tracings or flow-volume loops for later evaluation.

Histamine Challenge

Aerosolized histamine extract (histamine phosphate) may be used for inhalation challenge in a manner similar to methacholine challenge. Histamine produces bronchoconstriction by an uncertain pathway. The response to histamine can be blocked by antihistamines or H_1 receptor antagonists. Histamine-induced bronchospasm is also partially blocked by most classes of bronchodilators. Histamine differs from methacholine in its side effects, half-life, and cumulative effects. Flushing and headache are two common side effects of histamine inhalation. The peak action of histamine occurs within 30 seconds to 2 minutes, which is similar to that observed in methacholine. Recovery of baseline function is significantly shorter for histamine than for methacholine. The action of histamine, unlike methacholine, is thought to be less cumulative.

Subject preparation for histamine challenge is similar to that used for methacholine (see Table 8–2). Antihistamines and H_1 receptor antagonists should be withheld for 48 hours prior to testing.

The usual dosing protocol for histamine challenge is:

Histamine Dosing Schedule
0.03 mg/mL
0.06 mg/mL
0.12 mg/mL
0.25 mg/mL
1.00 mg/mL
2.50 mg/mL
5.00 mg/mL
10.0 mg/mL

These increments approximately double the concentration of drug at each level. The same criteria as used for baseline spirometry in methacholine challenge are observed. Diluent is administered first to determine a control value for FEV_1. If the FEV_1 does not fall by more than 10%, then 5 breaths of the first dilution is administered. Spirometric measurements are performed immediately, then repeated at 3 minutes. A positive response is considered if the FEV_1 falls by 20% or more below the control at 3 minutes. If there is a negative response, the next dilution is given and the measurements repeated.

The results of histamine challenge are reported in a manner similar to that described for methacholine. The concentration of histamine that produced a 20% fall in FEV_1 is called the PD_{20} (i.e., provocative dose). Response also may be reported by graphing the percent change in FEV_1 against the concentration (or its logarithm) of the drug. This type of plot is commonly referred to as a dose-response graph. It permits extrapolation of a precise concentration of drug that elicited the 20% decrease (see Fig. 8–2).

Histamine, like methacholine, is relatively safe if the technologist follows the procedures described. Baseline and control values should always be established. Bronchial challenge should always begin with a low concentration of drug. The range of concentrations used should be appropriate for the type of subjects tested. For adult subjects in whom airway hyperreactivity is the suspected diagnosis, the dosing schedules described previously are recommended. Subjects who have a positive response to histamine challenge are found to recover more quickly than if tested with methacholine. Histamine challenge can be repeated within 2 hours after the subject has returned to the baseline level of function.

Eucapnic Hyperventilation

Airway hyperreactivity may be assessed by having the subject ventilate at a high level. Heat and/or water loss from the upper airways has been demonstrated to provoke bronchospasm in susceptible individuals. These physiologic changes are most pronounced when the subject inspires cold, dry gas, but also can be demonstrated with gas at room temperature. In order to prevent respiratory alkalosis (i.e., true hyperventilation), CO_2 is mixed with air. This gas mixture allows high levels of ventilation with little effect on the pH.

In subjects to be tested using eucapnic hyperventilation, bronchodilators should be withheld as suggested in Table 8–2. Baseline spirometry is performed.

If cold gas is to be used, the mixture is passed through a heat exchanger or over a cooling coil. These devices lower the temperature and remove water vapor from the gas. Gas temperatures are typically reduced to a subfreezing level. Temperatures in the range of -10 to $-20°$ C are typical. The relative humidity is usually very near 0%.

The subject breathes the gas at an elevated level of ventilation. One method has the subject breathe at a level that represents a fraction of the MVV (i.e., 30% to 70% of the MVV). Carbon dioxide is added to the gas to maintain a stable $P_{ET CO_2}$. This is accomplished either by titrating CO_2 into the mixture, or by using a gas composed of 5% CO_2 and the balance air. The subject maintains this level of ventilation for 4 to 6 minutes. Spirometry, or SGaw, is then measured at fixed intervals following the hyperventilation (e.g., 1, 3, 5, 7, and 9 minutes). A second method has the subject breathe at increasing levels of ventilation up to the MVV (e.g., 7.5, 15, 30, 60 L/min, and MVV). Again CO_2 is added to the inspired gas to maintain eucapnia (i.e., Pa_{CO_2} of approximately 40 mm Hg).

Eucapnic hyperventilation with room-temperature gas also provides a ready stimulus for bronchospasm. In this technique, the subject breathes a mixture of 5% CO_2 and air at room temperature. The gas is used to fill a "target" bag or balloon of approximately 5 L. The subject is connected to the bag via a nonrebreathing valve (see Chapter 9) and large-bore tubing. A noseclip is worn by the subject. A high-output flow meter is used to fill the target bag. The flow meter is adjusted to deliver gas at approximately 70% of the subject's MVV. The subject breathes from the bag and tries to match his/her ventilation to the bag to keep it partly deflated. The high level of ventilation is continued for 5 minutes. Spirometry is performed immediately following the period of hyperventilation, and then at 5-minute intervals.

For both the cold-air and room-temperature protocols, if no fall in FEV_1 occurs within 20 minutes following hyperventilation, the test may be considered negative. The percentage of decrease is calculated just as for methacholine challenge testing, described previously. A fall of 5% to 10% is consistent with some degree of airway hyperreactivity. Some asthmatic subjects may experience decreases of FEV_1 greater than 20%. Bronchospasm should be reversed with inhaled bronchodilators, and the reversal documented with spirometry.

Both cold-air and room-temperature hyperventilation tests can be used when airway conductance (SGaw) is measured. Because the stimulus may be applied once, the subject can then be transferred to the body plethysmograph for measurements at defined intervals. Cold-air testing requires specialized equipment to refrigerate and dry the inspired gas. Testing with cold air is slightly more sensitive and specific than testing with room-temperature gas. Both techniques correlate well with the results of methacholine challenge tests, although they are slightly less specific. If multiple levels of ventilation are evaluated, a dose-response curve can be constructed. However, the single challenge is less complicated and can be used to evaluate subjects suspected of airway hyperreactivity.

Exercise Challenge

Exercise-induced asthma (EIA) is typified by bronchospasm during or immediately following vigorous exercise and is related to heat/water loss from the upper airway that accompanies increased ventilation during exercise. Evaluation of exercise-induced bronchospasm may be helpful in quantifying the extent of reversible airway obstruction in the following instances:

1. In subjects who have shortness of breath on exertion, but exhibit normal resting pulmonary functions.
2. In symptomatic subjects in whom other bronchial provocation tests produce negative or ambiguous results.
3. In subjects with known EIA in whom therapy is being evaluated.
4. In screening subjects when some risk to asthmatics might be involved (athletics, etc.).

Subjects referred for exercise challenge should be evaluated by means of an appropriate history and physical examination. The evaluation should include a resting ECG to ascertain potential contraindications to exercise testing (see Chapter 7). Bronchodilators should be withheld as for methacholine challenge, described previously (see Table 8–2). Before exercise, the subject's FEV_1 should not be less than 65% of the predicted value. Subjects with overt obstruction typically do not require an exercise challenge to demonstrate airway hyperreactivity.

Either a treadmill or cycle ergometer may be used, depending on the type of physiologic measurements being made. The exercise should be vigorous enough to elicit work rates between 60% and 85% of the subject's predicted maximal oxygen consumption for 6 to 8 minutes. The subject's response to an increasing work load should be monitored via continuous ECG and blood pressure. Ventilatory parameters (such as $\dot{V}_E$ and V_T) may be helpful in assessing the pulmonary response to exercise. A spirometer that meets the American Thoracic Society requirements (see Chapter 11) is necessary. The device should allow for multiple recordings of either volume-time tracings or flow-volume curves, or both. Some systems provide software specifically for challenge testing (either by inhalation or exercise) with capability for superimposing MEFV curves. Resuscitation equipment, as described in Chapter 7, should be available.

One to two minutes of low-intensity exercise allow evaluation of ventilatory and cardiovascular responses to work. As soon as a normal cardiovascular response is observed, the work load should be increased up to a level that will allow the subject to attain 85% of the predicted maximum HR or predicted maximum $\dot{V}_{O_2}$. In most instances, a short period of moderately heavy work is all that is required to trigger exercise-induced bronchospasm. Bronchospasm usually occurs immediately following the exercise, not during it, unless the test is extended over a longer interval. Repeated testing within 2 hours may result in a "refractory period," during which the severity of the bronchoconstriction lessens. This response presumably results from the buildup of catecholamines. An extended warm-up period before the actual exercise also may protect the airways and lessen the subsequent bronchoconstriction.

Baseline spirometry values are established prior to testing. Following exercise, measurements should be taken at 1 to 2 minutes, and then every 5 minutes as the selected parameter (usually FEV_1 or SGaw) decreases to a minimum. The highest value of duplicate measurements is recorded. Testing is continued until the parameter returns to baseline. Maximal decreases are typically seen in the first 5 to 10 minutes following cessation of exercise. A fall in the FEV_1 of 10% to 20% is usually consistent with increased airway reactivity. Spontaneous recovery occurs within 20 to 40 minutes. Severe bronchospasm may be reversed using an inhaled bronchodilator. Ambient temperature, relative humidity, and P_B should be recorded because of their influence on airway muscle tone.

Several methods of reporting the response to exercise are in common use:

1. Maximum percent of decrease of baseline function:

$$\frac{X - Y}{X} \times 100$$

where:

$$X = \text{baseline value (FEV}_1)$$

$$Y = \text{lowest postexercise value}$$

2. Maximum decrease as a percentage of the predicted value:

$$\frac{X - Y}{P} \times 100$$

where:

$$X = \text{baseline value (FEV}_1)$$

$$Y = \text{lowest postexercise value}$$

$$P = \text{subject's predicted value}$$

3. Lowest value as a percent of predicted value:

$$\frac{Y}{P} \times 100$$

where:

$$Y = \text{lowest postexercise value}$$

$$P = \text{subject's predicted value}$$

The advantage of the first method is that the baseline parameter is included in both the numerator and denominator and provides a unit that is independent of the absolute values. This makes it useful for comparisons between subjects. The first method also is used in assessing percent of change in other bronchial challenge methods. The second method relates the postexercise decrease to the subject's predicted value. Baseline values should always be reported, particularly if the third method is used.

The symptom of exercise-induced bronchospasm may be evaluated using one of the hyperventilation techniques described previously. These techniques eliminate the need for the more complicated exercise test. Eucapnic voluntary hyperventilation may be more sensitive in detecting airway hyperreactivity than exercise testing.

PREOPERATIVE PULMONARY FUNCTION TESTING

Preoperative pulmonary function testing is one of several means available to clinicians to evaluate surgical candidates at risk for developing respiratory complications. Preoperative testing, in conjunction with history and physical examination, ECG, and chest X-ray films, is indicated for one or more of the following reasons:

1. To determine the level of risk involved in the surgical procedure (i.e., morbidity and mortality).
2. To plan perioperative care, including preoperative preparation, type and duration of anesthetic during surgery, and postoperative care to minimize complications.
3. To estimate postoperative lung function in candidates for pneumonectomy or lobectomy.

The surgical candidate who needs preoperative pulmonary function testing is determined by the type of surgical procedure and the individual's risk factors. Many investigations, both prospective and retrospective, have identified that the risk of postoperative pulmonary complications are highest in *thoracic procedures,* followed by *upper abdominal* and *lower abdominal* procedures. Increased incidence of complications appears in both healthy subjects and those who have pulmonary disorders. Subjects who have pulmonary disease are at higher risk in proportion to the degree of pulmonary impairment.

Preoperative pulmonary function testing is *definitely* indicated in:

1. Subjects who have a smoking history.
2. Subjects who have symptoms of pulmonary disease (i.e., cough, sputum production, shortness of breath).
3. Subjects who have abnormal physical examination findings, particularly of the chest (i.e., abnormal breath sounds, ventilatory pattern, respiratory rate).
4. Subjects who have abnormal chest radiographs.

Preoperative testing also may be indicated in:

1. Subjects who are morbidly obese (i.e., greater than 30% above ideal body weight).

2. Subjects advanced in age, usually older than 70 years.
3. Subjects who have current or recent respiratory infections or a history of respiratory infections.
4. Subjects who are markedly debilitated or malnourished.

In each of these subjects, the primary purpose of pulmonary function testing is to uncover pre-existing pulmonary disease. The VC may decrease more than 50% from the preoperative value in thoracic or upper abdominal procedures. This places individuals with compromised function at high risk of developing atelectasis and pneumonia. Postoperative decreases in the FRC and increases in closing volume (CV) may lead to $\dot{V}/\dot{Q}$ abnormalities and hypoxemia. Abnormal ventilatory function related to the central control of respiration or to the ventilatory muscles also may play a role in postoperative complications.

Certain tests of pulmonary function appear to be better predictors of postoperative complications. These tests should be used for both risk evaluation and to assist in planning the perioperative care of the individual.

1. *Spirometry.* FVC, FEV_1, $FEF_{25\%-75\%}$, MVV. Obstructive disease can be easily identified with simple spirometry. A significant percentage of subjects who might develop postoperative problems can be detected with minimal screening. Subjects who have a reduced FVC, with or without airways obstruction, typically have an impaired ability to cough effectively when the VC decreases further during the immediate postoperative period. The MVV, although dependent on subject effort, appears to be uniquely suited to detecting postoperative risk. This may result in part because the MVV tests lung parenchyma, airway function, ventilatory muscle function, and subject cooperation. The measured MVV correlates better with the incidence of postoperative problems than the estimated MVV (i.e., $FEV_1 \times 35$ or 40). This may be attributable to measurement of both inspiratory and expiratory flow during the MVV, whereas the FEV_1 assesses only expiration. Because the ventilatory muscles may be involved in the development of postoperative complications, the MVV may be a more sensitive predictor than forced expiratory flows.

2. *Bronchodilator Studies.* Operative candidates who have airways obstruction also should be tested with bronchodilators. Postbronchodilator values for FVC, FEV_1, $FEF_{25\%-75\%}$, and MVV may be used in estimating the surgical risk. There may be significantly less risk if the subject's airway obstruction is reversible. Bronchodilator studies are similarly helpful in planning perioperative care. Bronchodilator therapy may improve the subject's bronchial hygiene preoperatively as well as postoperatively.

3. *Blood Gas Analysis.* In subjects who have documented lung disease, arterial blood gas analysis is helpful in assessing the response to the pulmonary changes known to occur postoperatively. The Pao_2 itself is not a good prognosticator of postoperative problems. Individuals with hypoxemia at rest

usually also have abnormal spirometry, and hence are at risk. The Pa_{O_2} actually may improve postoperatively in subjects undergoing thoracotomy for lung resection, if the resected portion was contributing to $\dot{V}/\dot{Q}$ abnormalities. The Pa_{CO_2} appears to be the most useful blood gas indicator of surgical risk. If the Pa_{CO_2} is above 45 mm Hg, there is a marked increase in postoperative morbidity and mortality. Elevated Pa_{CO_2} values are most commonly encountered in subjects with significant airways obstruction.

4. *Exercise Testing.* Exercise studies can accurately predict subjects at risk. Individuals who cannot tolerate moderate work loads typically have airways obstruction, or similar ventilatory limitations. Subjects who can attain an oxygen uptake of greater than 20 mL/min/kg typically have a low incidence of cardiopulmonary complications. Those unable to attain a $\dot{V}_{O_2}$ of 15 mL/min/kg almost always have complications.

Lung volumes, even though they may be reduced dramatically in the immediate postsurgical phase, do not correlate well preoperatively with postoperative complications, and do not enhance the estimate of complications. Diffusion studies, like lung volume determinations, do not appear to improve the prediction of postoperative complications.

In addition to routine pulmonary function studies, several other tests are employed specifically in predicting postoperative lung function in candidates for pneumonectomy or lobectomy. These procedures are normally used in addition to spirometry and blood gas analysis.

1. *Perfusion and $\dot{V}/\dot{Q}$ Scans.* Lung scans (see Chapter 4) are particularly useful in estimating the remaining lung function in patients who are likely to require removal of all or part of a lung. Split function scans are performed. These allow partitioning of lungs into right and left halves, or into multiple lung regions. Although ventilation/perfusion scans give the best estimate of overall function, simple perfusion scans yield similar information. Lung scan data, in the form of regional function percentages, is used in combination with simple spirometric indexes to calculate the patient's postoperative capacity. For example:

$$\text{postop } FEV_1 = \text{preop } FEV_1 \times \% \text{ perfusion to unaffected portions}$$

Subjects whose postoperative FEV_1 is calculated to be less than 800 mL are typically not considered surgical candidates.

2. *Pulmonary Artery Occlusion Pressure.* In some candidates for pneumonectomy, the development of postoperative pulmonary hypertension may be a limiting factor. In order to estimate the effect of redirecting the entire right ventricular output to the remaining lung, a catheter is inserted into the pulmonary artery of the affected lung and blood flow occluded by means of a

TABLE 8–3.

Preoperative Pulmonary Function

Test	Increased Postoperative Risk	High Postoperative Risk	Candidate for Pneumonectomy*
FVC	Less than 50% of predicted	Less than 1.5 L	—
FEV_1	Less than 2.0 L or 50% of predicted	Less than 1.0 L	Greater than 2.0 L
$FEF_{25\%-75\%}$	Less than 50% of predicted	—	—
MVV	—	Less than 50 L/min or 50% of predicted	Greater than 50 L/min or 50% of predicted
Pa_{CO_2}	—	Greater than 45 mm Hg	—
Predicted postoperative FEV_1	—	—	Greater than 0.8 L/min
Pulmonary artery occlusion	—	—	Less than 35 mm Hg

*Values in this column determine if the subject is to be considered a candidate for lung resection (see text).

balloon. The resulting pressure increase in the remaining lung is then measured. A pressure increasing to less than 35 mm Hg is usually considered consistent with acceptable postoperative pressures. The effect of redirected blood flow on oxygenation also may be a consideration. This also can be examined during occlusion to estimate postoperative Pa_{O_2}.

These tests to predict the effects of resection on the remaining lung normally are used in series, with spirometry done first, followed by split function lung scans if the spirometry is acceptable, and then pulmonary artery occlusion pressure, if the development of cor pulmonale is a concern. Table 8–3 summarizes some general ranges of values used for preoperative pulmonary function testing.

PULMONARY FUNCTION TESTING FOR DISABILITY

Pulmonary function tests are one of several means of determining a subject's inability to perform certain tasks. Respiratory impairment and disability, however, are not synonymous. Respiratory impairment relates to the failure of one or more of the functions of the lungs, which is what pulmonary function studies measure. Disability is the inability to perform tasks required either for employment or everyday activities. Those pulmonary function tests used to determine impairment leading to disability should characterize the type, extent, and cause of the impairment. Pulmonary function testing may not completely describe all the factors involved in the disabling impairment. Other factors involved may be the age, educational background, and motivation of the subject. The energy requirements of the task in question also affect a subject's level of disability.

Determination of the level of impairment resulting from pulmonary disease usually consists of the following:

1. *Physical examination* does not allow measurement of disabling symptoms, but is useful in grading shortness of breath. Shortness of breath is the most prominent feature of respiratory impairment. Shortness of breath, like pain, is subjective. Tachypnea, cyanosis, and abnormal respiratory patterns are not indicative of the extent of impairment, but may be helpful in interpretation of pulmonary function studies.
2. *Chest x-ray studies* do not correlate well with shortness of breath or pulmonary function studies, except in advanced cases of pneumoconioses (i.e., "dust" diseases). Absence of usual findings in the pneumoconioses may be helpful in excluding occupational exposure as part of the impairment.
3. *Pulmonary function studies* should be objective and reproducible, and most importantly, specific to the disorder being investigated.
   a. *FVC and FEV_1.* Spirometry is the most useful index for the assessment of impairment from airway obstruction. A permanent record of the tracings should be kept. The volume-time tracing should have the time sensitivity marked on the horizontal axis and the volume sensitivity marked on the vertical axis. The paper speed should be at least 20 mm/sec and the volume excursion at least 10 mm/L. The three largest FVC values and FEV_1 values should be within 5%. Each maneuver should be continued at least 10 seconds. The largest FVC and FEV_1 of three acceptable maneuvers is reported. An FEV_1 reported when only a flow-volume curve is recorded is not acceptable. A volume-time tracing from which the FEV_1 can be measured is required. Spirometry is normally repeated following bronchodilator therapy.
   b. *MVV.* The maximal voluntary ventilation is influenced by subject effort, which may be in question in disability determinations. The test also may be affected by muscular coordination, cardiac disease, neurologic function, and chest wall compliance. One satisfactory MVV maneuver is required (see Chapter 11), but it should not be calculated from the FEV_1. The tracing should show both inspiratory and expiratory excursions, rather than just accumulated volume. The recording should be continued for 10 to 15 seconds.
   c. *Lung volumes.* Lung volume determinations correlate poorly with shortness of breath and disability, but may be necessary to assess the extent

of restriction present. The VC may be required for disability determination, but other lung volumes are not.

d. DL_{CO}. The diffusing capacity is useful in determining impairment in restrictive disorders such as pulmonary fibrosis. Either single-breath or steady-state methods may be used. The reference value for the method also should be reported.

e. *Arterial blood gas analysis.* Although blood gas results are objective, they are largely nonspecific in determining impairment. The A-a$_{O_2}$ gradient may not be reliable because it can be affected by hyperventilation. Blood gas analysis may be required in diffuse pulmonary fibrosis, and should include both the Pao$_2$ and the Paco$_2$. Blood gases (and A-a gradient) are helpful if measured during exercise. The requirement for supplementary O$_2$ also may be quantified by exercise blood gas analysis.

f. *Exercise testing.* Exercise testing may be indicated if the results of simple spirometry, diffusing capacity, or blood gases are uncertain regarding the extent of respiratory impairment. The $\dot{V}_{E_{max}}$, compared with the MVV, helps to determine the ventilatory reserve, if any, that remains (see Chapter 7). Similarly, the HR$_{max}$, if much less than predicted for the work load, may indicate a ventilatory rather than cardiovascular limitation. Ventilatory equivalents for O$_2$ and CO$_2$ ($\dot{V}_E/\dot{V}_{O_2}$ and $\dot{V}_E/\dot{V}_{CO_2}$) are most useful if measured during sustained exercise. They may be used to estimate functional limits that can be compared with the job requirements of the individual. The dyspnea index (see Chapter 7) is considered normal if less than 12% of the MVV. Values between 35% and 50% are equivocal, and values greater than 50% are almost always considered abnormal.

Limits for determining disability on the basis of respiratory impairment have been set for the United States by the Social Security Administration. Criteria are set according to the disease category (Table 8-4).

In reporting impairment for disability purposes, the remaining functional capacity is as important in determining the subject's ability to carry out a certain task as the percentage of lost function. Some statement of the subject's ability to understand and cooperate with the pulmonary function measurements should accompany the tabular and graphic data.

PULMONARY FUNCTION TESTING IN CHILDREN

Pulmonary function testing in children employs many of the same basic tests as testing of adults. Differences between adult and pediatric testing exist not only in the absolute dimensions of the developing pulmonary system but also in two main areas concerning the testing regimens themselves:

TABLE 8–4.
Disease Category Criteria

COPD
FEV_1 less than 1.0 to 1.4 L (heights of 57 to 73 inches, respectively)
MVV less than 32 to 48 L/min (heights of 57 to 73 inches, respectively)

Asthma
(Same as for COPD)
or
Episodes of severe attacks in spite of treatment every 2 months
or
6 times per year with wheezing between attacks

Diffuse Pulmonary Fibrosis
VC less than 1.2 to 2.0 L (Heights of 57 to 73 inches, respectively)
or
$D_{L_{CO}}SS$ less than 6 mLCO/min/mm Hg
$D_{L_{CO}}SB$ less than 9 mLCO/min/mm Hg
or
Pa_{O_2} less than 65 mm Hg (at a Pa_{CO_2} of 30 mm Hg)
Pa_{O_2} less than 55 mm Hg (at a Pa_{CO_2} of 40 mm Hg)

Other Restrictive Ventilatory Disorders (kyphoscoliosis, thoracoplasty, lung resection)
VC less than 1.0 to 1.4 L (heights of 59 to 70 inches, respectively)

Pneumoconioses (demonstrated by chest x-ray)
Nodular focal fibrosis evaluated as for COPD
or
Interstitial disseminated fibrosis evaluated as for pulmonary fibrosis

1. Newborns, infants, and very young children cannot strictly perform those tests that require and depend on subject cooperation. Such tests include VC, FVC maneuvers, MVV, and $D_{L_{CO}}SB$.
2. Young children and adolescents may perform variably on those tests that are effort dependent or that require considerable cooperation.

Testing Infants and Young Children

Tests of lung function in infants and very young children can be used to assess lung volumes, flows, and mechanical factors, including compliance and resistance. Inability to perform maximal efforts eliminates such parameters as FVC, FEV_1, or maximal expiratory flow-volume curves. A number of new techniques have recently emerged that are particularly applicable to young children.

Partial Expiratory Flow-Volume Curves (PEFV)

The partial expiratory flow-volume (PEFV) curve is a record of the maximal flow developed over a portion of the VC. In infants, the forced exhalation is obtained by applying either a positive pressure to the thorax and abdomen, or a negative pressure to the airway. In an infant who is intubated, and usually deeply sedated, the lungs can be inflated to TLC. The airway is then connected to a source of negative pressure. As the lungs empty, expiratory flow is plotted against volume to derive the usual flow-volume curve. This technique is usually reserved for the measurement of flows in infants in the critical care setting, and is not performed routinely in the infant laboratory. In infants who are not intubated, the pressure necessary to produce a forced exhalation may be generated by an inflatable jacket that encircles the infant's chest and abdomen. The PEFV curve is obtained by rapidly applying a pressure around the thorax and abdomen at end-inspiration. This increases the pleural pressure and generates the forced expiratory maneuver. The pressure jacket must reach 95% of the peak pressure within approximately 100 msec. The pressure jacket must be connected to a reservoir that has a volume 10-times greater than the jacket. The pressure reservoir assures a relatively constant pressure. Flow is usually measured using an infant facemask sealed with lubricant and attached to a low dead space pneumotachometer. The infant is evaluated after falling asleep spontaneously or after mild sedation with chloral hydrate. Chloral hydrate should be used with caution if the child has clinical signs of wheezing. The flow-volume curve may be either displayed on a storage oscilloscope or digitized for computerized storage (Fig. 8–3).

In young children (i.e., ages 3 to 6 years), cooperation is essential to obtain reliable PEFV curves. Some children in this age group who have a good attention span and coordination may be capable of performing full MEFV curves. The child must be relaxed and must be able to follow instructions. The technologist's ability to elicit cooperation and to motivate the child are crucial. Several attempts may be necessary to generate an adequate, reproducible effort. The young child is tested breathing through a mouthpiece with a noseclip in place. Flow is measured by a pneumotachometer and volume determined by analog or digital integration of the flow signal. The tracing may be displayed on a storage oscilloscope or computer screen. Tidal breathing is recorded to obtain a consistent end-expiratory point (FRC) on the volume axis. The child is then instructed to exhale forcefully from end-inspiration, and to continue exhaling past the end-expiratory level to produce the PEFV curve.

The primary measurement derived from the PEFV curve is the flow at FRC (see Fig. 8–3). The highest flow obtained is reported as the $\dot{V}_{max}FRC$. In infants, the pressure in the reservoir attached to the inflatable jacket is increased with each maneuver until a maximal flow is reached. Theoretically, when no further increase in flow results from increasing the jacket pressure, flow limitation has been reached. It is not clear, however, whether the applied pressure can be directly related to the pleural pressure under dynamic conditions. Flow limitation may not be achieved in a reproducible fashion. PEFV curves in young children very likely do represent maximal flows (i.e., flow limitation) if two or

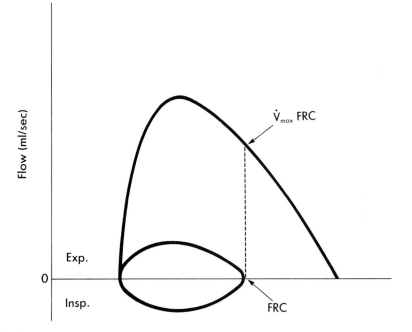

FIG 8–3.
Partial expiratory flow-volume curve (PEFV). A flow-volume curve typical of that which might be obtained in a normal infant or child. The term *partial* refers to the fact that flow is plotted only over a portion of the vital capacity (VC) rather than over the entire VC, as is normally done. This maneuver can be performed in young children who may not be able to inspire to total lung capacity or exhale completely to residual volume by having them exhale forcefully after a normal inspiration. In infants, PEFV curves may be obtained by applying positive pressure to the thorax and abdomen using a pressure jacket. The primary flow measurement is the $\dot{V}_{E_{max}}$FRC. The flow at functional residual capacity *(FRC)* is determined by recording tidal breathing (small loop) to identify the end-expiratory point, and then reading the maximal flow at that volume from the PEFV tracing. Abnormal PEFV curves show a concave appearance much like those in adults with airways obstruction (see Chapter 3).

more reproducible curves can be obtained. Infants with obstructive disease (i.e., severe airflow limitation) have intrathoracic obstruction, suggesting that true flow limitation is reached during external compression. In normal infants, inspiratory efforts or upper airway resistance such as closure of the glottis may impede forced expiratory flow. This causes the flow at FRC to appear less than it would if true flow limitation occurred. Flow limitation occurs, but not in an effort-independent manner.

In order to standardize measurements, the $\dot{V}_{max}$FRC may be divided by the absolute FRC determined either by He dilution, by N_2 washout, or by plethysmograph (V_{TG}). The maximal flow at FRC is expressed as FRC/sec. The $\dot{V}_{max}$FRC displays a variability similar to flow measures at low lung volumes

($\dot{V}_{max50}$, $\dot{V}_{max25}$) in older children or adults. The intersubject variability (approximately 30%) makes the $\dot{V}_{max}FRC$ less sensitive than the FEV_1 for detecting differences between healthy children and those with asthma.

Partial expiratory flow-volume curves in infants and young children have been used to assess normal lung growth and development. Asthma, cystic fibrosis, and bronchopulmonary dysplasia all show reduced $\dot{V}_{max}FRC$ values. Inhalation challenge studies using methacholine, histamine, or cold air as the stimulus and $\dot{V}_{max}FRC$ as the dependent variable have shown that a significant number of infants and young children have nonspecific airway hyperreactivity. Because young children and infants typically cannot perform a forced expiratory maneuver to determine FEV_1, the $\dot{V}_{max}FRC$ may be helpful in tracking the effectiveness of bronchodilators or related therapies. The FEV_1 is still the parameter of choice for detecting airway reactivity in older children and adolescents.

Lung Volumes

Lung volume determinations, specifically the FRC, in infants and young children are usually accomplished using the closed-circuit He dilution, open-circuit N_2 washout, or body plethysmograph techniques. Special procedures are typically required to adapt the general methods for each of these techniques to the pediatric patient. In the commonly used He dilution technique, a small-volume spirometer is used for infants with special attention to reduction of system volume and dead space components to accommodate the small FRC volumes commonly encountered. Infant plethysmography is accomplished using a small constant-volume chamber in which the infant reclines. The infant's nose and mouth rest against a cuffed opening in the plethysmograph. Flows can be measured by a close-fitting facemask as is done for PEFV curves. The airway is occluded at end-expiration for determination of V_{TG} and airways resistance. Plethysmographic lung volume measurements are possible in young children by allowing a parent to hold the child on their lap while sitting in the plethysmograph. The adult is instructed to hold their breath while the child breathes through a pneumotachometer, and the mouth shutter is closed at end-expiration. Nonpanting V_{TG} maneuvers are normally obtained, but some children can be coached to perform the closed-shutter panting acceptably. Corrections for the gas displacement of both the child and parent based on their combined weights are used in the calculation of the V_{TG} (see Sample Calculations in the Appendix).

Because VC may not be obtained in infants or young children, FRC is often the only reproducible lung volume that can be determined. The FRC in infants is a function not only of the recoil forces of the lung and chest wall, but is dynamically maintained by the laryngeal "braking" (of flow) and by shortening of the expiratory time. Because of these mechanisms, FRC may change rapidly from breath to breath, confounding measurements by the foreign-gas techniques. The variability of the FRC may lead to errors in measurements that use lung volumes such as $\dot{V}_{max}FRC$ or compliance. The problem of variability of the FRC may occur in young children as well as infants. Despite the mechanisms by which the FRC can change dynamically, the FRC has been shown to be reproducible in sedated children.

Pulmonary Mechanics

Measurements of lung compliance and resistance are of greatest importance in infants with abnormal pulmonary physiology. The compliance of the respiratory system (C_{rs}) can be determined noninvasively by one of several methods. The infant may breathe spontaneously into a small-volume (approximately 1 L) water-filled spirometer, while two or more weights are added to the bell. The weights produce pressure changes in the circuit which are measured and related to the change in end-expiratory lung volume on the breathing tracing. The C_{rs} is then calculated as the slope of the pressure-volume changes. The C_{rs} also may be derived by occlusion of the airway at end-inspiration and recording of the pressure plateau that occurs as the respiratory muscles relax. By recording the difference between the relaxed volume of expiration and the volume at end-inspiration, a pressure-volume slope (i.e., compliance) can be determined. This technique may be modified to allow multiple occluded breaths. The slope of the pressure-volume points at the end of each breath is then measured.

Dynamic compliance or resistance determinations require measurement of flow, volume, and esophageal pressure. These tests are usually reserved for infants requiring ventilatory support. Two problems that interfere with these groups of measurements are long time constants and the effects of changes in the upper airway. Measurement of a stable pressure during airway occlusion may be impossible in infants with marked differences in the compliance/resistance characteristics in different lung units (i.e., long time constants). This phenomenon occurs if equilibration of pressures within the lung is incomplete when a subsequent breath begins. Because the infant chest wall is extremely compliant, distortion of pleural pressure within the thorax may occur during inspiration, also affecting measurements of esophageal pressure. Similarly, the upper airway (i.e., the larynx) may influence the time constants by its contribution to the total resistance.

Testing in Older Children and Adolescents

Pulmonary function testing in older children and adolescents is often directed toward diagnosis and evaluation of the most common disease states in this group of pediatric subjects. These are asthma, cystic fibrosis, and chest deformities. In each of these diseases, the tests utilized are basically the same as might be used in adults with either obstructive or restrictive disorders.

The presence and severity of *asthma* in children is evaluated using a method similar to that used for testing the extent of reversible obstructive lung disease in adults.

1. *Lung volume measurements* (VC, TLC, RV, FRC, RV/TLC) provide information concerning air trapping and/or hyperinflation, particularly in acute asthmatic episodes.

2. *Flow measurements* (FEF_X, FEV_T, $FEV_{T\%}$, MEFV curves,and PEF) help to quantify the degree of obstruction and determine the effectiveness of bronchodilators. The PEF may be particularly useful as it can be measured conveniently at the bedside with a portable peak-flow meter, providing serial measurements for planning and evaluating therapy. The PEF should be correlated with the FEV_1 or other flow measurements in order to detect changes that may result from obstruction and not just effort.

3. *Blood gas analysis* may be indicated in acute asthmatic episodes to detect hypoxemia and hypercapnia. Impending respiratory failure may be signaled by worsening hypoxemia which is accompanied by hypocapnia progressing to hypercapnia.

4. *Exercise and/or bronchial challenge testing* may be used to determine the presence of exercise-induced bronchospasm and to evaluate the effectiveness of particular therapeutic regimens.

The alterations in lung function in children who have *cystic fibrosis* may be followed using the same group of tests as used in adults with COPD.

1. *Lung volumes* (VC, FRC, RV, TLC, RV/TLC) are most useful in detecting increases in FRC and RV associated with air trapping typical of advanced obstruction.

2. *Flow measurements* (FEF_X, FEV_T, $FEV_{T\%}$, MEFV curves, and PEF) assess the extent of obstruction caused by mucus plugging, bronchospasm, and edema. The efficacy of bronchodilators, aerosol therapy, chest physical therapy, and other therapeutic modalities aimed at management of secretions is determined largely by the change in FEV_1 and FVC before and after treatment.

3. *Arterial blood gas studies* may provide information concerning the degree of respiratory insufficiency, particularly the effects of $\dot{V}/\dot{Q}$ mismatching on oxygenation.

Chest deformities that are commonly evaluated by pulmonary function studies include kyphoscoliosis and pectus excavatum. Measurements include those parameters that are useful in assessing restrictive ventilatory patterns, such as lung volumes and $D_{L_{CO}}$. Flow studies, such as FEV_1 and MEFV curves, may provide additional information if the chest deformity contributes to large airway abnormalities. Spirometry, lung volumes, and blood gas analysis all may be used to follow postoperative changes if surgical intervention is employed. Calculation of predicted values based on height should be performed using the "wing-tip" method (i.e., arm-span distance) instead of standing height.

Normal values of lung function for children in all cases depend on height (length in infants), sex, and age. Lung function predicted values in children vary mainly with height, and some parameters change dramatically at the onset of puberty. For spirometric variables (i.e., FVC, FEV_1) lung function increases in up to about age 18 years in boys and about age 16 in girls. After these ages, volumes and flows plateau and then begin to decline. Because of this "peaking" of lung function in the late teens to early twenties, separate regression equations are often used for young children, adolescents, and adults. Problems can arise if gaps occur in the ranges over which the predicted normals are valid. For example, regressions from a study of children might include ages 6 to 17 years, and regressions from a study of adults from 20 to 80 years. It may not be valid to extrapolate either set of equations to determine expected values in 18- or 19-year-old persons. Rather, reference equations should be selected that eliminate these gaps. Nomograms and regression equations for common lung volumes and flows in children are included in the Appendix.

CRITICAL CARE MONITORING

Measurement of selected pulmonary function parameters is often indicated in subjects who are critically ill, particularly those who require mechanically supported ventilation. Some of these parameters, such as the VC, are similar to tests used in day-to-day pulmonary function evaluation. Others, such as capnography and reflective spectrophotometry, are highly specific for patients in an intensive care setting. Monitoring of the respiratory system includes the broad areas of pulmonary mechanics and gas exchange.

Pulmonary Mechanics

Ventilation ($\dot{V}_E$, V_T, f). Assessment of minute ventilation and its components, tidal volume (V_T) and respiratory rate (f), is usually accomplished by means of a flow-sensing spirometer attached to the patient's airway. The range of flows measured in spontaneously breathing subjects is usually much narrower than maximal flows (i.e., 0 to 12 L/sec). Some bedside spirometers may not accurately measure very low or very high flows. In subjects who are breathing spontaneously, a mouthpiece and noseclip, or close-fitting facemask, may be used. A low-resistance, unidirectional valve is normally employed so that only expired gas is collected. In subjects who are intubated, the valve and spirometer combination may be attached directly to the artificial airway. The patient then breathes normally while the expired volume, respiratory rate, and time are recorded. The interval for measuring expired volume may be dictated by the patient's condition and ability to cooperate. If the respiratory pattern is stable, a 1-minute interval usually provides an acceptable estimate of the resting ventilation. The V_T is derived by dividing the $\dot{V}_E$ by the rate (see Chapter 2). Most subjects change their breathing pattern when a mouthpiece/noseclip or mask are applied. Measurements of resting ventilation should be continued long enough to ensure a stable pattern. The dead space of the valve system (i.e., valve plus mouthpiece or mask) also may influence the resting ventilation. Subjects with very small tidal volumes (i.e., V_T less than 200 mL) may not tolerate the addition of a valve system with a dead space in excess of 100 mL. The addition of a significant dead space volume also may result in a pattern of ventilation that differs markedly from the subject's true resting level. Low dead space systems may offer higher resistance because their values have smaller apertures. Increased resistance to breathing may be a consideration in subjects with high resting respiratory rates.

Measurements of resting ventilation also can be accomplished indirectly by means of inductive plethysmography (see Chapter 9). The respiratory inductive plethysmograph records the motion of the rib cage and abdomen. After appropriate calibration, the volume and timing of individual breaths can be derived. The advantage of this approach is that no connection to the airway is required. The disadvantage is that calibration must be done carefully and checked often.

Patients receiving supplementary O_2 or being mechanically supported pose special problems for measurements of ventilation. Many mechanical ventilators incorporate volume-displacement or flow-sensing spirometers as an integral part of their monitoring/alarm systems. When practical, these built-in spirometers should be used to assess ventilation. The patient may remain connected to the ventilator support system if it allows spontaneous breathing through the ventilator circuit. Some systems that allow spontaneous ventilation (i.e., intermittent mandatory ventilation, or IMV) may have inappropriately high resistance and/or dead space. This may result in patient discomfort or inability to reach a stable ventilatory level. In such patients, ventilation measurements may require a separate spirometer and removal of the patient from the support system for the test. Subjects receiving supplementary O_2 should have an appropriate Fio_2 maintained while ventilatory parameters are measured. This may require addition of O_2 to the inspiratory side of the one-way valve. Care should be taken that the flow of supplementary O_2 does not directly enter the spirometer in order to avoid falsely elevated $\dot{V}_E$.

Minute ventilation is usually interpreted by comparing it with the patient's $Paco_2$. A normal or elevated $Paco_2$ with a markedly elevated $\dot{V}_E$ usually indicates increased physiologic dead space. A less common cause of increased $Paco_2$ is increased $\dot{V}co_2$. Patients who have limited ventilatory reserves may not be able to compensate for increased CO_2 production. Adjustment of the source of caloric intake from high carbohydrates to high fat (see Metabolic Studies, this chapter) may be necessary to reduce the CO_2 load to a level that can be accommodated by the patient. An elevated Pa_{CO_2} with a low minute ventilation suggests decreased respiratory drive or neuromuscular dysfunction. Inability to wean from mechanical ventilation often accompanies low V_T values (i.e., less than about 300 mL) and high respiratory rates (i.e., 22 to 30 per minute). Subjects who are disconnected from mechanical support for the purpose of measurement of ventilation or other spontaneous parameters may show markedly different patterns as the time off the ventilator increases. Respiratory muscle fatigue, worsening hypoxemia or hypercapnia, and anxiety may cause deterioration of the pattern of breathing. These changes may make interpretation of rate, tidal volume, and minute ventilation difficult.

Vital capacity, flows, and MVV. The VC is routinely measured in the management of patients who require ventilatory support or who have impending ventilatory failure. The VC is usually measured using a portable spirometer, often employing a pneumotachometer or other flow-sensing device (see Chapter 9). The spirometer should meet the American Thoracic Society's recommendation for volume accuracy (i.e., $\pm 3\%$ or 50 mL, whichever is greater). Accuracy for flow measurements may be unnecessary if the device is used only for VC determinations. Patients who are alert and cooperative can often perform reproducible VC maneuvers, usually by inspiring to TLC and expiring slowly to RV.

Measurement of the MVV also requires patient cooperation and effort. In addition, the spirometer must be accurate over the range of flows developed. Healthy subjects may generate flows in excess of 200 L/min during the MVV maneuver. Patients who are critically ill seldom achieve such high levels. The measuring device should have a low resistance, particularly over the flow range of 0 to 50 L/min.

The VC may be reduced in critically ill patients because of obstruction, restriction, or neuromuscular disease. Poor effort or inability to perform the VC maneuver also may result in low values. Healthy adults have VC values in excess of 50 mL/kg. The ability to move a VC of 10 to 12 mL/kg is usually required to maintain unsupported ventilation. Values less than 10 mL/kg are typical in patients who are difficult to wean from mechanical support of ventilation. The MVV maneuver helps to estimate the ventilatory reserve available in the patient. If the resting $\dot{V}_E$ exceeds approximately 50% of the MVV, the subject probably will not be able to ventilate spontaneously for an extended period.

Measurements of FVC and flow rates in the critical care setting provide a quantitative basis for therapy in obstructive airway processes, particularly asthma. Portable spirometers allow serial measurements on a daily or even hourly basis. Spirometry can be used at the bedside to assess the effectiveness of bronchodilators, aerosol therapy, or chest physical therapy. If the FVC and

FEV_1 are to be measured in the intensive care setting, the spirometer should meet the minimum ATS requirements (see Chapter 11) for volume as well as for flows.

Peak expiratory flow (PEF), though used commonly, may not quantify the reversibility of obstruction. Normal peak flows may be developed early in a forced expiration even though the FEV_1 or FEF_x values are decreased. Ideally, PEF should be correlated with the FEV_1. Peak flows, as measured with a small portable device, may be beneficial in evaluating the control of asthma in subjects who use the device routinely and for whom conventional spirometric measurements are well documented. Serial measurements, daily or more often, can serve as an index for evaluation of therapeutic maneuvers to control bronchospasm.

Respiratory pressures. Respiratory muscle strength is assessed by measuring the maximal pressure that can be generated at the airway. Negative inspiratory force (NIF) is similar to the maximal inspiratory pressure (MIP, see Chapter 3). The NIF is measured by connecting a pressure manometer to an occluded airway and noting the maximum negative pressure that can be developed. While the MIP is normally measured by having the subject inspire from RV, the NIF is measured at or near FRC. The NIF (sometimes referred to as the maximum inspiratory force) is used in obtunded individuals in whom a VC measurement cannot be obtained. Occlusion of the airway produces maximal values within 10 to 20 seconds. Airway occlusion may not be tolerated well by subjects with unstable cardiovascular status. A VC of 15 mL/kg requires development of approximately -20 cm H_2O. This value is considered the minimum below which a subject usually will not be able to maintain adequate spontaneous ventilation over an extended period. Values greater than -80 cm H_2O are observed in healthy individuals. However, negative pressures exceeding -20 cm H_2O are not predictive of a specific VC.

Gas Exchange

Capnography.   Continuous analysis of expired CO_2 (see Chapter 6) may be used as a respiratory monitor in patients who are intubated, as well as those who are not. Carbon dioxide is analyzed either by means of an infrared analyzer or mass spectrometer. Most infrared analyzers withdraw a small continuous flow of gas from the patient and direct it into a sample cell. Accurate analysis depends on a constant flow and adequate removal or compensation for water vapor. The CO_2 analyzer is usually zeroed by sampling room air and spanned by sampling a 5% CO_2 mixture. Some analyzers are specially designed for use with mechanical ventilators. These analyzers feature a heated infrared chamber that is placed directly in the gas flow, usually near the artificial airway. The infrared light passes through the gas in the breathing circuit without the necessity of a sample pump. Response time of in-line analyzers is very rapid, and there are no changes in sample flow rate to alter calibration. As described in Chapter 6, capnography may be used to monitor end-tidal CO_2, to calculate the Pa-$P_{ET_{CO_2}}$ gradient, and to estimate dead space. Exhaled CO_2 analysis can detect acute reductions in cardiac output, as dead space usually increases as cardiac output falls. Simple CO_2 trend monitoring of respiratory rate can detect disconnection from the mechanical ventilator.

Pulse oximetry.   Noninvasive oximetry to measure Sa_{O_2} is widely used to monitor patients on mechanical ventilation or being supported by supplementary O_2. The measurement of oxygen saturation by means of two-wavelength pulse oximetry is described in Chapter 6. In the critical care setting, pulse oximetry is used for continuous monitoring, employing probes located on either the ear or finger. Most pulse oximeters currently available utilize a microprocessor to analyze arterial pulsations in a capillary bed. Computerization allows the oximeter to adjust light output to accommodate different tissues and conditions in order to obtain an optimal signal. In addition, the microprocessor permits alarms to be triggered when saturation or pulse rate exceeds preset limits. Many instruments provide digital and/or analog outputs for connection to recorders or computerized central monitoring systems.

Oxygen saturation by pulse oximetry (Sp_{O_2}) is particularly well suited for detecting changes in saturation across the physiologic range often encountered in critically ill patients, namely 75% to 95%. Clinical decisions regarding changes in mechanical ventilator settings or O_2 therapy are often made when the saturation falls below 90%. Conversely, pulse oximetry is relatively insensitive to changes in oxygen content when the Pa_{O_2} is greater than 100 mm Hg. This results from the relatively flat upper portion of the oxyhemoglobin dissociation curve. Though the accuracy of many oximeters differ, confidence limits of $\pm 4\%$ are realistic for most instruments. At low saturations (i.e., less than 75%), most pulse oximeters tend to become less accurate (see Chapter 9). Despite this large imprecision, detection of acute changes in oxygen saturation can be made if pulse oximetry is compared with blood oximetry. In addition, careful attention must be paid to those factors that can affect the accuracy of the pulse oximeter. COHb, MetHb, jaundice, cardiac output dyes, high-intensity light, skin pigmentation, and hypoperfusion are all interfering substances that are not uncommon in the critical care setting. Motion artifact, particularly shivering, interferes with the detection of the pulse waveform necessary to distinguish arterial absorption from venous and tissue absorption. Decreased local perfusion, resulting from hypothermia or vasopressor drugs, is known to result in an Sp_{O_2} that is less than the Sa_{O_2}. Response times of some oximeters may also present problems, particularly if saturation falls rapidly, as sometimes occurs with bradycardia.

Transcutaneous blood gases.   Transcutaneous electrodes for measuring Po_2 ($tcPo_2$) and Pco_2 ($tcPco_2$) are used in some intensive care units. Transcutaneous gas monitoring, specifically the $tcPo_2$, is used widely in neonatal units because the gradients between arterial blood and the skin tend to be smaller. Transcutaneous Po_2 monitors utilize a Clark electrode (see Chapter 9). The attachment site is heated by the electrode itself to produce local hyperemia. The hyperemia helps to "arterialize" the capillary flow in the skin, but also necessitates periodic repositioning of the electrode to prevent burns. Transcutaneous Po_2 electrodes that can be attached to the conjunctiva of the eye and to the mucous membranes of the oropharynx also have been designed but are not widely used. The $tcPco_2$ is monitored by a modified Severinghaus electrode, attached in a manner similar to the $tcPo_2$ electrode. The $tcPco_2$ electrode has a slower response time than the $tcPo_2$, and is somewhat more tedious to calibrate. A combination $tcPo_2$ and $tcPco_2$ electrode is available.

The $tcPo_2$ correlates well with Pao_2 in patients who have a stable cardiovascular status. Decreases in cardiac output normally result in a reduction in cutaneous blood flow and localized hypoxia. In adults, because of the thickness of the keratin layer of the skin, the $tcPo_2$ tends to be about 20% less than the Pao_2 when the subject is at rest. This gradient widens in the face of reduced blood flow, either systemically or locally. The transcutaneous oxygen tension is useful for detecting large swings in Po_2. Such fluctuations sometimes occur when lung function changes as supplementary oxygen is being administered. The $tcPo_2$ may be particularly valuable in distinguishing abrupt increases in oxygen tension in susceptible patients such as neonates.

The $tcPco_2$, like $tcPo_2$, depends largely on the local perfusion and metabolism. The $tcPco_2$ usually exceeds the $Paco_2$ because of the increased CO_2 production caused by the heated electrode.

Mixed venous oxygen saturation.   The use of a fiberoptic pulmonary artery catheter employing reflective spectrophotometry (see Chapter 9) allows continuous measurement of mixed venous saturation. This catheter uses a fiberoptic bundle to transmit light at either 2 or 3 wavelengths to blood flowing in the pulmonary artery. The reflected light returns via a second fiberoptic pathway to a photodetector. A microprocessor then calculates the $S\bar{v}o_2$ based on the absorption of light by O_2Hb and reduced Hb, and displays the value continuously. All of the other data normally obtained from a pulmonary artery catheter (i.e., mixed venous blood samples, pulmonary artery pressure, wedge pressure) are available.

Mixed venous oxygen saturation is useful in monitoring cardiac status and oxygen delivery. The $S\bar{v}o_2$ is the average of the venous blood returning from all parts of the body. It may be affected by oxygen consumption, cardiac output, and the content of the arterial blood. Normal subjects have an $S\bar{v}o_2$ of 75% to 85%. The mixed venous oxygen saturation may fall if the cardiac output decreases and the tissues continue to consume the same amount of oxygen. An $S\bar{v}o_2$ in the range of 60% to 70% represents a slightly reduced cardiac output. Values less than 60% are usually associated with a significant reduction in cardiac output. However, a low $S\bar{v}o_2$ also may result from increased O_2 extraction by the tissues. This typically occurs during exercise while the cardiac output is actually increasing. Redistribution of the cardiac output to organs that have a high O_2 consumption also may reduce the $S\bar{v}o_2$ without an actual decrease in cardiac output. Conversely, the $S\bar{v}o_2$ may increase if the tissue O_2 consumption decreases, as sometimes occurs with sepsis. Arterial content, as determined by the Sa_{O_2} and Hb, also may influence the $S\bar{v}o_2$. If arterial content falls because of pulmonary disease or anemia and cardiac output and O_2 consumption remain constant, mixed venous saturation will decrease. Interpretation of changes in $S\bar{v}o_2$ should always be considered in the context of the multiple factors that influence it.

Metabolic Measurements (Indirect Calorimetry)

Description

Measurements of $\dot{V}o_2$ and $\dot{V}co_2$, and their ratio (RER), may be used to determine the caloric energy expenditure. These measurements also allow partitioning the calories among the various substrates (i.e., fat, carbohydrate, protein). In combination with measurements of caloric intake and other laboratory values such as urinary nitrogen, indirect calorimetry allows nutritional assessment and management.

Technique

Indirect calorimetry may be performed using either an open-circuit or closed-circuit system to measure O_2 consumption, CO_2 production, and RER.

Open-circuit calorimetry. Exchange of O_2 and CO_2 may be measured by recording $\dot{V}E$ and the fractional differences of O_2 and CO_2 between inspired and expired gas. These measurements are accomplished using either a mixing-chamber or breath-by-breath system similar to those used for expired gas analysis during exercise (see Chapter 7). The $\dot{V}o_2$ and $\dot{V}co_2$ are measured as described for exercise testing. The $\dot{V}E$, V_T, and f (respiratory rate) also may be measured. Connection to the subject may be made by a standard unidirectional valve with mouthpiece and nose clips. A ventilated hood or canopy (Fig. 8–4) also may be used. Many metabolic measurement systems provide for connection to a mechanical ventilator circuit.

A hood or canopy allows long-term measurements without direct connection to the patient's airway. The hood is ventilated by drawing a flow of gas that exceeds the patient's peak inspiratory demand through it (40 L/min is usually adequate). By measuring the change in flow into and out of the hood during breathing ("bias" flow), ventilation can be calculated.

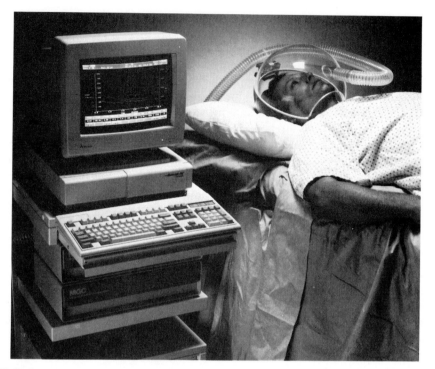

FIG 8–4.
Canopy for metabolic measurements. Resting energy expenditure (REE) may be measured by assessing the changes in gas flow and fractional concentrations of expired air drawn from a hood or canopy. A continuous or "bias" flow of gas is drawn through the canopy. Changes (i.e., increases or decreases) in the bias flow are measured to determine ventilation. Fractional gas concentrations are determined either breath by breath or after passing the gas through a mixing chamber. The canopy offers the advantage of not requiring direct connection to the subject's airway, which may affect ventilation and the measurement of REE. Although useful for spontaneously breathing subjects, the hood cannot be used with patients requiring mechanical support of ventilation. (Courtesy of Medical Graphics Corporation, St. Paul, Minn).

Connection to a ventilator requires a means of measuring exhaled volume along with both the inspired and expired fractional gas concentrations. Breath-by-breath metabolic measurement systems usually sample gas at the patient/ventilator connection.

Closed circuit calorimetry.   The simplest type of closed-circuit calorimeter is one that measures $\dot{V}O_2$ volumetrically. The subject rebreathes gas from a closed system containing a spirometer that has been filled with oxygen. Carbon dioxide is scrubbed from the circuit and a recording of the decrease in system (i.e., the spirometer) volume equals the rate of O_2 uptake or $\dot{V}O_2$. A similar approach uses a closed spirometer system that allows measured amounts of oxygen to be added as the subject rebreathes and removes oxygen. The $\dot{V}_{O_2}$ is then equal to the volume of O_2 that must be added per minute to maintain a constant volume. Carbon dioxide production cannot be measured using a closed-circuit system unless a CO_2 analyzer is added to the device. Minute ventilation, V_T, and respiratory rate all may be determined from volume excursions of the spirometer. Closed-circuit systems may be used with spontaneously breathing patients by means of a simple breathing valve and mouthpiece. Use of a closed-circuit calorimeter with a mechanical ventilator requires that the spirometer system be connected between the patient and ventilator. The ventilator then "ventilates" the spirometer which in turn ventilates the patient. This technique usually requires a bellows-type spirometer in a fixed container so that the bellows can be compressed by the positive pressure generated by the ventilator. The volume delivered by the ventilator (i.e., V_T) must be increased to compensate for the volume of gas compressed in the closed-circuit spirometer during positive-pressure breaths.

The purpose of indirect calorimetry is primarily to estimate resting energy expenditure (REE) over an extended period, usually 24 hours. In order to extrapolate the values obtained during the sampling period, the subject's condition during the measurement is critical. The following guidelines help assure that measurements are made under steady-state conditions:

1. The subject should be recumbent or supine for 20 to 30 minutes before beginning measurements and should stay quiet during the test. The testing apparatus should not cause discomfort or exertion on the part of the subject.

2. The subject should be fasting for 2 to 4 hours before the test starts. If the subject is receiving feedings, either enteral or parenteral, they should be continuous rather than in bolus form.

3. The subject should be in a neutral thermal environment. Special corrections may be required for subjects who are febrile or who are hypothermic.

4. Drugs or substances that alter metabolism should be avoided. Substances related to caffeine and nicotine are particularly common stimulants. Theophylline-based drugs also may increase metabolic rate.

5. Data collection should continue long enough so that a stable baseline is established and steady-state conditions can be verified (Fig. 8–5). Common indicators of steady-state conditions are the parameters assessed as part of the metabolic study itself. The $\dot{V}_{O_2}$, $\dot{V}_{CO_2}$, $\dot{V}_E$, and HR should not change by more than $\pm 5\%$ during the testing interval. If the subject does not demonstrate steady-state conditions, a longer test interval may be required to average representative periods of metabolic activity.

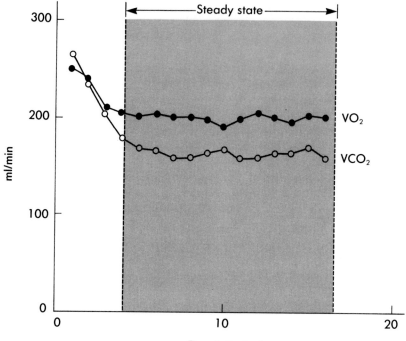

FIG 8–5.
Indirect calorimetry. Typical tracing of continuous measurement of $\dot{V}_{O_2}$ and $\dot{V}_{CO_2}$ as performed during open-circuit indirect calorimetry. The subject's expired gas is analyzed to determine O_2 consumption, CO_2 production, and RQ during a resting state. The measurements are observed until a metabolic steady state can be determined. During the steady-state interval, values representative of resting energy expenditure can be measured. From these measurements, the daily caloric requirements can be estimated, and the percentages of energy derived from fats, carbohydrates, and proteins calculated.

6. Patients on ventilators should be in a stable condition. No ventilator adjustments should be made for 1 to 2 hours preceding the test period. Modifications in minute ventilation or Fi_{O_2} settings can cause gross changes in the patterns of gas exchange, particularly in subjects with pulmonary disease.

Metabolic calculations.

1. *Harris-Benedict equations* for estimating resting energy expenditure:
Males:

$$REE \text{ (kcal/24 hours)} = 66.47 + 13.75W + 5.00H - 6.76A$$

Females:

$$REE \text{ (kcal/24 hours)} = 655.10 + 9.56W + 1.85H - 4.68A$$

where:

$$W = \text{weight in kilograms}$$

$$H = \text{height in centimeters}$$

$$A = \text{age in years}$$

The REE by these formulas was originally described as the basal metabolic rate (BMR). These equations may be used to estimate the caloric expenditure in normal subjects under conditions of minimal activity. The basal metabolic rate in these circumstances is related to lean body mass. To determine the optimum level of caloric intake, the BMR must be adjusted upward, as trauma, surgery, infections, and burns all cause the REE to increase.

2. *Weir equation* for calculating REE from respiratory gas exchange and urinary N_2:

$$REE \text{ (kcal/24 hours)} = 1.44(3.941\dot{V}_{O_2} + 1.106\dot{V}_{CO_2}) - 2.17(UN)$$

where:

$$\dot{V}_{O_2} \text{ is expressed in mL/min}$$

$$\dot{V}_{CO_2} \text{ is expressed in mL/min}$$

$$UN = \text{urinary nitrogen (g/24 hours)}$$

$$1.44 = \text{correction from mL/min to L/24 hours}$$

Indirect calorimetry by the open-circuit method provides measures of both oxygen consumption and CO_2 production. The RER is the ratio of $\dot{V}_{CO_2}/\dot{V}_{O_2}$. Under steady-state conditions, the RER approximates the mean respiratory quotient (RQ) at the cell level. The RQ normally varies from 0.71 to 1.00 depending on the substrates being metabolized. Carbohydrate oxidation produces an RQ near 1.0, fat oxidation produces an RQ near 0.71, and protein oxidation produces an RQ of 0.82. The RQ attributable to carbohydrates and fats may be determined by subtracting the $\dot{V}_{CO_2}$ and $\dot{V}_{O_2}$ derived from protein. This form of the RQ is called the nonprotein RQ or RQ_{NP} and is calculated:

$$RQ_{NP} = \frac{(\dot{V}_{CO_2} \text{ (in L/24 hours)} - 4.8 \text{ UN})}{(\dot{V}_{O_2} \text{ (in L/24 hours)} - 5.9 \text{ UN})}$$

where:

$$\dot{V}_{CO_2} \text{ (in L/24 hours)} = 1.44 \, \dot{V}_{CO_2} \text{ (in mL/min)}$$

$$\dot{V}_{O_2} \text{ (in L/24 hours)} = 1.44 \, \dot{V}_{O_2} \text{ (in mL/min)}$$

Because CO_2 production varies with O_2 uptake, deviations of the RQ from the average value of 0.85 result in differences of less than 5% in the calculation of REE if the $\dot{V}_{O_2}$ and RQ are used. Indirect calorimetry by the closed-circuit (volumetric) method takes advantage of this small difference by assuming a fixed RQ (usually 0.85) and measuring only $\dot{V}_{O_2}$. Urinary N_2 is obtained from a 24-hour collection. Because protein metabolism accounts for only a small proportion of the total calories per day (about 12%), omission of the UN in the Weir equation changes the calculated REE by only 2%.

3. *Consolazio equations* for determination of energy expenditure from gas exchange ($\dot{V}_{O_2}$, $\dot{V}_{CO_2}$), urinary N_2 (UN), and the caloric equivalents of carbohydrates, fats, and proteins:

$$\text{carbohydrates (in g)} = (4.12\dot{V}_{O_2}) - (2.91\dot{V}_{CO_2}) - (1.94UN)$$

$$\text{fat (in g)} = (1.69\dot{V}_{O_2}) - (1.69\dot{V}_{CO_2}) - (2.54UN)$$

$$\text{protein (in g)} = (6.25UN)$$

From the grams of each substrate utilized, the kilocalories derived from that source can be computed:

$$\text{carbohydrates (in kcal)} = 4.18 \text{ carbohydrates (in g)}$$

$$\text{fat (in kcal)} = 9.46 \text{ fat (in g)}$$

$$\text{protein (in kcal)} = 4.32 \text{ protein (in g)}$$

$$\text{total (in kcal)} = \text{carbohydrate} + \text{fat} + \text{protein (in kcal)}$$

The percentage of calories attributable to each of the substrates also may be calculated by dividing the kilocalories derived from the substrate by the total kilocalories. Because the Consolazio equations are intended for analysis of normal substrate partitioning, RQ values outside of the range of 0.71 to 1.00 will result in negative values for either carbohydrates or lipids (fat). These negative values are erroneous if the RER does not equal the RQ (i.e., the patient is not in a metabolic steady state).

Significance and Pathophysiology

Indirect calorimetry is most often used to assess nutritional status of patients whose daily energy expenditure is altered by disease, injury, or therapeutic interventions. The REE accounts for approximately two-thirds of the daily energy requirements in healthy subjects. The Harris-Benedict equations (see above) or similar predictive equations are commonly used to estimate the REE. Various "factors" have been added to the basic equation to account for the extra requirements imposed by the patient's clinical status. The metabolic requirements of patients who are critically ill varies widely. Indirect calorimetry can be used to detect undernourishment, overnourishment, or the utilization of inappropriate substrates.

Undernourishment or starvation can occur during illness. It may be detected by caloric expenditure in excess of caloric intake (negative energy balance). Both fat stores and protein from muscle breakdown may contribute to metabolism during periods of undernourishment. Indirect calorimetry is often used along with measurement of body weight, triceps skinfold measurements, and other approximations of energy reserves. These measurements allow planning of nutritional therapy to replete diminished reserves.

Overnourishment occurs when any substrate is supplied in excess of the energy requirements. Overfeeding is most deleterious when the patient's nutritional status is already adequate. Excess lipid or carbohydrate calories are stored as fat, which may place stress on one or more organ systems.

Patients with pulmonary disease present a special dilemma. Excessive carbohydrate intake results in increased CO_2 production because the RQ of carbohydrates is 1.00. In patients who have respiratory failure, this excess production of CO_2 places an increased ventilatory load on the respiratory system. Adjustments in substrate utilization can be made after the nonprotein RQ is determined by indirect calorimetry. Lipids (i.e., fats) are typically substituted for glucose so that the RQ can be reduced while the caloric intake is maintained. Patients with respiratory failure also may experience atrophy of ventilatory muscles. Substrate analysis can be used to assess nitrogen balance which is related to the breakdown of muscle protein. Substrate analysis permits the nutritional requirements necessary to maintain nitrogen balance to be measured.

Technical considerations involved in indirect calorimetry include the accuracy of gas analysis and measurement of expired volume during the test interval. The most common problem related to gas analysis during metabolic measurements is attainment of a true steady state. Only if the measurements are made under steady-state conditions is the metabolic rate representative of the caloric expenditure over 24 hours. Hyperventilation resulting from connection to a mask or mouthpiece or from a ventilator manipulation is a frequent occurrence. Head hoods or continuous-flow canopies can eliminate much of the stimulation associated with connection to the metabolic measurement system (see Fig. 8–4), but cannot be used for patients on mechanical ventilators. An RER greater than 1.00 should always be evaluated in relation to the $\dot{V}_E$ and end-tidal CO_2. Abnormally high $\dot{V}_E$ and low end-tidal CO_2 values may indicate hyperventilation. RER values in excess of 1.00 that cannot be explained as hyperventilation may be the result of the storage of excess calories as fat (lipogenesis). RER values below 0.70 may occur in ketosis caused by extreme fasting or diabetic ketoacidosis. More commonly, however, low RER values signal improper calibration of the gas analyzers or hypoventilation. Inaccurate calibration or improper performance of either the CO_2 or O_2 analyzers can result in RER values outside of the usual metabolic range of 0.70 to 1.00.

Special problems may be encountered in performing metabolic measurements on patients requiring mechanical ventilatory support. The most common difficulty relates to measurements of O_2 consumption when the patient is receiving supplementary oxygen. Measurement of $\dot{V}o_2$ by respiratory gas exchange requires analysis of the difference between inspired and expired O_2 and the minute ventilation. In subjects breathing room air, the inspired Fio_2 is constant. Many oxygen blending systems, such as those used on ventilators, may not provide a constant fraction of inspired O_2. Large differences in the calculated $\dot{V}o_2$ can result from small fluctuations in the Fio_2, even if the Feo_2 remains relatively constant. Small differences in the inspired and expired volumes (resulting from the respiratory exchange ratio) are corrected by adjusting the inspired fraction of oxygen according to the following equation:

$$\frac{(1 - Feo_2 - Feco_2)}{(1 - Fio_2)} \times Fio_2$$

This correction of inspired Fio_2 for gas balance in the lung (i.e., the Haldane transformation; see $\dot{V}o_2$, Chapter 7) limits the accuracy of the open-circuit method of determining $\dot{V}o_2$. As the Fio_2 is increased, the value in the denominator of the equation becomes smaller. Even with very accurate gas analyzers, measurement of differences between the Fio_2 and Feo_2 when the Fio_2 is above 0.50 is quite variable. Indirect calorimetry by the volumetric method (i.e., a closed system) avoids this problem by measuring the actual volume of O_2 removed during rebreathing. Measurement of $\dot{V}o_2$ and $\dot{V}co_2$ in spontaneously breathing patients who require supplementary O_2 can usually be accommodated by allowing the subject to breath from a high flow Venturi device or from a reservoir bag containing an increased Fio_2.

Other considerations involved in metabolic measurements on ventilated patients include the effects of positive pressure on gas analysis and on volume determination. Analysis of O_2 and CO_2 in the ventilator circuit must take into account the effect of positive pressure breaths on the gas analyzers. Depending on the sampling method employed, positive pressure swings during each breath may generate falsely high partial pressure readings. Closed-circuit calorimetry places a volumetric device in the breathing circuit between the ventilator and the patient. The volume delivered by the ventilator must be increased to accommodate the higher compressible gas volume in the circuit, approximately 1 mL/cm H_2O for each liter of added volume.

SELF-ASSESSMENT QUESTIONS

1. Clinical information provided by the patient's history is particularly important:
   a. When the subject has severe COPD
   b. When the subject is unable to perform the test
   c. When the test results are borderline normal
   d. If only lung volumes are measured

2. A before- and after-bronchodilator study (spirometry) produces these values in a subject who complains of shortness of breath on exertion:

		Predrug	**Postdrug**	**Predicted**
FVC	(L)	3.30	3.70	4.40
FEV_1	(L)	1.77	1.87	3.20
FEV_1		54	51	—

   The percent improvement following bronchodilator administration is:
   a. -3%
   b. 3%
   c. 6%
   d. 12%

3. Which of the following are true concerning withdrawal of bronchodilators before bronchial challenge testing:
   I. Cromolyn sodium should be withheld for 6 hours
   II. Beta-adrenergic agents should be withheld for 12 hours
   III. Sustained action theophylline should be withheld for 48 hours
   IV. Anticholinergic aerosols should be taken as prescribed
   a. I, II, III
   b. I, II, IV
   c. II, III
   d. I, IV

4. A subject performing a methacholine challenge test has the following reproducible results:
   FEV_1 (baseline)   3.3 L
   FEV_1 (control)   2.8 L
   The technologist should do which of the following:
   a. Administer methacholine 0.075 mg/mL
   b. Administer methacholine 2.50 mg/mL
   c. Repeat the diluent control
   d. Stop, the test is positive

5. Following 5 minutes of hyperventilation of cold air, a subject's FEV_1 has fallen by 9% from the pretest values. This indicates that:
   a. The subject has hyperreactive airways
   b. The air was not cool enough to provoke a response
   c. A further 5 minutes of hyperventilation is required
   d. Inadequate CO_2 was added to the inspired gas

6. The use of a pressure jacket to produce PEFV curves in infants requires a large reservoir in order to:
   a. Accurately measure expiratory flow
   b. Maintain a relatively constant pressure
   c. Regulate the end-expiratory lung volume
   d. Reduce the noise during jacket inflation

7. In addition to a flow-sensing spirometer, which of the following are needed to measure V_T in a spontaneously breathing patient who is not intubated:
   I. Mouthpiece, noseclips
   II. Low-resistance one-way valve
   III. Supplementary O_2
   IV. Capnograph or CO_2 analyzer
   a. I, III, IV
   b. I, II
   c. II, III
   d. III, IV

8. A subject on mechanical ventilation has a pulmonary artery catheter in place. The mixed venous O_2 saturation as measured by reflective spectrophotometry through the catheter is 75%. This finding is consistent with:
   a. Normal cardiopulmonary function
   b. Mildly reduced cardiac output
   c. Severely reduced cardiac output
   d. Incorrect location of the catheter tip

9. The vital capacity (VC) may decrease as much as _____ following thoracic or upper abdominal surgery.
   a. 10%
   b. 20%
   c. 50%
   d. 5 L

10. Which of the following blood gas values suggests significant postoperative complications:
    a. A pH of 7.46
    b. A Pao_2 of 49

    c. A Pa_{CO_2} of 70

    d. A COHb of 2%

11. In order for spirometric tracings to be acceptable for determining respiratory impairment for disability, the recording must have a:
    a. Paper speed of 10 mm/sec, volume sensitivity of 20 mm/L
    b. Paper speed of 20 mm/sec, volume sensitivity of 10 mm/L
    c. Paper speed of 20 mm/sec, volume sensitivity of 20 mm/L
    d. Paper speed of 50 mm/sec, volume sensitivity of 20 mm/L

12. A subject's REE is estimated from $\dot{V}_{O_2}$ measured while he breathed from a spirometer that had been filled with O_2. This technique is described as:
    a. Closed-circuit calorimetry
    b. The Consolazio method
    c. Open-circuit calorimetry
    d. The bias-flow technique

13. A patient has a metabolic study performed with the following results:

$\dot{V}_{O_2}$	300 mL/min
$\dot{V}_{CO_2}$	270 mL/min

    If the patient's 24 hour urinary nitrogen (UN) is 22 g/24 hours, approximately what is his REE?
    a. 1480 kcal/24 hours
    b. 2084 kcal/24 hours
    c. 2132 kcal/24 hours
    d. 2666 kcal/24 hours

14. A patient with chronic obstructive pulmonary disease has been difficult to wean from mechanical ventilation. In order to minimize CO_2 production, the caloric intake of the patient should consist mainly of:
    a. Protein
    b. Carbohydrate
    c. Fat
    d. Glucose

SELECTED BIBLIOGRAPHY

TESTING REGIMENS

American Thoracic Society: Lung function testing: selection of reference values and interpretive strategies. *Am Rev Respir Dis* 144:1202, 1991.

Becklake MR, Permutt S: Evaluation of tests of lung function for screening for early detection of chronic obstructive lung disease. In Macklem, et al: *The lung in transition between health and disease.* New York, 1979, Marcel Dekker.

Cotes JE: Lung function throughout life; determinants and reference values. In Cotes, JE, editor: *Lung function: assessment and application in medicine.* Oxford, 1979, Blackwell Scientific Publications.

BEFORE- AND AFTER-BRONCHODILATOR STUDIES

Dales RE, Spitzer WO, Tousignant P, et al: Clinical interpretation of airway response to a bronchodilator: epidemiologic considerations. *Am Rev Respir Dis* 138:317, 1988.

Guyatt GH, Townsend M, Nogradi S, et al: Acute response to bronchodilator, an imperfect guide for bronchodilator therapy in chronic airflow limitation. *Arch Intern Med* 148:1949, 1988.

Light RW, Conrad SA, George RB: The one best test for evaluating the effects of bronchodilator therapy. *Chest* 72:512, 1977.

Sourk RL, Nugent KM: Bronchodilator testing: confidence intervals derived from placebo inhalations. *Am Rev Respir Dis* 128:153, 1983.

BRONCHIAL CHALLENGE

Aquilina AT: Comparison of airway reactivity induced by histamine, methacholine, and isocapnic hyperventilation in normal and asthmatic subjects. *Thorax* 38:766, 1983.

Bhagat RG, Grunstein MM: Comparison of responsiveness to methacholine, histamine, and exercise in subgroups of asthmatic children. *Am Rev Respir Dis* 129:221, 1984.

Chai H, Farr RS, Froelich LA, et al: Standardization of bronchial inhalation challenge procedures. *J Allergy Clin Immunol* 56:323, 1975.

Cockcroft DW, Berscheid BA: Standardization of inhalational provocation test: dose vs concentration of histamine. *Chest* 82:572, 1982.

Cockcroft DW, Killian DN, Mellon JJA, et al: Bronchial reactivity to inhaled histamine: a method and clinical survey. *Clin Allergy* 7:235, 1977.

Cropp GJA, Bernstein IL, Boushey HA, et al: Guidelines for bronchial inhalation challenges with pharmacologic and antigenic agents. ATS News, Spring, 11–19, 1980.

Eggleston PA, Rosenthal RR: Guidelines for the methodology of exercise challenge testing of asthmatics. *J Allergy Clin Immunol* 64:642, 1979.

Eliasson AH, Phillips YY, Rajagopal KR, et al: Sensitivity and specificity of bronchial provocation testing: an evaluation of four techniques in exercise induced bronchospasm. *Chest* 102:347, 1992.

Michoud MC, Ghezzo H, Amyot R: A comparison of pulmonary function tests used for bronchial challenges. *Bull Eur Physiopathol Respir* 18:609, 1982.

Pepys G, Hutchcroft BJ: Bronchial provocation tests in etiologic diagnosis and analysis of asthma. *Am Rev Respir Dis* 112:829, 1975.

Phillips YY, Jaeger JJ, Laube BL, et al: Eucapnic voluntary hyperventilation of compressed gas mixture. *Am Rev Respir Dis* 131:31, 1985.

Scott GC, Braun SR: A survey of the current use and methods of analysis of bronchoprovocational challenges. *Chest* 100:322, 1991.

PREOPERATIVE PULMONARY FUNCTION TESTING

Boysen PG: Preoperative pulmonary function tests and complications after coronary artery bypass. *Anesthesiology* 57:A499, 1982.

Cain HD, Stevens PM, Adaniya R: Preoperative pulmonary function and complications after cardiovascular surgery. *Chest* 76:130, 1979.

Olsen GN, Block AJ, Swenson EW, et al: Pulmonary function evaluation of the lung resection candidate: a prospective study. *Am Rev Respir Dis* 111:379, 1975.

Reichel J: Assessment of operative risk of pneumonectomy. *Chest* 62:570, 1972.

Tisi GM: Preoperative evaluation of pulmonary function: validity, indications, and benefits. *Am Rev Respir Dis* 119:293, 1979.

RESPIRATORY IMPAIRMENT FOR DISABILITY

Gaensler EM, Wright GW: Evaluation of respiratory impairment. *Arch Environ Health* 12:146, 1966.

Harber P, Schnur R, Emery J, et al: Statistical 'biases' in respiratory disability determinations. *Am Rev Respir Dis* 128:413, 1983.

Morgan WKC: Pulmonary disability and impairment: can't work? won't work? Basics of RD. *Am Thorac Soc* 10:No. 5, 1982.

Social Security Regulations: Rule for determining disability and blindness, US Dept of Health and Human Services, SSA Pub No. 64-014, 1981.

PULMONARY FUNCTION TESTING IN CHILDREN

England SJ: Current techniques for assessing pulmonary function in the newborn and infant: advantages and limitations. *Pediatr Pulmonol* 4:48, 1988.

Falliers CJ: Why test function in children routinely. *J Respir Dis* 3(1):37, 1982.

Hanrahan JP, Tager IB, Castile RG, et al: Pulmonary function measures in healthy infants: variability and size correction. *Am Rev Respir Dis* 141:1127, 1990.

Kanner RE, Schenker MB, Munoz A, et al: Spirometry in children: methodology for obtaining optimal results for clinical and epidemiologic studies. *Am Rev Respir Dis* 127:720, 1983.

LeSouef PN, Hughes DM, Landau LI: Shape of forced expiratory flow-volume curves in infants. *Am Rev Respir Dis* 138:590, 1988.

Morgan WJ, Geller DE, Tepper RS, et al: Partial expiratory flow-volume curves in infants and young children. *Pediatr Pulmonol* 5:232, 1988.

Polgar G, Promadhat V: Pulmonary function testing in children: techniques and standards. Philadelphia, 1971, WB Saunders.

Stocks J, Nothen U, Sutherland P, et al: Improved accuracy of the occlusion technique for measuring total respiratory compliance in infants. *Pediatr Pulmonol* 3:71, 1987.

Taussig LM: Standardization of lung function testing in children. *J Pediatr* 97:668, 1980.

Tepper RS, Pagtakhan RD, Taussig LM: Noninvasive determination of total respiratory compliance in infants by the weighted spirometer method. *Am Rev Respir Dis* 130:461, 1984.

Wall MA, Misley MC, Dickerson D: Partial expiratory flow-volume curves in young children. *Am Rev Respir Dis* 129:557, 1984.

CRITICAL CARE MONITORING

Fahey PJ, Harris K, Vanderwarf C: Clinical experience with continuous monitoring of mixed venous oxygen saturation in respiratory failure. *Chest* 86:748, 1984.

MacNaughton PD, Morgan CJ, Denison DM, et al: Pulmonary function testing in the intensive care unit. *Respir Med* 84:437, 1990.

Marini JJ: Monitoring during mechanical ventilation. *Clin Chest Med* 9:73, 1988.

Maunder RJ, Hudson LD: Respiratory monitoring in the intensive care unit. In Shoemaker WC, Abraham E, editors: *Diagnostic methods in critical care.* New York, 1987, Marcel Dekker.

Rebuck AS, Chapman KR: Measurement and monitoring of exhaled carbon dioxide. In Nochomovitz ML, Cherniack NS, editors: *Non-invasive respiratory monitoring.* New York, 1986, Churchill-Livingstone.

Taylor MB, Whitman JG: The current status of pulse oximetry: clinical value of continuous noninvasive oxygen saturation monitoring. *Anaesthesia* 41:943, 1986.

Tobin MJ: Respiratory monitoring in the intensive care unit. *Am Rev Respir Dis* 138:1625, 1988.

Tobin MJ, Perez W, Guenther SM, et al: The pattern of breathing during successful and unsuccessful trials of weaning from mechanical ventilation. *Am Rev Respir Dis* 134:1111, 1986.

Tremper KK, Waxman KS: Transcutaneous monitoring of respiratory gases. In Nochomovitz ML, Cherniack NS, editors: *Non-invasive respiratory monitoring.* New York, 1986, Churchill-Livingstone.

Yamanaka MK, Sue DY: Comparison of arterial-end-tidal P_{CO_2} difference and deadspace/tidal volume ratio in respiratory failure. *Chest* 92:832, 1987.

METABOLIC MEASUREMENTS (INDIRECT CALORIMETRY)

Askanazi J, Nordenstrom J, Rosenbaum SH, et al: Nutrition for the patient with respiratory failure: glucose vs fat. *Anesthesiology* 54:373, 1981.

Consolazio CF, Johnson RE, Pecora LJ: *Physiological measurements of metabolic functions in man.* New York, 1963, McGraw-Hill.

Feurer I, Mullen JL: Bedside measurement of resting energy expenditure and respiratory quotient via indirect calorimetry. *Nutr Clin Prac* 1:43, 1986.

Harris JA, Benedict FG: Biometric studies of basal metabolism in man. Carnegie Institute of Washington, Publication #279, 1919.

Weir JB: New methods for calculating metabolic rate with special reference to protein metabolism. *J Physiol* 109:1, 1949.

Weissman C, Damask MC, Askanazi J, et al: Evaluation of a non-invasive method for the measurement of metabolic rate in humans. *Clin Sci* 69:135, 1985.

Weissman C, Kemper M, Elwyn D, et al: The energy expenditure of the mechanically ventilated critically ill patient—an analysis. *Chest* 89:2, 1986.

9

Pulmonary Function
Testing Equipment

The forerunner of the modern spirometer was introduced by Hutchinson in the mid-19th century. Some signs of the original device are still evident in today's spirometers. Analysis of respiratory gases by volumetric methods was pioneered by Haldane in the early part of the 20th century. Modern gas analyzers utilize indirect means of assessing the partial pressures of gases. Many of the instruments in the pulmonary function laboratory today combine physical transducers, analog signal generators, and computerized representations of those signals. Some devices, such as the pulse oximeter, are based almost entirely on electronic components whose technology is less than 10 years old. The use of microcomputers (see Chapter 10) has eliminated many tedious calculations. Sophisticated data processing is available, even at the bedside.

This chapter generalizes the principles of some common pulmonary function equipment in relation to specific testing applications. Included are volume-displacement and flow-sensing spirometers, peak flow meters, gas analyzers, blood gas electrodes and oximeters, body plethysmographs, the respiratory inductive plethysmograph, breathing valves, and recording devices.

VOLUME-DISPLACEMENT SPIROMETERS

Water-Sealed Spirometers

For many years, the basic tool in the determination of lung volumes and flow rates was the water-sealed spirometer. The water-sealed spirometer consists of a large bell (7 to 10 L) suspended in a container of water with the open end of the bell below the surface of the water (Fig. 9–1). A system of breathing tubes into the interior of the bell allows for the accurate measurement of gas volumes. The subject breathes into the spirometer and in so doing moves the bell a

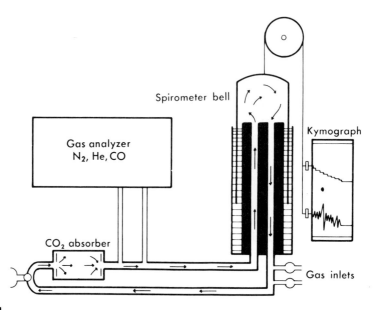

FIG 9–1.
Water-seal type spirometer. Typical water-seal spirometer apparatus based on bell counter-weighted with a pulley. Also included are a one-way breathing circuit with free breathing valve, CO_2 absorber, inlets for addition of gases, outlets for sampling by gas analyzers, and recording kymograph. (From Clinical spirometry, Warren E. Collins, Inc., Braintree, Mass.)

proportional distance. Each spirometer has a "bell factor" representing the vertical distance moved per unit of volume (milliliters or liters). The movement of the bell can be used to move a pen across a rotating drum or kymograph. By using paper that incorporates the bell factor for the spirometer, volumes can be measured directly from the kymograph tracing. The spirometer bell also can activate one of several types of potentiometers to produce an analog DC voltage signal. A potentiometer is a device that produces a variable voltage depending on its position, much like a dimmer switch connected to a light. The analog output provided by the potentiometer (in volts) is proportional to the movement of the bell. The analog signal can be used to drive a mechanical recorder, such as a strip-chart recorder. More commonly, however, the analog signal is digitized using an analog-to-digital (A/D) converter (see Chapter 10). The digitized signal from the spirometer then can be manipulated directly by computer.

For simple spirometry, a single large-bore tube carries both inspiratory and expiratory gases. For rebreathing studies, the breathing circuit incorporates a CO_2 absorber (soda lime), and separates inspiratory and expiratory circuits by means of one-way valves to eliminate dead space. Water-seal spirometers are typically used for spirometry. They also may be used for measurements of ventilation, including $\dot{V}_E$, V_T, and respiratory rate. In conjunction with an appropriate potentiometer and recording device, water-sealed spirometers can be used to record flow-volume curves. By including the rebreathing apparatus described previously, lung volumes by helium dilution can be obtained. In combination with an appropriate reservoir for the test gas, water-sealed spirometers can be used to perform diffusing capacity tests, both single breath and rebreathing. The water-sealed spirometer itself can be used as a reservoir for special gas mixtures such as those used for diffusing capacity tests or for helium-air flow-volume curves.

Two types of water-sealed spirometers, the *Collins* and the *Stead-Wells*, have been widely used. Only the Stead-Wells spirometer is in common use today. Although it is no longer used commonly, the Collins spirometer was the basic tool of pulmonary function testing for many years (see Fig. 9–1). This water-sealed spirometer was available in a variety of sizes. Older models featured a 9- or 13.5-L bell, and the later modular units were available with interchangeable 7- and 14-L bells. The spirometer employed a metal bell counterweighted by means of a pulley-and-chain assembly, which served to move two recording pens, and a variable speed kymograph (paper drum). One pen recorded respiratory excursions during inspiration as well as expiration, the other during inspiration only, thus tracing accumulated volumes such as $\dot{V}_E$ and MVV. The pen of the Collins spirometer moved in the opposite direction from the bell itself. When the bell rose during expiration, the pen moved downward. Many computerized spirometers still depict the expired volume tracing with downward deflection, mimicking the Collins tracing. The kymograph had rotational speeds of 32, 160, and 1920 mm/min. These speeds allowed various timed capacities such as the FEV_1 or MVV to be recorded using a single device. The Collins type water-sealed spirometer also was fitted with a rotary potentiometer on the pulley that supported the chain assembly. The potentiometer provided analog output signals for flow as well as volume.

The Stead-Wells type of water-sealed spirometer (Fig. 9–2) operates on principles similar to those described for the Collins spirometer. The Stead-Wells spirometer employs a lightweight plastic bell that is not counterweighted or supported by pulleys. The plastic bell "floats" in the water well, rising and falling with breathing excursions. The Stead-Wells spirometer carries a recording pen mounted against a variable speed (i.e., 32, 160, and 1920 mm/min) kymograph. However, unlike the Collins spirometer, respiratory excursions deflect the pen in the same direction as the bell. Expiration is traced upward on the volume-time graph (see Fig. 3–1). The Stead-Wells spirometer bell can also be directly attached to a linear potentiometer. The linear potentiometer provides analog signals proportional to volume and flow, allowing either analog recording or analog-digital conversion of the signals.

The primary advantages of the water-sealed spirometer are its simplicity and its accuracy. Because the spirometer bell can be used to drive a pen against the chart drum directly, direct mechanical tracings can be obtained. These tracings

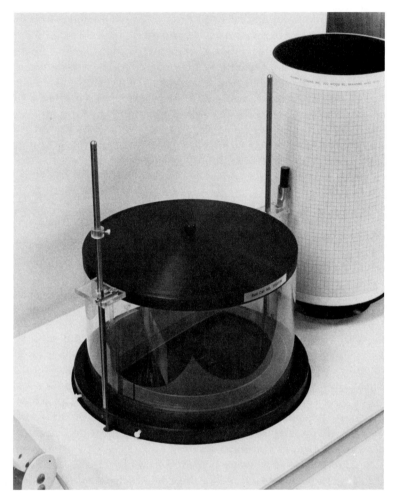

FIG 9–2.
Stead-Wells dry-seal spirometer. The conventional Stead-Wells spirometer uses a light weight plastic bell that is not counterweighted but floats in water. This version of the Stead-Wells uses a silicon seal similar to that found in the dry rolling-seal spirometer. The spirometer bell carries a pen that traces directly on a rotating kymograph. The bell also moves a linear potentiometer to generate analog signals for computerized measurements. With appropriate circuitry and gas analyzers, He dilution functional residual capacity determinations and $D_{L_{CO}}$ measurements are easily performed. (Courtesy of Warren E. Collins, Inc., Braintree, Mass.)

can be used for manual calculation of volumes and flows. The tracings also can be used for comparison with results derived by computer or from the analog recordings. Measurements of volumes and flows can be taken from the kymographic tracings if the bell factor and paper speed are known. The bell factor is simply the volume displacement per unit of vertical movement, usually expressed in milliliters per millimeter. Although most laboratories use computer-derived measurements, the capability to perform tests manually may be useful for quality assurance or for calibration.

A recent innovation combines the Stead-Wells concept with the principle of the dry rolling-seal spirometer (see next section). This combination produces a "waterless" spirometer (see Fig. 9–2), with other characteristics remaining basically unchanged. Eliminating water from the water-sealed design allows the device to be transported more easily. In addition, periodic draining is eliminated and cleaning of the spirometer is simplified.

The Collins water-sealed spirometer is no longer widely used for measuring FVC or flow parameters derived from that maneuver. The inertia of the counterweighted bell limits its ability to faithfully record the change in flows occurring during forced expiration, particularly in healthy subjects. The Stead-Wells design, however, is capable of meeting the minimum requirements for flow and volume accuracy as outlined by the American Thoracic Society (ATS) (see Chapter 11). For manual measurements from kymograph tracings, corrections from ATPS to BTPS are necessary.

The problems encountered with water-sealed spirometers usually arise from leaks in the bell or in the breathing circuit. Gravity causes the spirometer to lose volume in the presence of such leaks. Leaks in the spirometer, tubing, or valves can be detected by raising the bell and plugging the patient connection. By recording the spirometer volume over a period of several minutes, any change in volume can be easily detected. Weights can be added to the top of the bell to enhance detection of small leaks. Improper positioning of the spirometer, either too high or too low, can cause inaccurate measurements. If positioned too high, the bell can rise out of the water or reach the top of its travel range. This causes the volume-time tracing to become abruptly flattened. The pattern observed may be mistaken for a normal end of expiration. If the Stead-Wells spirometer is positioned too low, it may empty completely. This results in water being drawn into the breathing circuit, gas analyzer, or other system components. Inadequate water in the device also may lead to erroneous readings that are sometimes difficult to detect. The size of the water-sealed spirometer and the weight when it is filled with water make it somewhat difficult to transport. The waterless version of the spirometer eliminates the last two considerations.

Maintenance of water-sealed spirometers includes routine draining of the water well and checking for cracks or leaks in the bell itself. Chemical absorbers for water vapor must be routinely checked. Water absorbers are rapidly exhausted because the gas in the spirometer is almost completely saturated with water vapor. Cleaning of water-sealed spirometers typically involves replacing breathing hoses and mouthpieces after each subject. Although the subject's expired gas comes into direct contact with the water in the spirometer, cross contamination is not common. Some systems allow the use of low-resistance bacteria filters to protect those parts of the breathing circuit not changed after each use from contamination. Such filters should be used only for maneuvers that are not flow dependent. The volume of these filters may need to be taken into account when calculating system volume or system dead space.

Dry Rolling-Seal Spirometers

Another widely used volume-displacement spirometer is the dry rolling-seal spirometer. A typical unit consists of a lightweight piston mounted horizontally in a cylinder. The piston is supported by a rod that rests on frictionless bearings (Fig. 9–3). The piston is coupled to the cylinder wall by a flexible plastic seal. The seal rolls on itself rather than sliding as the piston moves. A similar type of rolling-seal also is used with a vertically mounted, lightweight piston that rises and falls with breathing. The maximum volume of the cylinder with the piston fully displaced is usually 10 to 12 L. The piston has a large diameter so that excursions of just a few inches are all that is necessary to record large volume changes. The piston is normally constructed of lightweight aluminum to reduce inertia. Mechanical resistance is kept to a minimum by the bearings supporting the piston rod, and by the rolling seal itself.

Some dry rolling-seal spirometers employ a mechanically driven graphing device in which the piston rod has a pen attached. The pen moves across graph

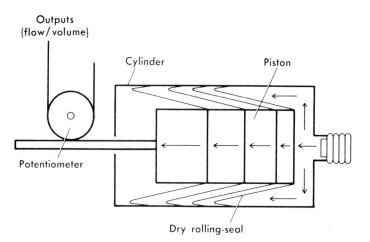

FIG 9–3.
Cutaway view of the main components of a dry rolling-seal spirometer. The figure gives an exaggerated view of the rolling-seal, which actually fits closely between the piston and cylinder wall. The piston has a large surface area so that its horizontal movement is minimized. This allows recording of normal breaths and maximal respiratory excursions with only a small amount of mechanical movement, and thus little resistance. The piston is supported by a rod that activates a rotary potentiometer. The rotational movement of the potentiometer is translated into analog signals for both flow and volume. Alternately, the rod may carry the recording pen across moving graph paper for direct tracing of volume-time curves. (From Form 370, Ohio Medical Products, Madison, Wisc.)

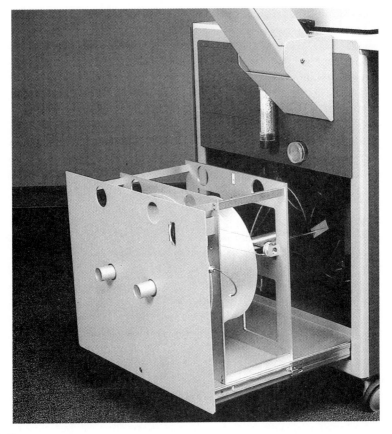

FIG 9–4.
Dry rolling-seal spirometer. A typical dry-seal spirometer consisting of a large aluminum piston mounted in a cylinder, with two ports to accommodate simple spirometry, as well as rebreathing maneuvers with a CO_2 absorber (see Fig. 9–3). (Courtesy of Gould Medical Instruments, Inc., Dayton, Ohio.)

paper or a strip chart recorder as the subject inspires and expires. Most dry rolling-seal spirometers, however, utilize a linear or rotary potentiometer. The potentiometer responds to the movement of the piston to produce a DC voltage output for volume and flow. A typical system might employ a 10 volt potentiometer attached to a 10 L spirometer with an output of 1 volt/L. On the flow channel, a flow of 1 L/sec might produce an output of 1 volt. These analog outputs for volume and flow are usually directed to an analog-to-digital converter (see Chapter 10) so that the data can be stored by computer. The piston of the standard dry rolling-seal spirometer (Fig. 9–4) travels horizontally, eliminating the need for counterbalancing. The vertically mounted spirometer depends on the lightweight piston and the rolling seal to reduce resistance to breathing. Temperature corrections (i.e., from ATPS to BTPS) are made either by adjusting the analog signal or by modifying the digital value stored in the computer. One-way circuits and CO_2 scrubbers can be added to the inlets of the device so that dry rolling-seal spirometers can be used for rebreathing tests in the same way as water-sealed spirometers. In order to perform studies in which gas volumes larger than the spirometer itself are measured, such as the open-circuit nitrogen washout, a "dumping" mechanism is attached to the spirometer. The dumping device empties the spirometer after each breath or after a predetermined volume has been reached. Addition of an automated valve and sampling device allows the dry rolling-seal spirometer to be used for single-breath diffusion studies. Dry rolling-seal spirometers are typically capable of meeting the minimum standards of accuracy for volume and flow set by the ATS (see Chapter 11).

As with most volume displacement–type spirometers, the dry rolling-seal spirometer can be used for manual or computerized testing. Manual testing, using a mechanical recorder, may be used for bedside or screening tests. Despite their large size, most dry rolling-seal spirometers can be transported rather easily. However, the addition of a computer, gas analyzers, or recorder may make the system too bulky for bedside testing. Common problems encountered with dry rolling-seal spirometers are sticking of the rolling-seal and increased mechanical resistance in the piston-cylinder assembly. These difficulties usually can be avoided by adequate maintenance of the spirometer. Cleaning of the dry rolling-seal involves disassembling the piston-cylinder. The interior of the cylinder and the face of the piston are usually wiped with a mild antibacterial solution. The rolling-seal itself also is wiped with disinfectant. Alcohol or similar drying agents may cause deterioration of the seal and should not be used. The seal may be lubricated with corn starch to prevent sticking, but care must be taken to avoid leaving excessive powder in the spirometer. The seal should be checked routinely for leaks or tears. After reassembly, the piston should be positioned at the maximum volume position. When the rolling-seal is completely extended, the material of the seal is less likely to develop creases that can result in uneven movement of the piston.

Bellows-Type Spirometers

A third type of volume-displacement spirometer is the bellows or wedge bellows. Both of these devices consist of collapsible bellows that fold or unfold in response to breathing excursions. The conventional bellows design is a flexible accordion-type container. One end is stationary while the other end is displaced in proportion to the volume inspired or expired. The wedge bellows operates similarly, except it expands and contracts like a fan (Fig. 9–5). One side of the bellows remains stationary, the other side moves with a pivotal motion around an axis through the fixed side. Displacement of the bellows by a volume

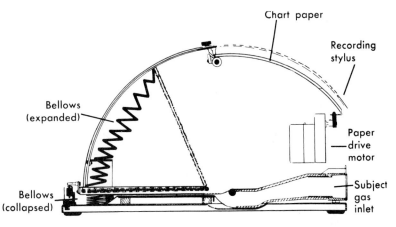

FIG 9–5.
Cross-sectional diagram of a wedge-bellows type of spirometer. The fan-like movements of the wedge bellows produce mechanical movement, which is usually translated directly to a recording device. Some manufacturers suspend the bellows so that the primary movement is in a horizontal rather than vertical direction. Large wedge bellows offer little mechanical resistance and are comparable to dry-seal or water-seal spirometers in accuracy and linearity. (Modified from Vitalograph Medical Instrumentation, Product Brochure, Lenexa, Kan.)

of gas is translated either to movement of a mechanical recording device or to a potentiometer. For mechanical recording, chart paper moves at a fixed speed under the pen while a spirogram is traced. For computerized testing, displacement of the bellows is transformed into a DC voltage by a linear or rotating potentiometer. The analog signal is routed to an A/D converter.

The conventional and wedge bellows may be mounted either horizontally or vertically. Horizontal bellows are mounted so that the primary direction of travel is on a horizontal plane. This design minimizes the effects of gravity on bellows movement. Horizontal bellows, either conventional or wedge, with a large surface area offer little mechanical resistance. This type of bellows is normally used in conjunction with a potentiometer to produce analog volume and flow signals. Several types of small (i.e., approximately 7 L), vertically mounted bellows are currently available and are used widely for portable spirometry and bedside testing. Most of these offer simple mechanical recording and/or digital data reduction by means of a small dedicated microprocessor.

Both types of bellows (Fig. 9–6, A and B) are suitable for measurement of the VC and its subdivisions, as well as the FVC, FEV_1, expiratory flow rates, and the MVV. Some bellows-type spirometers, especially those that are mounted vertically, are designed specifically for measurement of expiratory flows. These types expand upward when gas is injected, then empty spontaneously under their own weight. Horizontally mounted bellows usually can be set in a mid-range to record both inspiratory and expiratory maneuvers such as the

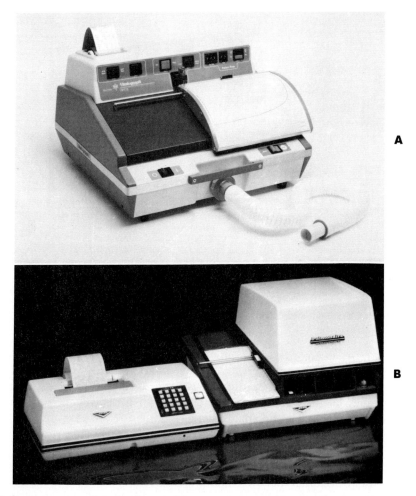

FIG 9–6.
Two types of bellows spirometers. **A,** a wedge-bellows spirometer with direct writing recorder, digital displays, and built-in printer for automated data reduction. (Courtesy of Vitalograph Medical Instrumentation, Lenexa, Kan.) **B,** a conventional bellows-type spirometer, with the bellows mounted horizontally and driving a pen across moving graph paper. A potentiometer allows analog output to a dedicated microprocessor with built-in printer for automatic data reduction. (Courtesy of Jones Medical Instrument Co., Oakbrook, Ill.)

flow-volume loop. In conjunction with the appropriate gas analyzers and breathing circuitry, bellows systems may be used for lung volume determinations and $D_{L_{CO}}$ measurements. Most bellows-type spirometers meet the ATS minimum requirements for flow and volume accuracy.

A problem that can occur with bellows spirometers is inaccuracy resulting from sticking of the bellows. The folds of the bellows may adhere because of dirt or moisture or aging of the bellows material. Some bellows-type spirometers require the bellows to be partially distended when not in use. This technique allows moisture from exhaled gas to evaporate and prevents deterioration of the bellows. Leaks also may develop in the bellows material or at the point where the bellows is mounted. Leaks usually can be detected by filling the bellows with air, plugging the breathing port, and attaching a weight or spring to pressurize the gas inside. Cleaning bellows-type spirometers depends on their construction. With some instruments, the bellows can be entirely removed, while with others, the interior of the bellows must be wiped clean. Many bellows are made from rubberized or plastic-based material that can be cleaned with a mild detergent and dried thoroughly before reassembly.

Flow-Sensing Spirometers

In contrast to the volume-displacement spirometers described above is the flow-sensing spirometer, or pneumotachometer. The term *pneumotachometer* describes a device that measures flow. Flow-sensing spirometers use various physical principles to produce a signal proportional to gas flow. This signal is then integrated to allow measurement of volumes in addition to flow. Integration is a process in which flow (i.e., volume per unit of time) is divided into a large number of small intervals (i.e., time) and the volume from each interval summed (Fig. 9–7). Integration can be performed quite easily by an electronic circuit. Accurate determination of volumes by integration of flow requires accurate flow signals, accurate timing, and sensitive detection of low flows. One type of device that responds to bulk flow of gas is the turbine or impeller. Integration is unnecessary because the turbine flow device directly measures gas volumes. Some flow-sensing spirometers produce volume pulses, in which each "pulse" equals a fixed volume. These spirometers incorporate very accurate counters to count the pulses. The remaining types of flow-sensing spirometers all use tubes through which laminar air flow is possible (see Useful Equations in Appendix). Although a wide variety of flow-sensing spirometers is presently available, four basic designs are commonly used: turbines, pressure differential, heated wire, and ultrasonic flow sensors.

Turbines. The simplest type of flow-sensing device is the turbine or respirometer. This instrument consists of a vane connected to a series of precision gears. Gas molecules flowing through the body of the instrument rotate the vane which registers a volume (Fig. 9–8). The respirometer can be used for measurement of the VC. It also can be used for ventilation tests such as V_T and $\dot{V}_E$. One typical device, the Wright respirometer, can be used to measure volumes at flows between approximately 3 and 300 L/min. At flows above 300 L/min, the vane is subject to distortion. Because of this limitation, it should not be used to

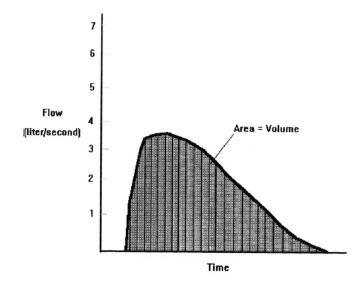

FIG 9–7.
Volume measurement by flow integration. The flow signal from many types of flow-sensing spirometers is integrated to compute volume. Flow is measured against time. The area under the flow-time curve is subdivided into a large number of small sections *(rectangles)*. Volume is the sum of the areas of all the rectangular sections. By dividing the curve into a large number of sections, even irregular flow curves can be accurately integrated. Integration is usually performed by a dedicated electronic circuit.

measure FVC when the subject is capable of flows greater than 300 L/min (i.e., 5 L/sec). At flows less than 3 L/min (i.e., 0.05 L/sec) the inertia of the vane-gear system may cause erroneous measurements. The special advantages of the respirometer are its compact size and usefulness at the bedside. Most respirometers register a wide range of volumes, from 0.1 to 1 L on one scale and up to 100 L on another scale. Turbine devices also are widely used for bulk measurements in various dry gas meters.

An adaptation of the turbine flow device includes a photo cell and light source that is interrupted by the movement of the vane or impeller. A pulsing of the light beam is caused by the interruption of the rotating vane, with each of the pulses equivalent to a fixed gas volume. The pulse count is summed and is proportional to the volume of gas flowing through the tube. The signal produced may not be linear at high or low flows because of inertia or distortion of the rotating vane.

Pressure-differential flow sensors.   The most common type of flow-sensing device consists of a tube containing a resistive element. The resistive element allows gas to flow through it, but causes a pressure drop. The pressure difference across the resistive element is measured by means of a sensitive pressure transducer, with pressure taps on either side of the element. The pressure differential across the resistive element is proportional to the flow of gas as long as the gas flow is laminar (Fig. 9–9, A). The flow signal from the pneumotachometer is electronically integrated to derive volume measurements. Turbulent gas flow either upstream or downstream of the resistive element may interfere with the development of true laminar flow. Most pneumotachometers attempt to reduce turbulent flow by tapering the tubes in which the resistive elements are mounted.

Two types of resistive elements are commonly employed. The Fleisch-type pneumotachometer uses a bundle of capillary tubes as the resistive element. Laminar flow is generally assured by size and arrangement of the capillary tubes. The cross-sectional area and length of the capillary tubes determines the actual resistance to flow through the Fleisch pneumotachometer. The dynamic range of the Fleisch device must be matched to the range of flows to be measured. Different sizes (i.e., resistances) of pneumotachometers may be used to accurately measure high or low flows.

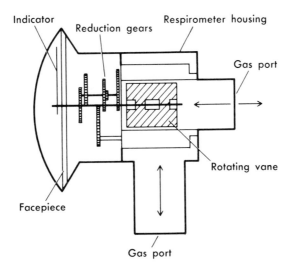

FIG 9–8.
Turbine-type flow sensor. A cutaway diagram of the Wright respirometer. A large rotating vane mounted on jeweled bearings drives reduction gears connected to the main indicator arm. Two gas ports allow flow through the body for measurements of volume. Although the vane turns in only one direction, gas can either be inspired through the respirometer, or expired into it. Not pictured is a small indicator arm that marks volumes larger than 1 L on the face so that accumulated volumes can be measured. The instrument also features controls for engaging or disengaging the vane and for resetting the indicators to zero. (From the British Oxygen Co., Ltd. Operating Instructions, Wright Respirometer, print No. 630207, Issue 3:6, August 1971).

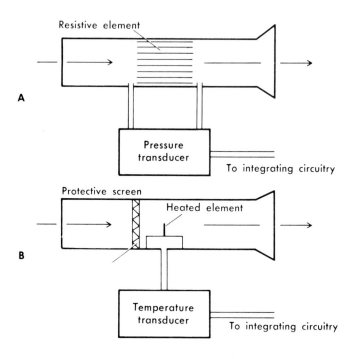

FIG 9–9.
Two common flow-sensing devices (pneumotachometers). **A,** pressure-differential type of pneumotachometer in which a resistive element causes a pressure drop proportional to the flow of gas through the tube. A sensitive pressure transducer monitors the pressure drop across the resistive element and converts the differential into a signal that varies as the flow changes. The volume passing through the pneumotachometer can be calculated by integrating the flow over the time interval during which the flow occurred. The resistive element may be a mesh screen or capillary tubes. The resistive element is usually heated to 37°C or higher to prevent condensation of water from expired gas. **B,** a heated-wire type of pneumotachometer in which a heated element of small mass responds to gas flow by heat loss. An electrical current heats the element. Gas flow past the element causes cooling. A greater current is needed to maintain a constant temperature. The current change is proportional to gas flow, and a continuous signal is supplied to an integrating circuit as for the pressure differential flow sensor.

The other common variety of the pressure-differential flow sensor is the Silverman, or Lilly, type. The Silverman pneumotachometer uses one or more screens to act as a resistive element. A typical arrangement has three screens mounted parallel to one another. The middle screen acts as the resistive element with the pressure taps on either side, while the outer screens protect the middle screen and help to assure laminar flow. The Silverman pneumotachometer has a somewhat wider dynamic flow range than the Fleisch type, making it better suited to measuring varying flows and volumes. Most Fleisch and Silverman pneumotachometers employ a heating mechanism to warm the resistive element to 37°C or higher. Heating the resistive element prevents accumulation of moisture from exhaled gas on the element. Condensation, or other debris, lodging in the resistive element changes the resistance across it and changes the calibration of the device.

Some spirometers utilize other types of resistive elements, such as porous paper, so that the flow sensor itself is disposable. Typically, these devices have a single pressure tap upstream of the resistive element and the pressure in front of the resistive element is referenced against ambient pressure. The accuracy of these types of spirometers is often dependent on how carefully the disposable resistive elements are manufactured. If the resistance varies widely from sensor to sensor, accurate measurement of flows or volumes requires individual calibration of each unit.

Heated-wire flow sensors.   A third commonly used type of flow-sensing spirometer is based on the cooling effect of gas flow. A heated element, usually a platinum wire or small bead of metal called a thermistor, is situated in a laminar flow tube (Figs. 9–9,B and 9–10). Gas flow past the element causes a temperature drop, so more current must be supplied to maintain the preset

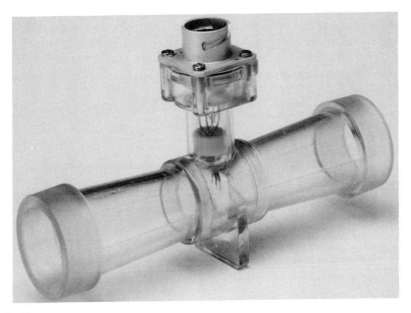

FIG 9–10.
A heated-wire type of flow sensor. A tube contains very thin, paired stainless steel wires. The wires are maintained at two different temperatures exceeding body temperature connected by a Wheatstone bridge. The tube streamlines gas flow into laminar flow. The temperature of the wires decreases in proportion to the mass of the gas and its flow. Two wires are used, one measuring flow and the other serving as a reference. (Courtesy of SensorMedics, Corp., Yorba Linda, Calif.)

temperature of the element. The amount of current needed to maintain the temperature is proportional to the magnitude of the gas flow. The heated element usually has a small mass so that very slight changes in gas flow can be detected. The flow signal is integrated electronically to derive volume measurements. The heated element is usually protected behind a screen to prevent impaction of debris on the element. Debris or moisture droplets on the element can change its thermal characteristics. Some systems employ two matched thermistors. One measures gas flow while the second serves as a reference. Most thermistor-type flow sensors have their elements heated to a temperature in excess of 37°C so that condensation does not interfere with sensitivity of the element.

   Ultrasonic flow sensors.   A fourth type of flow-sensing spirometer is designed to utilize the principle of vortex shedding. A flow tube is constructed with struts placed in the airstream. Gas flowing over the struts is broken up into waves called vortices. An ultrasonic crystal downstream of the strut transmits high-frequency sound waves through the turbulent gas flow to a receiving crystal on the opposite side of the tube (Fig. 9–11). The size of the strut and flow tube determine the size of the vortices. This allows the device to be calibrated so that each vortex passing through the ultrasonic beam produces a pulse. Each pulse is proportional to specific volume, for example, 1 mL/pulse. The pulses are counted and summed electronically, providing a measurement of volume. The ultrasonic flow-sensing spirometer is relatively insensitive to gas temperature or humidity, although accumulation of moisture on the struts or ultrasonic

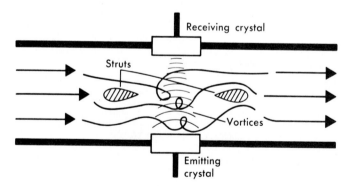

FIG 9–11.

Ultrasonic flow sensor. A beam of ultrasonic waves is emitted by one crystal and received by another crystal on the opposite side of the flow tube. Gas flowing in streamline passes over struts in the tube and forms vortexes. This is called *vortex shedding*, and changes the frequency of the transmitted ultrasound waves in proportion to the volume of gas forming the vortexes. Each vortex causes a "pulse." The pulses are summed electronically to obtain volume measurements. Volume can be measured for gas moving in either direction.

transducers can cause erroneous readings. The crystals are usually heated to prevent condensation.

Pulmonary function testing with the flow-sensing spirometer offers some advantages over volume-displacement spirometry systems. When combined with appropriate gas analyzers and breathing circuits, flow-sensing spirometers can be used to perform lung volume determinations by the open- or closed-circuit methods. Diffusing capacity can be measured with flow-sensing spirometers as well. Pressure differential pneumotachometers are widely utilized for measurement of flows and volumes in body plethysmographs, exercise testing systems, and metabolic carts. Because of their small size, flow-sensing devices are often incorporated into spirometers designed for portability. Because most of the sensors described require electronic circuitry for integration of the flow signal or summing of volume pulses, flow-based spirometers are usually microprocessor controlled. Some flow-sensing spirometers permit direct connection of the analog signal (flow, volume, or both) to a strip chart or X-Y recorder. However, most flow-sensors utilize computer-generated graphics to produce volume-time or flow-volume tracings.

Many flow-sensing spirometers have been designed to interface directly with small personal computers (Fig. 9–12, A and B). These devices incorporate an A/D converter that plugs directly into the user's personal computer. By installing the appropriate software, spirometry can be performed. Some of these devices contain the electronic hardware in the flow-sensor head. This implementation allows the sensor to be connected to a serial port, which is standard on most small computers. Direct interface to a small computer allows users to define the system according to their individual needs. Laptop or portable computers can be used to provide powerful spirometry systems in very small packages.

Most flow sensors can be easily cleaned and disinfected. Some sensors can be immersed in a disinfectant without disassembly. As noted previously, many systems use inexpensive, disposable sensors based on the pressure-differential type, which can be discarded after a single patient use. The use of filters to prevent contamination of flow-based spirometers may result in changes in the operating characteristics of the spirometer. This is particularly true if the filter increases resistance because of contamination with moisture.

There are some disadvantages associated with flow-sensing spirometers. Most of the flow sensors described operate on the premise that a given flow will generate a proportional signal. However, at extremes of flow, either low or high, the signal generated may not be proportional (i.e., not linear). Almost every type of flow-sensing device displays some nonlinearity. Some systems use two separate flow sensors, one for high flows as in the FVC and another for lower flows as in V_T excursions. Better accuracy is obtained for flows and volumes by reducing the range of the flow sensor to match the physiologic signal. Most flow-based spirometers "linearize" the flow signal electronically or by means of software corrections. In many systems, a flow "table" is stored in the computer.

A

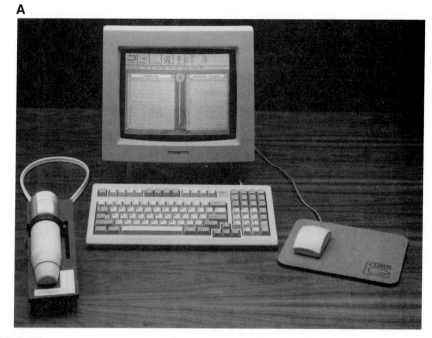

FIG 9–12.
Flow-sensing spirometers interfaced to personal computers. **A,** a flow-based spirometer consisting of a pressure-differential pneumotachometer. The pneumotachometer plugs into an interface card located in the PC. PC-based software is then used to perform and record spirometry. The pneumotachometer–interface card combination may be used with any compatible personal computer. (Courtesy of Vitalograph, Lenexa, Kan.)

As long as the flow table matches the flow sensor in use, flows across a wide range can be accurately measured. The flow or derived volume is typically corrected before any parameters are measured so that the values will be accurate within acceptable limits.

Turbines, pressure-differential, and heated-wire flow-sensing spirometers may be particularly affected by the composition of the gas being measured. Changes in gas density or viscosity most often require special corrections to the output of the transducer in order to obtain accurate volumes. In most systems, these corrections are performed by computer software using a stored table. A flow-sensing spirometer may be calibrated with air, but then used to analyze mixtures containing helium, neon, oxygen, or other test gases, provided that the software is designed to correct for differences in gas composition for each individual test.

Results from any measurement done with a flow-sensing spirometer depend on the electronic circuitry that converts the raw signal into an actual volume or flow. Pulmonary function parameters measured on a time base, such as FEV_T or MVV, require precise timing mechanisms as well as accurate flow measurements. The timing mechanism in flow-based spirometers is critical in the detection of the start or end of the test. Timing is usually triggered by a minimum flow or pressure change. Integration of flow signal begins when the flow through the spirometer reaches a threshold limit, usually around 0.1 to 0.2 L/sec. Instruments that initiate timing in response to volume pulses usually have a similar threshold that must be achieved to begin recording the input signal. Contamination of resistive elements, thermistors, or turbine vanes by moisture or other debris can alter the flow-sensing characteristics of the transducer and interfere with the spirometer's ability to detect the start or end of the test.

Problems related to electronic "drift" often require flow-sensors to be calibrated frequently. Many systems "zero" the flow signal immediately before a measurement. Zeroing corrects for much of the electronic drift that occurs. A true zero requires no flow through the flow-sensor. Most systems utilize a 3-L syringe for calibration. By calibrating with a known volume signal, the accuracy of the flow-sensor and the integrator can be checked with one input. Calibration

B

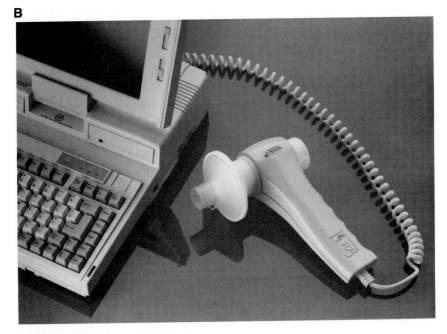

FIG 9-12–cont'd.
B, a flow-based spirometer in which the interface electronics are mounted in the handle of the pneumotachometer. A cable connects to the serial port of the PC. This type of device is useful for performing spirometry with a laptop or portable computer, which may not accept a full-size interface card. (Courtesy of Pulmonary Data Services, Louisville, Colo.)

and quality control techniques for volume-displacement and flow-sensing spirometers are included in Chapter 11.

Peak Flow Meters

Peak expiratory flow (PEF) can be measured easily with most types of spirometers, either volume-displacement or flow-sensing types. Several devices are available that measure PEF exclusively. The PEF has become a recognized means of monitoring patients who have asthma (see Chapter 3). By incorporating a simple design into an inexpensive package, portable peak flow meters allow monitoring of airway status in a variety of settings.

Most of the peak flow meters available utilize similar designs. The subject expires forcefully through a resistor that has a movable scale attached. The resistance in most devices is provided by an orifice. The movable scale is deflected in proportion to the velocity of air flowing through the device. The PEF is then read directly from the scale indicator (Fig. 9–13, A and B). Because these devices are nonlinear, different flow ranges are usually available. High-range peak flow meters typically measure flows as high as 600 to 800 L/min. Low-range meters measure up to 300 or 400 L/min. Low-range peak flow meters are useful for small children or for subjects who have marked obstruction.

The absolute accuracy of portable peak flow meters is less of a concern than proper use by the subject. These devices are intended to provide serial measurements of peak flow as a guide to treatment. Subjects who are carefully instructed should be able to reproduce their peak flow measurements within 10%. Although their simple design allows them to be used repeatedly, moisture or other debris can cause sticking of the movable indicator. Some instruments can be cleaned, but may require periodic replacement.

Breathing Valves

Several types of valves are commonly used with both volume-displacement and flow-sensing spirometers. These valves direct inspired and expired gas through the measuring transducer as well as provide sampling for gas analysis.

Free breathing valves. The simplest type of valve is that which allows the subject to be switched from breathing room air to breathing gas contained in a spirometer or special breathing circuit. Free breathing valves are routinely employed in both the open- and closed-circuit methods of FRC determination. The free breathing valve is designed so that the subject can be "switched in" to the system either manually or by computer control at any point in the breathing cycle. The typical free breathing valve consists of a body with two or more ports. A drum in the valve body rotates to connect different combinations of ports.

Because these types of valves are used mainly for tidal breathing or slow VC maneuvers, resistance to flow is not critical. Most have ports with diameters of 1.5 to 3 cm. For studies involving gas analysis, such as the FRC determination, the valve must be leak free.

Directional (one-way, two-way) valves. Directional valves are used in many types of breathing circuits to assure gas flow either to the subject or to the measuring device. The simplest type consists of a flap or diaphragm that opens in only one direction. The diaphragm is mounted in a rigid tube that can be

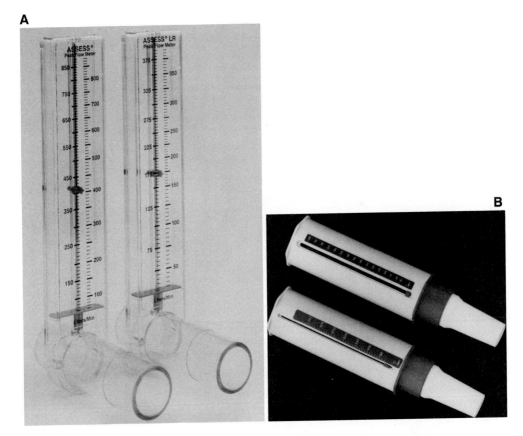

FIG 9–13.
Portable peak flow meters. **A,** portable peak flow meters for measuring peak expiratory flow outside of the pulmonary function laboratory. The subject exhales forcefully through the mouthpiece at the bottom. Pressure generated by the flow of gas deflects the movable indicator up the scale. Two flow ranges are available, for normal and reduced peak flows (Courtesy HealthScan Products Inc., Cedar Grove, NJ). **B,** portable peak flow meters in which exhaled flow is directed against a movable indicator. Separate flow ranges are provided. (Courtesy of Clement Clarke Inc., Columbus, Ohio.)

inserted in a breathing circuit. Because gas is only permitted to flow in one direction, these valves are referred to as one-way valves.

A more common design is that used to separate inspired from expired gas, often referred to as a two-way nonrebreathing valve. This type of directional valve consists of a T-shaped body with three ports and two separate diaphragms (Fig. 9–14). The diaphragms allow gas to flow in only one direction with the subject connection between the diaphragms, effectively separating inspired and expired gas. These types of devices are commonly used in exercise testing, metabolic studies, or any procedure requiring collection, measurement, or analysis of exhaled gas. The valve body may contain a tap for connection of gas-sample tubing. This tap typically is placed between the diaphragms so that both inspired and expired gas can be sampled.

Two variables must be considered in the selection of appropriate directional valves: dead space volume and flow resistance. In one-way valves, only flow

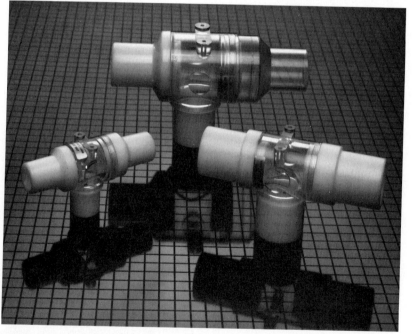

FIG 9–14.
Two-way breathing valves. Three different sizes of two-way valves as employed for studies involving collection or measurement of expired gas. Each valve consists of a T-shaped body that contains two diaphragms that separate inspired and expired gas. The smaller valves have less dead space but higher flow resistance, while the large valve has low flow resistance but more dead space. The small- and medium-sized valves are used for studies in which low flows are encountered, such as metabolic measurements. The large valve is appropriate for high flow rates such as those occurring during maximal exercise testing. (Courtesy of Hans Rudolph Inc., Kansas City, MO)

resistance is a concern. In the gas-collection type of valve just described, the dead space consists of the volume contained between the two diaphragms along with the volume of any connectors (i.e., mouthpiece). Most manufacturers supply information on the dead space of particular valves and some have the value printed on the valve body. Unknown dead space usually can be readily determined by blocking two of the three ports and measuring the water volume required to fill the dead space portion of the valve.

Low–dead space valves (i.e., less than 50 mL) are required for studies in which the subject's ventilatory status is already compromised, particularly if only tidal breathing is being assessed. Valves with larger dead space volumes may be required to accommodate large-bore ports and low-resistance diaphragms. The valves used during exercise testing to minimize resistance at high flow rates typically have a large dead space volume. The valve dead space should be accurately determined in order to incorporate corrections in calculations involving gas analysis, such as physiologic dead space measurements.

Low-resistance to flow is also a critical characteristic of directional valves, whether they are one-way or two-way valves. Resistance to flow through most valves is nonlinear and dependent on the cross sectional area of the valve leaflets or diaphragms (Fig. 9–15). Flow resistance is usually not critical in applications during which flows less than 1 L/sec are developed. Small-bore directional valves can be selected on the basis of an appropriate dead space volume. Most small-bore nonrebreathing valves have resistances in the range of 1 to 2 cm H_2O/L/sec at flows up to 1 L/sec (60 L/min). If the subject breathes through the valve for long intervals, even small resistances may result in respiratory muscle fatigue and changes in the ventilatory pattern. Applications such as exercise testing typically involve increased flow rates. Large-bore two-way valves are indicated in most situations when the subject can be anticipated to develop flows in excess of 1 L/sec (60 L/min). Pressures of less than 3 cm H_2O can be maintained, even at flows of 5 L/sec (300 L/min) with large-bore valves. Even appropriately selected valves can cause increased flow resistance if not properly maintained. Rubber, plastic, or silicon leaflets and diaphragms can all stick or become rigid with age. Valves should be disassembled and cleaned according to the manufacturers' directions after each use and allowed to dry thoroughly before reassembly. Care must be taken when reassembling valves to make sure that all diaphragms are oriented properly. Valves should be visually inspected to make sure diaphragms are seated correctly before being used.

Gas sampling valves. Specialized valves are used to obtain gas samples during procedures such as the single-breath $D_{L_{CO}}$ or CO_2 rebreathing cardiac output. Most gas-sampling valves utilize electrically activated solenoids to rapidly change the direction of gas flow to a spirometer or sample bag. Some devices employ pneumatically powered slide valves that can be triggered manually or by a DC voltage. The primary concern with gas-sampling valves is smooth operation

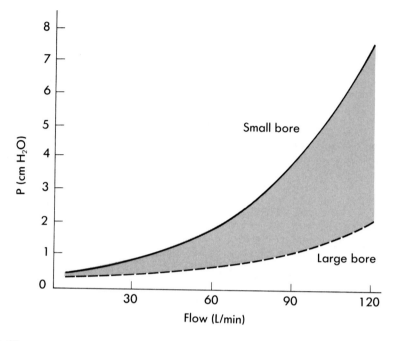

FIG 9–15.
Breathing valve resistance. A graph plotting pressure developed across two different size valves in relation to gas flow through them. For small-bore valves (see Fig. 9–14), pressures less than 1 cm H_2O are generated up to approximately 60 L/min (1 L/sec). Large-bore valves have less resistance (i.e., pressure per unit of flow) and are typically used for studies in which the subject develops high flow rates. Other factors affecting resistance include the design and material used for the diaphragms in the valve and whether the diaphragms move freely. Resistance increases nonlinearly in all types of valves and high resistance can occur even in large-bore valves if extremely high flow rates are attained.

with appropriate direction of the gas to be sampled. Electrically activated solenoids may deteriorate with age, particularly if exposed to high humidity conditions such as expired air. Replacement of O-rings or similar types of seals may be necessary to ensure uncontaminated gas samples. Some sampling valves employ balloons that inflate under high pressure to block or direct the flow of gas. These balloons require periodic replacement, as a small leak in a balloon can prevent the balloon from "seating." As a result gas may not be directed to the appropriate device.

PULMONARY GAS ANALYZERS

The types of gas analyzers used in pulmonary function testing are determined by the gases commonly analyzed. Oxygen and CO_2 are analyzed as part of patient monitoring, as well as during metabolic studies and exercise testing. Helium analysis is widely employed for closed-circuit FRC determinations and for several types of $D_{L_{CO}}$ tests. Nitrogen analysis is used in the open-circuit FRC method. Carbon monoxide measurements are integral to all of the diffusion capacity methods currently used. Analyses of neon, argon, methane, and acetylene are utilized in specialized tests for diffusion, lung volume measurements, and cardiac output determination.

Table 9–1 lists some of the types of O_2 analyzers available. Most of these are suitable for monitoring patients. Three types are used for rapid analysis of O_2: the polarographic electrode, zirconium fuel cell, and mass spectrometer. How rapidly a gas analyzer can detect and display a change in gas concentration is called the response time. Response time is commonly measured in seconds or milliseconds (thousandths of a second). Manufacturers of gas analyzers list response time as the interval required for an analyzer to measure some fraction of a step change in gas concentration. For example, an O_2 analyzer might require 2 seconds to respond to an increase in O_2 concentration from 21% to 100%. The response time would be listed as the time required for 90% of the total change to be detected. Response time of an analyzer often depends on the size of the change in gas concentration. Another important factor is transport time. Transport time is how long it takes to move the gas from the sample site to the analyzer itself. How rapidly a gas, such as O_2, can be analyzed depends on both the response time and the transport time of the instrument.

TABLE 9–1.

Oxygen Analyzers

Type	Applications	Advantages/Disadvantages
Paramagnetic	Monitoring	Discrete sampling only
Polarographic electrode	Monitoring, exercise testing, metabolic studies	Discrete or continuous sampling; requires special electronics for fast response (200 msec)
Galvanic cell (fuel cell)	Monitoring	Continuous sampling; similar to polarographic but does not require polarizing voltage
Zirconium cell	Breath-by-breath exercise and metabolic studies	Heated (700 to 800° C) fuel cell; fast response useful for continuous sampling; thermal stabilization required
Gas chromatograph	Exercise testing, monitoring, metabolic measurements	Discrete sampling; response time $\approx$ 30 seconds; very accurate; multiple gas analysis
Mass spectrometer	Breath-by-breath exercise and metabolic studies, multiple patient monitoring	Discrete or continuous sampling, fast response ($<$ 100 msec); multiple gas analysis; large and complex instrumentation

Polarographic Electrodes

The polarographic electrode is very similar to the blood gas O_2 electrode (see Blood Gas Electrodes section, this chapter). For routine gas analysis, the platinum cathode is not covered with a membrane. A pump draws the sample gas past the polarized electrode at a constant flow. By using special electronic circuitry, a response time of approximately 200 msec can be attained, and continuous analysis of oxygen is possible. Contamination of the electrode can degrade its response time and cause difficulty with calibration.

Zirconium Fuel Cells

An electrode is formed by coating a zirconium element with platinum. The zirconium, when heated to 700 to 800°C acts as a solid electrolyte between the platinum coating on either side. When the two sides of the electrode are exposed to differing partial pressures of O_2, the gas traverses the electrode, creating a voltage proportional to the difference in concentrations. The gas to be sampled is usually drawn past the element at a constant low flow. This allows rapid, continuous analysis without altering the temperature of the electrode. The electrode temperature must be held constant, so the electrode requires adequate insulation. A warm-up period of 10 to 30 minutes is typically required to reach thermal equilibrium at the elevated temperature. Response times of less than 200 msec are possible with the zirconium fuel cell. Both the zirconium fuel cell and the polarographic electrode measure partial pressure of oxygen. Changes in the pressure in the sampling circuit can affect the concentration measurement. Such pressure changes can be caused by gas flow in a breathing circuit, or by positive pressure in a mechanical ventilator circuit. The presence of water vapor in the sample affects both of these electrodes similarly (see Gas Conditioning Devices in this section). Oxygen concentration is measured accurately but is diluted in proportion to the water vapor pressure present in the sample.

Zirconium fuel cells eventually degrade in relation to the volume of O_2 analyzed. The cell may be refreshed by passing a current through it reversing the oxygen-uptake process.

Infrared Absorption

Several respiratory gas analyzers are based on the principle of absorption of infrared radiation to measure gas concentrations. Infrared analysis is used in CO analyzers for the $D_{L_{CO}}$ tests. Infrared CO_2 analyzers are used for exercise testing, metabolic studies, and bedside monitoring (capnography) in critical care (Fig. 9–16).

Certain gases, such as CO_2 and CO absorb infrared radiation. Two beams of

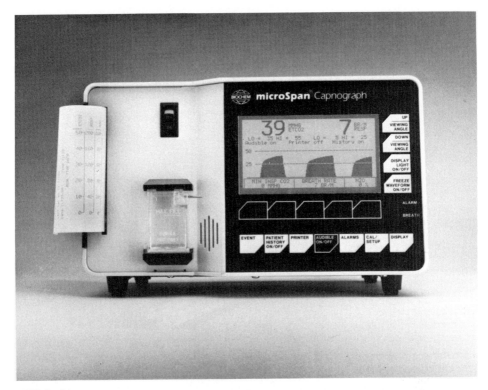

FIG 9–16.
Infrared CO_2 monitor. A microprocessor-controlled infrared CO_2 analyzer as used for critical care monitoring. A liquid crystal display allows presentation of end-tidal CO_2 values, breathing rate, and CO_2 waveforms. This capnograph includes a printer and alarms, along with a water trap to remove condensation from the sample line. (Courtesy of Biochem International Inc., Waukesha, Wisc.)

infrared radiation pass through parallel cells, one of which contains the gas to be sampled, and the other a reference gas. The two beams converge on a single infrared detector (Fig. 9–17). A small motor rotates an interrupter or "chopper" between the infrared source and the cells. The chopper blades alternately interrupt the infrared radiation passing through the sample and reference cells. If the sample gas and reference gas have the same concentration, the radiation reaching the detector is constant. However, when a sample gas with a different concentration is introduced, the amount of radiation reaching the detector varies in a rhythmic fashion. This causes a vibration in the detector that is translated into a pulsatile signal proportional to the difference between the two beams. Infrared analyzers are readily adaptable to measurements involving small changes in gas concentrations, such as differences between inspired and expired CO in tests of diffusing capacity. Gas can be sampled either continuously or discretely for use with infrared analyzers. For continuous sampling, the gas

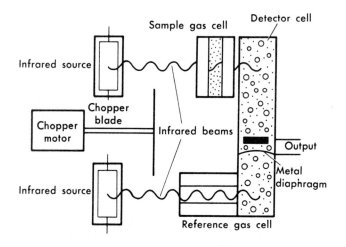

FIG 9–17.
Infrared absorption gas analyzer. Essential components of an infrared gas analyzer used for determination of CO_2 and CO concentrations. Infrared sources emit beams that pass through parallel cells. One cell contains a reference gas and the other the sample gas to be analyzed. A rotating blade "chops" the infrared beams in a rhythmic fashion so that when both the reference and sample cells contain the same gas, there is no variation in the radiation reaching either half of the detector cell. When the sample gas is introduced, it absorbs some of the infrared radiation. Different amounts of radiation reach the two halves of the detector cell, causing the diaphragm separating the compartments of the detector to oscillate. This oscillation is transformed into a signal proportional to the difference in gas concentrations. The infrared analyzer is ideal for determination of small changes in concentration in gas samples. (From Beckman Instruments, Inc., Medical gas analyzer LB-2: operating instructions, FM-149997-301, Schiller Park, Ill, 1972.)

flow rate must be constant and the analyzer calibrated at the same flow at which measurements are made. Condensation of water in the sampling circuit can significantly alter the flow rate and affect the accuracy of the measurement. Water vapor in the sample will dilute the gas being analyzed. Water vapor can be removed if response time is not critical. If response times are to be kept at a minimum, as required for breath-by-breath analysis, the effects of water vapor can be corrected mathematically by assuming that the expired gas is fully saturated.

The most common problems occurring with infrared analyzers involve the chopper motor, sample cell, and infrared detector. Motors turning the chopper blades typically wear out. Some analyzers employ a nonmechanical means of alternating the infrared beams, thus eliminating this problem. The sample cell can easily become contaminated. Water or other debris can partially occlude the "window" of the cell, interfering with the transmission of the infrared radiation. Infrared detector cells typically age over time, and become less sensitive. Both contamination of the sample cell and detector aging can reduce response time or make the analyzer impossible to calibrate.

Emission Spectroscopy

The single-breath and 7-minute N_2 distribution tests, as well as the open-circuit method of determining the FRC (see Chapter 1), require N_2 analysis. The Giesler tube ionizer is an N_2 analyzer based on the principle of emission spectroscopy (Fig. 9–18). This instrument consists of an enclosed ionization chamber that contains two electrodes and a photocell. A vacuum pump maintains a constant pressure in the ionization chamber by bleeding gas through a needle valve. The needle valve draws gas to be sampled from a breathing circuit. When a current is supplied to the electrodes, the N_2 between them is ionized and emits light. This light, after being filtered, is collected by a photodetector. The intensity of the light is directly proportional to the concentration of N_2 in the sample. The current, distance between electrodes, and gas pressure must remain constant. The photodetector converts the light signal into a DC voltage. This analog signal is then amplified, linearized, and directed to an appropriate meter or computing circuit. The Giesler tube ionizer allows continuous and rapid analysis of N_2 with response times less than 100 msec.

Analyzers utilizing emission spectroscopy typically require a vacuum pump. The vacuum pressure must be maintained at a stable level to insure accuracy and linearity. Leaks in the seals around the needle valve or in the pump itself may occur. Inability to zero and span the analyzer may be the first sign of a leak or faulty vacuum source. The photodetector, ionizing electrodes, and light filter all age with time. Periodic linearity checks allow adjustment for small changes in any of these components.

Thermal Conductivity Analyzers

The measurement of FRC by the closed-circuit method and the $D_{L_{CO}}sb$ each require He analysis. The thermal conductivity analyzer measures gas concentrations in a sample by detecting the rate at which different gases conduct heat. Heated wires or beads (thermistors) are exposed to the gas sample. By measuring the change in electrical resistance of the thermistors, the concentration of a specific gas can be detected. Two glass-coated thermistor beads serve as sensing elements connected by a Wheatstone bridge circuit (Fig. 9–19). Thermistors change temperature and their electrical resistance as a function of the molecular weight of the gases surrounding them. One thermistor serves as a reference. A difference in the concentration of gases between the two sensors can be detected because the differences in heat conducted away alters the electrical resistance in the circuit. Helium analyzers use a reference cell containing no helium. Other gases can be analyzed by means of thermal conductivity as long as interfering gases are not present. Thermal conductivity analyzers are used in conjunction with gas chromatography (see Gas Chromatography, this section) for just this reason. Water vapor and CO_2 are usually scrubbed before analysis when He

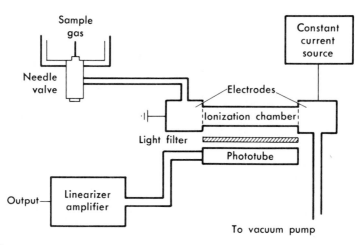

FIG 9–18.
Emission spectroscopy type gas analyzer. The optical emission analyzer (Giesler tube) is commonly used for N_2 analysis. A vacuum pump draws a gas sample into an ionization chamber, where the ionized gas emits light. All light except that from the desired gas is filtered out, and the remaining light is monitored by a phototube. The phototube transmits a signal proportional to the intensity of the light, allowing rapid gas analysis. (From Hewlett-Packard, Application not AN 729, San Diego, Calif, 1973.)

concentration is being measured. Thermal conductivity analyzers can be used for continuous or discrete measurements, but have a response time in the range of 10 to 20 seconds. Thermal conductivity analyzers cannot be used to detect rapid changes in gas concentration.

Thermal conductivity analyzers are very stable. Unless the thermistor in the sampling chamber is contaminated or physically damaged, the analyzer remains accurate for an extended period. Failure of water or CO_2 absorbers in the sample circuit commonly lead to errors with this type of analyzer. Some He analyzers use a water absorber in line with the reference thermistor, so that room air can be used to zero the analyzer. Exhaustion of this absorber can result in calibration errors.

Gas Chromatography

Gas chromatographs combine a means of separating a sample gas into its component gases and a detector mechanism. The detector is usually a thermal conductivity analyzer as described previously. Most chromatographs utilize the principle of column separation to segregate the component gases of the sample (Fig. 9–20). A column contains material that impedes the movement of gas molecules depending on their size. Some columns use materials that combine chemically with specific gases. A combination of columns allows a wide range of gases to be analyzed with a single detector. Helium is used as a carrier gas because of its high thermal conductivity. The sample gas, along with the He carrier gas, is injected into the column. The component gases exit the column at varying rates and are detected by the thermal conductivity analyzer. The concentrations of various gases can be determined by comparing the output of the thermal conductivity analyzer with a known calibration gas. Because He is used as the carrier gas, it cannot be used as an inert indicator for lung volume determinations or diffusing capacity measurements. Neon, which is relatively insoluble, may be substituted for helium in these tests. Water vapor and CO_2 are usually scrubbed from the sample to prevent contamination of the separator column. Gas chromatographs are well suited to applications requiring analysis of multiple gases such as $D_{L_{CO}}$ determinations. Chromatography is very accurate and is widely used for analysis of certified reference gases. Gas chromatographs

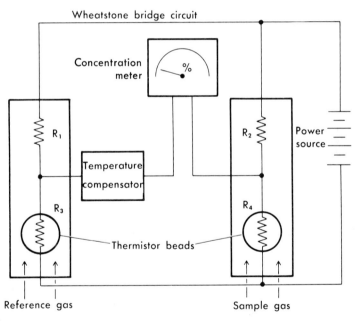

FIG 9–19.

Thermal conductivity analyzer. Thermal conductivity gas analyzer such as is used for analysis of He and in conjunction with gas chromatography. Two thermistor beads (temperature-sensitive electrical resistors) are connected in a Wheatstone bridge circuit. When the thermistors are subjected to the same gas concentrations, their electrical resistance decreases equally and the concentration meter registers zero (by calibration). When the sample gas is applied to the sample thermistor, R_4 in this example, and the reference thermistor submitted to a reference gas, a potential occurs and deflects the concentration meter by a proportional amount. (From Bourns, Inc., Life systems operations instruction manual, Model LS114-5, Riverside, Calif.)

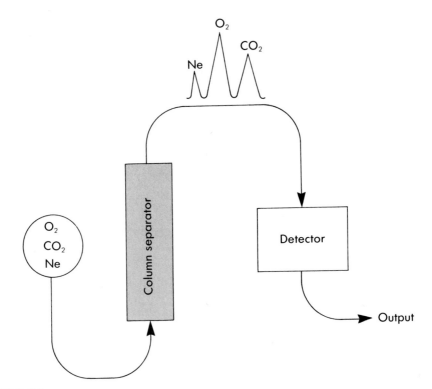

FIG 9–20.
Gas chromatograph. Diagrammatic representation of the components of a gas chromatograph for analysis of respiratory gases. The sample gas moves through a separator column via a carrier gas, usually He. Gases of different molecular sizes pass through the column at different rates and are monitored sequentially by a thermal conductivity–type detector. Most gases can be analyzed very accurately by means of appropriate columns.

can be used for discrete or continuous measurement. However, their response times are from 15 to 90 seconds depending on the gas to be detected.

As noted, gas chromatographs that are properly maintained are very accurate. Column material must be replaced when exhausted to maintain accuracy. Some chromatographs heat the column to enhance separation. Failure of the heating mechanism can lead to inaccurate analyses. Exhaustion of water and CO_2 absorbers also can cause the column to become contaminated.

Mass Spectrometry

Perhaps the most sophisticated means of measuring concentrations of respiratory gases is the mass spectrometer. A sample of gas is drawn into a capillary tube by a vacuum pump, which simultaneously reduces the pressure to a preset level. An ionization filament ionizes the sample gases. The ions are then directed into a beam by an electrostatic lens. The beam is passed through a magnetic field. The ions of the constituent gases separate according to their specific mass and electrical charge (Fig. 9–21). Ion detectors sense the various ions and amplify their charges into a usable signal for monitoring or analog computations. Mass spectrometers have response times of less than 100 msec. They are also capable of detecting multiple gases, making them ideally suited for breath-by-breath measurements. Not all gas combinations can be analyzed by mass spectrometry. Two gases having similar charge-to-mass ratios after being ionized will appear identical to the mass spectrometer.

Water vapor does not affect the mass spectrometer itself. However, condensation in the sampling circuit can block gas flow or increase the response time. Mass spectrometers are typically large and require a high level of maintenance. Common problems include failure of the vacuum system to pump down to an adequate level. The ionizer element also ages and may need to be replaced periodically to maintain accuracy. These instruments appear to be best suited for monitoring multiple patients simultaneously. In applications such as exercise testing or anesthesia, the ability to monitor multiple gases simultaneously may make the mass spectrometer the instrument of choice.

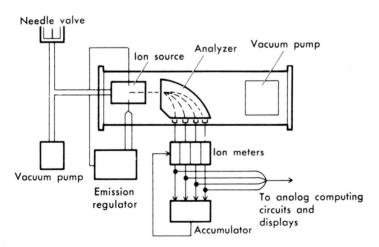

FIG 9–21.
Mass spectrometer. A mass spectrometer in which respiratory gases are analyzed. A vacuum pump draws a small sample of gas into an ionizing chamber, where a current sufficient to ionize the desired gases is supplied. A magnetic analyzer separates the ion beam into constituent gases according to their charge/mass ratio. The separated beams of ions are collected by distinct detectors and the relative concentration of each gas is determined in comparison to the total output of the detectors. The output signals are usually directed to computing and display circuits. (From Perkin-Elmer Medical Instruments, advertising brochure for Model 1100, Medical gas analyzer, Pomona, Calif.)

Gas Conditioning Devices

Interference from water vapor and CO_2 present in expired gas is common to many types of gas analyzers. These two gases are usually removed by chemical "scrubbers."

Carbon dioxide may be absorbed by passing the sample through granules containing either barium hydroxide (BaOH) or sodium hydroxide (NaOH). Granules containing NaOH have a light brown appearance that changes to white when saturated with CO_2. The BaOH (baralyme) scrubber is usually supplied with an indicator (ethyl violet) that changes from white to purple when saturated with CO_2. NaOH and BaOH are mildly corrosive and may generate heat if exposed to high concentrations of CO_2. Both generate water as a product of combination with CO_2, therefore they should be placed upstream of the water vapor absorber.

Water vapor is commonly absorbed by passing the wet gas over granules of anhydrous calcium sulfate ($CaSO_4$). The $CaSO_4$ usually contains an indicator that changes from blue to pink when exhausted. Some analyzers utilize silica gel to remove water vapor. Conditioning of gas containing water vapor also may be accomplished using special sample tubing. This tubing is permeable to water vapor. Sample gas passing through the tubing will typically equilibrate its water vapor pressure with that of the surrounding atmosphere. Water vapor is not removed, but remains constant at a known level. This allows corrections for water vapor pressure to be accurately applied when other gases are analyzed. Failure to adequately scrub water vapor or CO_2 from a gas sample will result in dilution of the remaining gases. Dilution lowers the fractional concentration of the gas being analyzed. Chemical scrubbers should always be used before the manufacturer's expiration date.

BLOOD GAS ELECTRODES, OXIMETERS, AND RELATED DEVICES

Measurements of arterial blood gases routinely include determination of Po_2, Pco_2, and pH. Calculation of Sao_2, HCO_3^-, total CO_2, base excess, and other parameters depend on measurements derived from one or more of the three primary electrodes.

pH Electrode

The *glass pH electrode* contains a solution of constant pH on one side of a glass membrane. The solution from which pH is to be measured is brought into contact with the other side of the pH-sensitive glass (Fig. 9–22, A and B). The difference in pH on either side of the glass causes a potential difference, or voltage. To measure this potential, two half-cells are used: one for the constant solution and one for the unknown solution. The constant solution half-cell (i.e., the measuring electrode) is usually a silver-silver chloride wire. The external

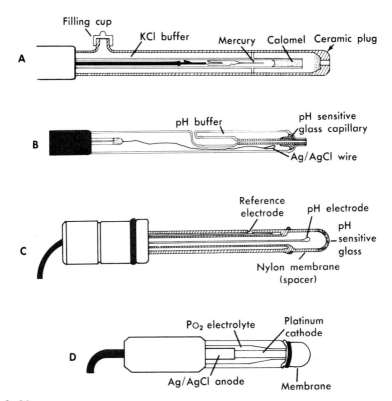

FIG 9–22.
pH, P_{CO_2}, and P_{O_2} electrodes. **A,** the reference pH electrode contains a potassium chloride buffer and a porous ceramic plug that allows electrical contact to the exterior. The reference wire develops a constant potential. **B,** the pH-measuring electrode contains a sealed-in buffer and a silver-silver chloride wire. A thin capillary tube (or similar surface) constructed of pH-sensitive glass allows a potential to develop, which varies with the pH of the unknown solution in contact with the glass. The difference between the variable potential and the constant potential of the reference electrode indicates the pH of the sample. **C,** the P_{CO_2} (Severinghaus) electrode is an adaptation of the pH electrode. The pH electrode contains a sealed-in buffer, while the reference electrode is the other half-cell and is in communication with a P_{CO_2} electrolyte of aqueous bicarbonate. The entire glass electrode is encased in a Lucite jacket (not shown) containing the electrolyte. The jacket is capped with a Teflon membrane that is permeable to CO_2. A nylon mesh covers the tip of the internal glass electrode acting as a spacer to keep electrolyte in contact with the pH-sensitive glass. CO_2 diffuses through the Teflon membrane, is hydrated in the electrolyte, and alters the pH. The pH change is displayed as partial pressure of CO_2. **D,** the P_{O_2} (polarographic or Clark) electrode contains a platinum cathode and a silver-silver chloride anode. The electrode is polarized by applying a slightly negative voltage. The tip is protected by a polyethylene or polypropylene membrane, which allows O_2 molecules to diffuse but prevents contamination of the platinum wire. Oxygen migrates to the cathode and is reduced by picking up free electrons that have come from the silver-silver chloride anode through a phosphate-potassium chloride buffer. Changes in the current flowing between the anode and cathode result from the amount of O_2 reduced in the electrolyte, and are proportional to partial pressure of O_2.

half-cell is usually a saturated calomel (i.e., approximately 20% KCl) electrode and is called the reference electrode. The reference electrode makes contact with the unknown solution by means of a permeable membrane or a liquid junction. These half-cells are connected to a millivolt display that is simply calibrated in pH units. The voltage difference between the two electrodes is proportional to the pH difference of the solutions. Because the pH of one solution is constant, the developed potential is a measure of the pH of the unknown solution.

Various means of implementing pH measuring systems are utilized. The measuring electrode may be constructed as in Figure 9–22, B, with the pH sensitive glass formed into a capillary through which the sample is drawn. Another design features a microelectrode with just the tip exposed to the sample. Electrical contact between the sample and the KCl electrolyte of the reference electrode may be formed by a liquid junction or by permeable membrane.

Protein contamination of the pH-sensitive glass is a common problem and depends on the number of specimens analyzed. Routine cleaning with a proteolytic agent helps to reduce the buildup of debris on the electrode. KCl depletion and blockage of the reference junction are also common problems associated with pH electrode malfunction. Contamination of buffers used for pH electrode calibration also can result in measurement errors. Daily (or more often) use of suitable quality control materials can detect these and other problems (see Chapter 11).

Pco_2 Electrode

The *Pco_2 electrode* (Severinghaus electrode) measures Pco_2 potentiometrically using an adaptation of the pH electrode (see Fig. 9–22, C). A combined pH glass and reference electrode is placed inside of a membrane-tipped plastic jacket. The jacket is filled with a bicarbonate-chloride buffer. The membrane is usually Teflon or a similar material that is permeable to CO_2 molecules. A spacer or wick made of nylon is usually placed between the pH-sensitive glass and the membrane. The spacer insures that a thin layer of bicarbonate electrolyte is in contact with the electrode. When the sample is introduced at the tip of the electrode, CO_2 diffuses across the membrane in proportion to partial pressure until equilibration between the electrolyte and the sample occurs. Carbon dioxide is hydrated in the electrolyte according to the equation:

$$CO_2 + H_2O \rightleftarrows H_2CO_3 \rightleftarrows H^+ + HCO_3^-$$

The change in H^+ concentration is proportional to the change in Pco_2. The electrode detects the change in Pco_2 as a change in pH of the electrolyte. The voltage developed is exponentially related to Pco_2. A tenfold increase in Pco_2 is approximately equal to a decrease of 1 pH unit. By calibrating the pH change when the electrode is exposed to gases with known P_{CO_2} values, partial pressure of CO_2 can be determined.

The most common problem with the P_{CO_2} electrode is degradation or contamination of the membrane. Protein or other debris deposited on the membrane slows down the diffusion of CO_2. Equilibrium may not be achieved during the time the sample is in the measuring chamber. Electrolyte depletion or exhaustion in the jacket around the electrode also may occur with extended use. Careful attention to shifts in electrode performance, either during calibration or control runs, can detect these common problems. Routine maintenance includes replacing the membrane and refilling the electrode with fresh electrolyte. Guidelines for quality control of blood gas electrodes are included in Chapter 11.

P_{O_2} Electrode

The *P_{O_2} electrode* (Clark electrode) consists of a platinum cathode that is usually a thin wire encased in plastic or glass, together with a silver/silver chloride (Ag/AgCl) anode (see Fig. 9–22, D). Both the anode and cathode are placed inside a plastic jacket tipped with a polypropylene or polyethylene membrane. The membrane is semipermeable and allows diffusion of oxygen molecules. The jacket is filled with phosphate-potassium chloride buffer. A polarizing voltage of -0.7 volts is applied to the electrode so that the cathode is slightly negative with respect to the anode. Because the electrode is polarized, it is often referred to as a "polarographic" electrode. Oxygen is reduced (i.e., takes up electrons) at the cathode according to the equation:

$$O_2 + 2H_2O + 4e^- \rightarrow 4OH^-$$

Electrons (i.e., e in the equation above) are supplied by the Ag/AgCl anode. Electrons flow from the anode to the cathode with a current proportional to the number of molecules of O_2 reduced. Each O_2 molecule can take up 4 electrons, and the greater the number of O_2 molecules present, the greater the current. The membrane causes a diffusion limitation to the number of molecules reaching the electrode. The greater the partial pressure on the sample side of the membrane, the higher the rate of diffusion. The measurement of the current developed within the electrode is therefore proportional to P_{O_2}.

As with the P_{CO_2} electrode, contamination or degradation of the membrane alters diffusion of O_2 and can result in erratic measurements. Most polarographic electrodes utilize a platinum wire of small diameter to reduce the actual consumption of O_2 at the tip of the electrode. The exposed surface of the platinum cathode gradually becomes plated with metal ions and must be periodically polished to maintain its sensitivity. The platinum wire can be polished by brushing or abrading with a coarse substance such as pumice.

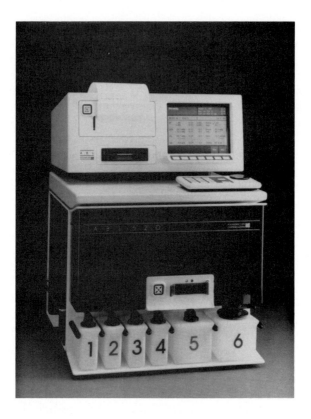

FIG 9–23.
Automated blood gas analyzer, including spectrophotometric oximeter. This system provides automatic flushing and calibration, and on-line display of results and calibrations using an attached computer and video display terminal. pH, P_{CO_2}, P_{O_2} are measured, while HCO_3^-, total CO_2, standard bicarbonate are calculated. This system also incorporates a spectrophotometric oximeter for analysis of Hb, O_2Hb, COHb, and MetHb. Base excess is calculated using the HCO_3^- from the blood gas analysis and the Hb measured by the oximeter. (Courtesy of Radiometer America, Westlake, Ohio.)

Because the membrane causes a diffusion limit to O_2 molecules reaching the cathode, the electrode performs differently when exposed to liquid vs. gas samples. Some blood gas systems use gas to calibrate the P_{O_2} electrode. Noticeable differences may result when the electrode is then used to analyze the tension of O_2 dissolved in a liquid. These differences are usually compensated by correcting the P_{O_2} using an empirically determined gas-to-liquid factor (see Chapter 11).

Although the gas measuring (P_{O_2} and P_{CO_2}) electrodes and the pH electrode system can each be used separately, all three are usually implemented together in a blood gas analyzer (Fig. 9–23). Most blood gas analyzers are microprocessor controlled. Such tasks as sample aspiration, rinsing, and calibration can all be done automatically under program control. The microprocessor can calculate a wide variety of parameters derived from pH, Pco_2, and Po_2, as well as from data received from other instruments. In addition, computerized analyzers can evaluate automated calibrations and track electrode performance to alert the technologist of existing or impending problems.

Transcutaneous Po_2 Electrode

The *transcutaneous O_2 electrode* (tcPo_2) operates on a principle similar to that of the polarographic (Clark) electrode. The tcPo_2 electrode consists of a ring-shaped silver anode that is heated by a coil to increase blood flow at the skin placement site. Inside the circular anode is a series of thin platinum cathodes (Fig. 9–24). All of the elements are enclosed in a plastic case, except for the face of the sensor, which is covered by a Teflon membrane. A KCl electrolyte is placed between the membrane and the sensor. A second layer of electrolyte and a cellophane membrane are added to form a double membrane. The electrical current between the silver and platinum electrodes is proportional to the partial pressure of O_2 diffusing through the skin and membrane. A feedback controller keeps the temperature constant at the skin site. This mechanism compensates for changes caused by capillary blood flow, thus stabilizing the measurement.

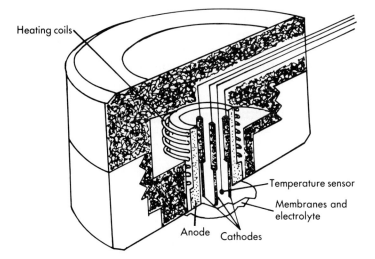

FIG 9–24.
Transcutaneous Po_2 electrode. A cross-sectional diagram of the components of the tcPo_2 electrode shows a circular anode around a series of cathodes and a temperature sensor. A heating coil causes local hyperemia so that surface Po_2 more closely resembles Pao_2. A double membrane separates the electrode proper from the skin.

tcP_{O_2} and Pa_{O_2} are not identical, but the gradient between them tends to be relatively constant in subjects with normal cardiac output. In neonates, there is a close correlation between transcutaneous and arterial P_{O_2}. In adult patients who are hemodynamically stable, the tcP_{O_2} is approximately 80% of the Pa_{O_2}. tcP_{O_2} can be valuable for trending oxygenation once the gradient has been established. In subjects who have a reduced cardiac output, the gradient between tcP_{O_2} and Pa_{O_2} widens. Conditions that affect perfusion to the skin also may alter the gradient between arterial and transcutaneous P_{O_2} (see Chapters 6 and 8).

Most transcutaneous electrodes heat the skin site in the range of 40 to 45°C. The increased temperature "arterializes" capillary blood flow in the skin. This process, however, necessitates movement of the electrode at 3- to 4-hour intervals to prevent burns. This is particularly important in neonates because of the reduced thickness of their epidermis. Periodic recalibration of the electrode is necessary even if the sensor site has not been changed. After placement of the electrode, an interval from 5 to 30 minutes may be required for equilibration to be reached.

The transcutaneous P_{CO_2} electrode (tcP_{CO_2}) consists of Severinghaus-type electrode that is mounted in a manner similar to the tcP_{O_2} device. Combination transcutaneous CO_2 and O_2 electrodes are available. In hemodynamically stable patients, tcP_{CO_2} reliably follows the trend of Pa_{CO_2}. However, tcP_{CO_2} is typically from 4 to 25 mm Hg higher than the corresponding Pa_{CO_2}. This gradient is the opposite of that observed with tcP_{O_2}. Like transcutaneous O_2 measurements, the difference between tcP_{CO_2} and Pa_{CO_2} is least in neonates and greatest in adults. Although tcP_{CO_2} electrodes can be used at 37°C, their response and equilibration times are prolonged unless they are heated to 42 to 44°C. Even when heated, stabilization of the electrode after placement may require 10 to 20 minutes. In addition, response to changes in Pa_{CO_2} may take from 1.5 to 4 minutes. This slow response time keeps tcP_{CO_2} monitors from being useful for detecting apnea or patient-ventilator disconnection. Like tcP_{O_2}, tcP_{CO_2} does not correlate with arterial values in the presence of reduced cardiac output or tissue hypoperfusion.

Intra-arterial Blood Gas Optodes

Devices capable of measuring pH, P_{CO_2}, and P_{O_2} via an indwelling catheter have recently become available. These sensors are referred to as optodes because of their principle of operation. Optodes specifically for pH and blood gas measurements are based on the concept of luminescence quenching.

When light strikes a photoluminescent dye, certain wavelengths are absorbed and electrons are excited to an elevated energy state. When the light source is removed, the electrons decay to a lower energy level and emit light at a different wavelength than was originally absorbed. The light emitted from the fluorescent dye also may be changed by the presence of substances that alter the dye's response to light. For example, certain photoluminescent dyes are inhibited from emitting light by the presence of O_2. This mechanism is called luminescence quenching. By utilizing dyes that respond to O_2 or CO_2 molecules, or to hydrogen ions (i.e., change with pH), an optical electrode may be created.

A fluorescent optode is composed of a fiberoptic element with a fluorescent dye at the tip. A membrane permeable to O_2, CO_2, or H^+ separates the dye from the subject's blood. An intermittent light source transmits light at an appropriate wavelength down the optical fiber. The resulting photoluminescence intensity is transmitted back up the fiber. The optode measures the difference between the excitation and emission energy of the light. If the excitation energy is kept constant, the light emitted from the dye is altered by the presence of the specific analyte (i.e., O_2, CO_2, or pH).

All three optodes can be combined into a probe small enough to be inserted through a 20-gauge arterial catheter. The catheter can be used simultaneously for monitoring blood pressure, withdrawing blood samples, and in vivo monitoring. The probe itself is coated with a special form of heparin to inhibit intravascular clotting. The probe assembly connects to an interface that routes the light beam and signals to an electronics module. Blood gas parameters are displayed digitally. The optode system requires approximately 15 seconds to compute a new set of blood gas data. During non–steady-state conditions, the monitor indicates simply that the desired parameter is changing, and in which direction.

The pH and P_{CO_2} optodes agree very closely with measurement using conventional electrodes. The differences in pH or P_{CO_2} measurements between optodes and a blood gas analyzer do not appear to be clinically significant. The accuracy of the Pa_{O_2} optode varies with the absolute value of the arterial O_2 tension. Optode luminescence and P_{O_2} appear to be inversely related. Low O_2 values produce higher optode signal intensities. The O_2 optode is potentially most accurate at low P_{O_2} levels. This is in contrast to the Clark (polarographic) electrode, in which the current produced by reduction of O_2 is directly proportional to the amount of the gas present. However, the variability of the Pa_{O_2} measured by optode reduces its usefulness for critical care monitoring. Further refinements of fluorescent optode technology may be able to improve the bias and precision of the O_2 optode.

Spectrophotometric Oximeter

The *spectrophotometric oximeter* (Fig. 9–25) uses the principle of light absorption to analyze the saturation of Hb with O_2. In addition, the concentration of carboxyhemoglobin (COHb) — the Hb bound with CO — or other forms of Hb (i.e., methemoglobin, sulfhemoglobin) can be determined. This type of spectrophotometer is sometimes referred to as a co-oximeter. The blood oximeter

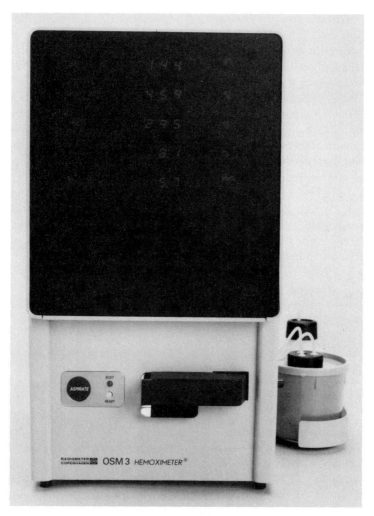

FIG 9–25
Automated spectrophotometric oximeter (co-oximeter). A small sample (approximately 0.2 mL) of blood is injected and hemolyzed ultrasonically. Spectrophotometric measurements are made to determine O₂Hb, COHb, MetHb, and total Hb. Oxygen content is calculated. Flushing and zeroing of the spectrophotometer are performed after each sample. (Courtesy of Radiometer America, Westlake, Ohio.)

analyzes the absorption of light at multiple wavelengths. At each of these wavelengths, two or more of the species of Hb have similar absorbances (Fig. 9–26). These common points are called isobestic points. A wavelength that is isobestic for oxyhemoglobin (O₂Hb), reduced Hb (RHb), and COHb is 548 nm. At this particular wavelength, the absorbance of a mixture of the three pigments is directly proportional to the total concentration of Hb. An isobestic point for O_2Hb and RHb is 568 nm. The absorbance of COHb at this point is considerably higher. Therefore, a change in absorbance at 568 nm compared with 548 nm indicates a change in the concentration of COHb relative to the sum of the concentrations of the other two species. Five hundred seventy-eight nm is the isobestic point for RHb and COHb, with O_2Hb absorbance being considerably greater. The difference in absorbance at 578 nm indicates the concentration of O_2Hb relative to the other two pigments. By analyzing the values for absorbance and solving simultaneous equations, the total Hb concentration, O_2Hb, COHb, and MetHb saturation can be determined.

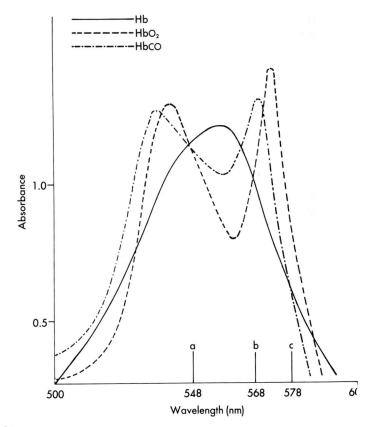

FIG 9–26.

Principle of spectrophotometric oximetry. Absorbance measurements are made at three or more distinct wavelengths (548, 568, 578 nm in this example) as light passes through a blood sample. At 548 nm, all three forms of Hb (Hb, Hbo₂ and COHB) have identical absorbances. At 568 nm, only Hb and Hbo₂ coincide; at 578 nm, Hb and COHb coincide. The solution of three simultaneous equations provides the relative proportions of each species, as well as the total Hb.

The spectrophotometric oximeter provides essential information regarding the O_2-Hb reaction. This is particularly important when increased concentrations of COHb, MetHb, or other abnormal species of Hb are present. Most automated blood gas analyzers calculate the saturation of Hb. Calculated saturation is based on the measured Pao_2 and pH at 37°C, and assuming that the Hb has a normal P_{50}. Normal adult Hb is 50% saturated at a Po_2 of 26 to 27 mm Hg. These approximations may significantly overestimate the true saturation in the presence of COHb or abnormal hemoglobins such as methemoglobin. The co-oximeter provides the most accurate estimate of the actual O_2 saturation of the blood. Combination blood gas analyzers and co-oximeters are available. These instruments combine the conventional pH and blood gas electrodes with spectrophotometric measurements of Hb saturation, all performed on the same blood sample.

The co-oximeter may give erroneously low Hb, O_2Hb, and COHb readings if large amounts of other pigments such as methemoglobin are present. Other substances that cause light scattering in the blood specimen, such as lipids resulting from lipid therapy, also may cause false readings. In order to function properly, the blood oximeter has to hemolyze the sample so that the hemoglobin molecules are evenly suspended in the solution rather than contained within the red cells. Hemolysis normally is accomplished by chemical or mechanical disruption of the red cell membranes. Incomplete hemolysis results in light scattering within the sample rather than simple absorption. Sickle cells are not easily disrupted, particularly by chemical lysis, and may result in false readings for O_2Hb and COHb.

Some newer co-oximeters feature microprocessor control that allows for specific errors such as incomplete hemolysis or abnormal light scattering to be detected and reported. Microprocessor-controlled oximeters also provide corrections so that specific varieties of hemoglobin such as fetal or animal Hb can be analyzed. In addition to measurements of O_2Hb, COHb, and MetHb saturations, the blood oximeter can be used to calculate oxygen content and to estimate the P_{50} of the blood. By measuring the actual saturation of a sample of blood (the saturation should be less than 90%) and comparing this value to the calculated saturation based on the Po_2 and pH of the same blood, a left or right shift of the O_2Hb curve can be determined and the P_{50} estimated. This simplified method compares favorably with the classic approach of tonometering the blood sample with gases of low oxygen concentrations and constructing a dissociation curve.

Pulse Oximeters

Pulse oximeters (Fig. 9–27, A and B) are the most recent development in the effort to assess oxygenation noninvasively. The pulse oximeter's immediate predecessor was a fiberoptic oximeter that passed multiple wavelengths of light

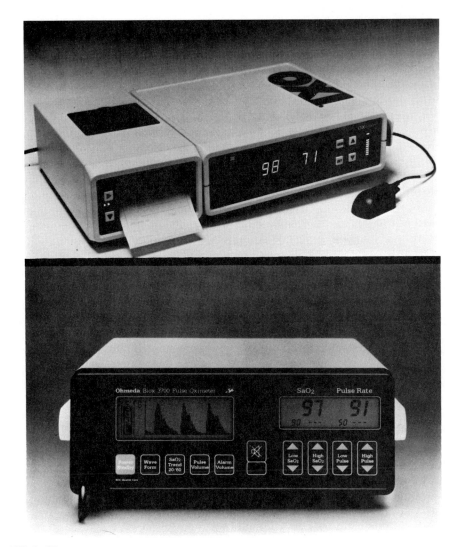

FIG 9–27.
Pulse oximeters. Two representative microprocessor-controlled pulse oximeters. Each provides a digital display of oxygen saturation measured by two wavelength oximetry along with pulse rate. Alarms for high and low saturations or pulse rates may be set. **A,** included with this pulse oximeter is a strip chart recorder useful for recording saturation and pulse rate trends. (Courtesy of Radiometer America, Westlake, Ohio.) **B,** a liquid crystal display included with this oximeter allows the operator to visualize the pulse waveform and to monitor signal quality, both of which may be helpful in detecting conditions that interfere with accurate saturation determinations. (Courtesy of Ohmeda, Louisville, Colo.)

through the pinna of the ear and measured the absorption to derive oxygen saturation of Hb.

The pulse oximeter treats Hb as a filter that allows only light in the red and near-infrared regions to pass. Beer's law relates the total absorption in a system of absorbers to the sum of their individual absorptions:

$$A_{total} = E_1C_1L_1 + E_2C_2L_2 + \ldots E_nC_nL_n$$

where:

A_{total} = the absorbance of a mixture of substances at a specific wavelength

E_n = the extinction of substance n

C_n = the concentration of substance n

L_n = the length of the light path through substance n

In principle, the pulse oximeter measures the absorption of a mixture of two substances, O_2Hb and reduced Hb (RHb). The concentration of either can be determined if their extinction is measured while the path length stays constant. The wavelengths of light used in pulse oximetry are about 660 nm in the red region of the spectrum and approximately 940 nm in the near-infrared portion. Extinction curves for O_2Hb and RHb show that reduced Hb has an absorption 10 times higher than oxyhemoglobin at 660 nm, while O_2Hb has a higher absorbance (2 to 3 times) at 940 nm. By calculating all the possible combinations of the two forms of Hb (i.e., varying the saturation from 0% to 100%), the ratio of absorbances at the two wavelengths can be determined. As a result, a calibration curve can be constructed. The capillary bed does not follow the optical principles exactly as described by Beer's law, so the calibration curve is derived empirically. The ratio of absorbances at the two distinct wavelengths is expressed:

$$R = A_{660nm}/A_{940nm}$$

A series of R values (i.e., the calibration curve) is determined by relating the ratio to actual saturation measurements. Unlike the spectrophotometric oximeter which measures absorption in a hemolyzed blood sample, the pulse oximeter measures light passing through living tissue. The transmitted light is not only absorbed but refracted and scattered, so the absolute accuracy of the pulse oximeter tends to be less than the blood oximeter.

The transmitted light output at each wavelength consists of two components, the *AC and DC components* (Fig. 9–28). The AC component varies with the pulsation of blood. The DC component is much larger than the AC and is a

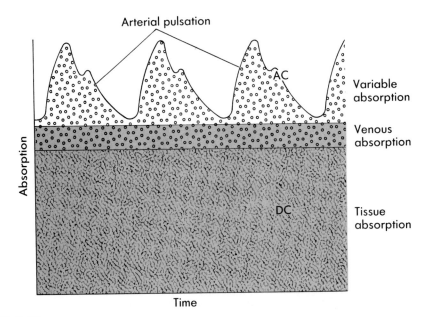

FIG 9–28.

AC and DC components in pulse oximetry. The transmitted light at each of two wavelengths (usually 660 nm and 940 nm) consists of two parts. A large fixed component, the DC component, represents the light passing through the tissue and venous blood without being absorbed. A second smaller portion is pulsatile in nature and represents the changing absorption as blood pulses through the arterioles; this is represented as the AC component. The pulse oximeter divides the AC signal by the DC signal at each wavelength, effectively cancelling the DC component. The ratio of the AC signals at the two wavelengths is then a function of relative absorptions of O_2Hb and RHb (see text).

constant output level. The DC component represents the light passing through the tissue without being absorbed or scattered. The amplitude of both the AC and DC levels depends on the intensity of the incident light. The AC component represents the arterial blood, as it is the arterioles that pulsate in the light path. By dividing the AC level by the DC level at each of the two wavelengths, the AC component is effectively corrected. The AC component then becomes a function of the extinction of O_2Hb and RHb. The ratio described above then becomes:

$$R = \frac{(AC_1/DC_1)}{(AC_2/DC_2)}$$

where:

1 = the red wavelength (660 nm)

2 = the near-infrared wavelength (940 nm)

Correcting the pulsatile component (AC) in this manner allows the pulse oximeter to "ignore" the absorbances caused by venous blood, tissue, and skin pigmentation.

The light source used in pulse oximetry is the light emitting diode or LED. The LEDs are capable of emitting a very bright light near the 660-nm and 940-nm wavelengths required for analysis of Hb saturation. The intensity of light is easily controlled by a feedback circuit that regulates the driving current to the diode. The greater the DC component resulting from pigmentation or venous blood, the greater the current supplied to the LED. A significant drawback to the use of LEDs is that the exact wavelength of light emitted varies with individual LEDs. Each LED has its own "center" wavelength that may differ from 660 or 940 nm by as much as 15 nm. In order to circumvent this variation, each oximeter must have a series of calibration curves programmed into it, so that it can accommodate different sensors. Because the extinction curves for RHb and O_2Hb are steep and quite different at 660 nm, 10 or more calibration curves are typically required for the red light range. Slight variations in center wavelength are less critical in the 940-nm region because the extinction characteristics of O_2Hb and RHb are the same from 800 to 1000 nm. A silicone photodiode is the detector for the transmitted light in the pulse oximeter. A single photodiode senses both the red and near-infrared light. The microprocessor that controls the oximeter cycles the LEDs on and off separately 400 to 500 times per second. The oximeter also turns both LEDs off during each cycle so that the photodiode can detect ambient light caused by scattering and can offset the LED signals. By having a short interval when both LEDs are off, the oximeter can measure ambient light levels and subtract them from the levels obtained when the LEDs are on.

Pulse oximeter accuracy tends to decrease at low saturations. Low saturations occur when the concentration of reduced hemoglobin (RHb) increases. Because RHb has a much higher absorbance at 660 nm than does O_2Hb, slight variations in the center wavelength of the red LED (as described above) exaggerate the error in measured saturation. This is one reason why pulse oximeters exhibit decreasing accuracy at lower saturations.

Because the AC, or pulsatile component is usually much smaller than the DC component, detecting it can sometimes cause problems. Very low perfusion or poor vascularity can cause the oximeter to be unable to measure the pulsatile component. The oximeter's microprocessor is usually programmed to display a warning message if the photodetector senses light levels that are inadequate. Motion artifact also can cause inaccuracy with most pulse oximeters. Motion artifact, especially shivering, often occurs in the same physiologic frequency range as the signal to be detected (i.e., arterial pulsations). If the motion is consistent and lasts long enough, it introduces a signal of approximately the same amplitude into both the red and infrared channels. The pulse oximeter senses the motion artifact as part of the DC component. This adds a large value to both the numerator and the denominator of the equation for R. The motion signal forces R toward a value of 1, which equates to a saturation of 85% on the typical oximeter calibration curve.

Most pulse oximeters use the AC signal from one channel, either 660 or 940 nm, to calculate the pulse rate. An algorithm implemented by the microprocessor locates the peaks in the waveform of the AC signal (see Fig. 9–28). Some oximeters use this signal to display graphic representations of the pulse waveform. Pulse detection can be enhanced by the addition of a single ECG lead, and the additional input may be necessary to allow the microprocessor to distinguish motion artifact or noise from the true signal.

Reflective Spectrophotometers

A specially designed pulmonary artery catheter (Swan-Ganz) that contains fiberoptic bundles makes it possible to continuously monitor mixed venous oxygen saturation $S\bar{v}_{O_2}$. The catheter has the regular proximal and distal pressure-sensing channels, a balloon tip for flotation through the right side of the heart, and a thermistor for thermodilution cardiac output determinations. In addition, it contains two fiberoptic bundles (Fig. 9–29). The catheter uses principles similar to both the co-oximeter and the pulse oximeter. Reflective spectrophotometry is based on the variable reflection of light by O_2Hb and RHb at different wavelengths. Just as the light absorbed by oxygenated and reduced hemoglobin is a function of wavelength, so is the intensity of reflected or

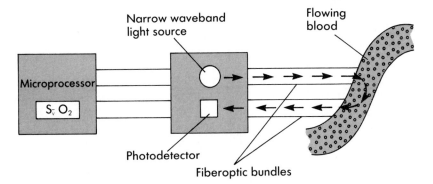

FIG 9–29.
Principle of reflective spectrophotometry. A diagrammatic representation of the components of the optical pulmonary artery catheter used for continuous monitoring of $S\bar{v}_{O_2}$. Light-emitting diodes (LEDs) provide a narrow-waveband light source that is transmitted along one fiberoptic filament to blood flowing past the tip of the catheter. Light reflected from the blood is transmitted back to a photodiode by the second fiberoptic bundle. The light intensity signals are then evaluated by a microprocessor to calculate light intensity ratios (usually two ratios are determined from three wavelengths), which are used to determine the $S\bar{v}_{O_2}$.

back-scattered light. Carefully spaced monofilament optical fibers are used as transmitting and receiving paths for light. Three LEDs, similar to those used in pulse oximeters, illuminate blood flowing past the tip of the catheter via one of the optical fibers. A photodetector receives the reflected light and converts its intensity into a signal. A microprocessor converts the data from the photodetector and calculates two independent ratios of reflected light intensities from the three wavelengths. Combining two reflected light intensity ratios reduces the instrument's sensitivity to physiologic phenomena such as pulsatile blood flow or hematocrit. This design also minimizes changes resulting from light scattering from red cell surfaces and the walls of the blood vessel. The $S\bar{v}_{O_2}$ is calculated from the light ratios using programmed calibration curves, as for the pulse oximeter. As in the pulse oximeter, the saturation measured is the saturation of *functional* Hb (see Chapter 6). The $S\bar{v}_{O_2}$ by this method will be higher than that measured by a co-oximeter, especially if large amounts of COHb or MetHb are present. The $S\bar{v}_{O_2}$ is then displayed and may be printed using a trend recorder (Fig. 9–30). The microprocessor also monitors the absolute intensity levels of the reflected light to allow detection of changes in catheter position or the integrity of the fiberoptics.

The reflective spectrophotometer has several advantages for monitoring patients in a critical care setting. The $S\bar{v}_{O_2}$ is measured continuously rather than discretely, as when mixed venous samples are withdrawn for routine analysis. A continuous indwelling monitor allows trending, as well as high and low alarms to detect large changes in mixed venous oxygen saturation. All of the other indices normally available from the pulmonary artery catheter, such as pulmonary artery pressures, pulmonary capillary wedge pressures, mixed venous blood samples, and thermodilution cardiac output can be measured while $S\bar{v}_{O_2}$ is being monitored. A change in mixed venous oxygen saturation, either an increase or a decrease, can result from multiple causes (see Critical Care Monitoring, Chapter 8).

The reflective spectrophotometer must be routinely calibrated in order to assure that observed changes in $S\bar{v}_{O_2}$ are the result of physiologic phenomena rather than instrument drift. The catheter is usually standardized by calibrating it against an absolute color reference before insertion. After the catheter is in place, calibration is accomplished by comparing the displayed values with saturation measured by a co-oximeter and adjusting the output of the indwelling device. This type of calibration is accurate at the time it is performed, but may change if there are shifts in the pH or hematocrit. Because the reflective spectrophotometer measures reflected light in whole blood that is flowing rather than transmitted light in a hemolyzed blood sample, its absolute accuracy tends to be less than that of the co-oximeter. Direct comparison of saturations by the two methods requires correction for COHb and MetHb as measured by the co-oximeter.

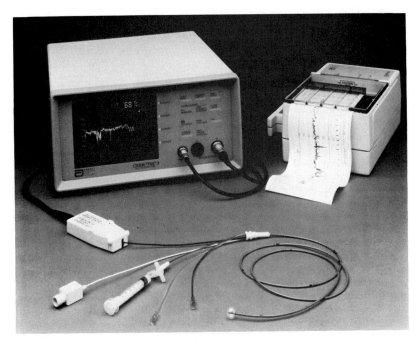

FIG 9–30.
Reflective spectrophotometer and pulmonary artery catheter. A microprocessor-controlled reflective spectrophotometer. The pulmonary artery catheter contains fiberoptic bundles for continuous measurement of the $S\bar{v}_{O_2}$, as well as the usual pressure-measuring ports and thermistor for thermodilution cardiac output. The instrument displays mixed venous saturation digitally and by means of a trend graph that can be optionally printed. High and low saturation alarms are included along with a "light intensity" alarm to detect artifact resulting from catheter motion or problems with the fiberoptics. (Courtesy of Abbott Critical Care Systems, Mountain View, Calif.)

BODY PLETHYSMOGRAPHS

Two types of body plethysmographs are in common clinical use: the constant-volume, variable-pressure plethysmograph, and the flow or variable-volume plethysmograph. These are commonly referred to as the pressure and flow plethysmographs, respectively. Both designs are employed for the measurement of VTG (see Chapter 1), and Raw and its derivatives (see Chapter 3).

The constant-volume plethysmograph is based on the principle that volume changes in a closed container can be determined from measured pressure changes as long as the temperature is constant. A sensitive pressure transducer monitors box pressure changes that are related to volume changes by calibration (see Chapter 11 for calibration techniques). Pressure fluctuations result from the compression and decompression of gas within both the subject's thorax and the box, as well as from thermal changes. If the temperature is constant, each unit of pressure change equals a specific volume change. For example, in many systems, 15 mL of volume change will result in a pressure change of 1 cm H_2O.

The pressure plethysmograph must be relatively free from leaks. A valving mechanism allows the technologist to vent the pressure plethysmograph to maintain thermal equilibrium. By making V_{TG} and Raw measurements at rapid breathing rates (panting), pressure changes resulting from thermal drift, leaks, or background noise are minimized. Some pressure plethysmograph systems use a "slow" leak to facilitate thermal equilibrium. A leak to allow thermal equilibration may be created by connecting a long length of small-bore tubing to the box. Similarly, connecting the atmospheric side of the box pressure transducer to a glass bottle within the box damps the effects of thermal drift. Both methods reduce the effect of temperature changes within the box while maintaining good frequency response. Pressure plethysmographs are best suited to maneuvers that measure small volume changes (i.e., 100 mL or less).

The flow plethysmograph employs a flow transducer in the box wall to measure volume changes in the box. Gas in the box is compressed or decompressed and the pressure change is measured as gas flows out of the box through the flow opening. Flow through the wall is integrated, corrections applied, and the volume change recorded as the sum of the volume passing through the wall and the volume compressed. In one implementation, the subject breathes through a pneumotachometer that is connected to the room (transmural breathing). The transmural pneumotachometer allows larger gas volumes (i.e., the VC or MEFV curves) to be measured while the subject is enclosed in the plethysmograph. The transmural flow is redirected to the plethysmograph for airway resistance measurements, so that the ratio of flow to box volume can be plotted. For V_{TG} measurements, the flow transducer in the plethysmograph wall is blocked so that the device works as a pressure box. The flow-type plethysmograph requires computerization so that the pressure, volume, and flow signals can be measured in phase. Although thermal changes must be accounted for, the flow plethysmograph does not need to be absolutely airtight.

In each type of plethysmograph (Fig. 9–31), a pneumotachometer is necessary for measuring air flow at the mouth for the Raw maneuver. The integrated flow signal (i.e., volume) is also used to determine the end-expiratory point for shutter closure in the V_{TG} measurement. The pneumotachometer must be linear across the range of flows typically measured (0 to 2 L/sec) for both spontaneous breathing and panting. Heated Fleisch or Silverman types of pressure-differential pneumotachometers are usually implemented in the plethysmograph. A mouth pressure transducer is normally coupled to an electronic shutter mechanism. The transducer records mouth pressures in the range of 0 to 20 cm H_2O when the airway is occluded. Some systems require the technologist to close the shutter by remote control at end-expiration. This is

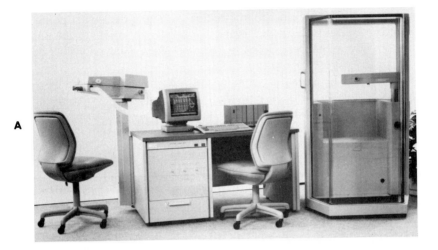

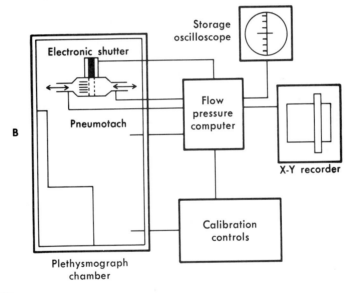

FIG 9–31.
Body plethysmograph. **A,** modern plethysmograph setup, with a highly transparent box, self-contained calibration equipment, and computerized data reduction and display. (Courtesy of Medical Graphics Corporation, St. Paul, Minn.) **B,** diagram of plethysmograph components: pneumotachometer with automatic shutter mechanism, body plethysmograph cabinet, interface/computer for reduction of pressure, flow, and volume signals, storage oscilloscope and X-Y recorder, and calibration instruments with controls.

accomplished by observing the tidal breathing maneuver on a display and actuating the shutter at end-expiration. Microprocessor-controlled systems allow the shutter to be closed automatically at a preselected point in the breathing cycle. The technologist initiates a sequence in which the computer analyzes the flow signal and closes the shutter when expiratory flow becomes zero.

Recording of the breathing maneuvers may be accomplished by one of several techniques. Some plethysmograph systems use a storage oscilloscope to record the breathing maneuvers. The scope may be erased as often as necessary to obtain acceptable tracings. The tracings then may be photographed or transferred to a plotter or X-Y recorder. Measurement of tangents or angles from the standard oscilloscope is usually performed by rotating a protractor to align its axes with those of the tracing and then reading the appropriate value.

Most commercially available systems are computerized. The breathing maneuvers may be stored in memory, analyzed, then displayed on the video screen. Computerized plethysmographs allow the technologist to select a "best-fit" line drawn by the computer, or to manipulate the tangent via the computer keyboard or mouse. Computerized plethysmographs offer the advantage of providing lung volume and airway resistance information immediately on completion of the maneuver. This aids the technologist in selecting appropriate maneuvers to report. In addition, the test can be repeated as required when questionable values are obtained. Comparison of lung volumes by alternate methods (i.e., He dilution or N_2 washout) to plethysmographically determined volumes is easily accomplished with computer-stored data. Computerization also allows panting frequency to be calculated and displayed. Measurements made at frequencies of 1 Hz or less may be more reliable in subjects who have severe obstruction.

Most plethysmographs include the necessary hardware to perform physical calibration (see Chapter 11). This hardware typically includes three signal-generating devices. A pressure manometer or U-tube may be mounted on the box for calibration of the mouth pressure transducer. A flow generator and rotameter (i.e., a flow meter) is included for pneumotachometer calibration. A volume-displacement device such as a 30- to 50-mL syringe driven by an electric motor allows box pressure or flow calibration. The motorized pump usually produces a sine-wave flow whose frequency can be varied. This allows checking of box calibration at various frequencies.

Computerized plethysmograph systems support automated calibration of transducers. In conventional calibration techniques, a signal such as pressure or flow is applied to a transducer. The output of the transducer (i.e., its amplified signal) is then adjusted to match the known calibration input. Computerized systems often bypass the physical adjustment of the output of the transducer. Instead of adjusting an amplifier zero or gain, the computer generates a software correction factor. This correction is then applied to every measurement made with the calibrated transducer. A few manufacturers also supply quality control devices such as the isothermal lung analog (see also Chapter 11). These devices serve as a control signal to check the calibration of transducers and software correction factors as well.

The ease with which the subject can enter the plethysmograph and perform the required maneuvers is an important feature. Some subjects may experience claustrophobia once inside the plethysmograph. Older boxes relied on solid materials, such as plywood, to provide the necessary rigidity for the cabinet so that pressure changes were not attenuated. Boxes made of durable plastics are largely transparent and less confining for the subject (see Fig. 9–31) while maintaining the necessary rigidity. Equally important is a communication system that allows both voice and visual contact with the subject. Panting against a closed shutter may be difficult for some individuals and continuous coaching is often necessary in order to elicit valid maneuvers.

RESPIRATORY INDUCTIVE PLETHYSMOGRAPHS

A noninvasive technique allowing measurement of pulmonary function is based on the principle of inductive plethysmography. The respiratory inductive plethysmograph (RIP) consists of two or more Teflon-insulated coils of wire sewn into elastic bands connected to oscillator circuits (Fig. 9–32). The elastic bands are then positioned around the chest and abdomen. Breathing excursions stretch the bands, causing a change in the inductance in the oscillator circuits. The distension of the coils within the elastic bands is proportional to the change in the cross-sectional areas of the rib cage and abdomen respectively. Measurement of volumes such as V_T is accomplished by summing the signals from the two compartments. The validity of this technique is based on the assumption that lung volume change is described with two degrees of freedom—change in thoracic volume plus change in abdominal volume.

The RIP must be calibrated so that changes in rib cage and abdominal cross-sectional areas may be translated into volumes. This is usually accomplished by measuring the relative contribution of the inductances of the two coils as the actual volume change is recorded by means of a spirometer or pneumotachometer. If volumes are measured with two different breathing patterns, a "best-fit" line can be generated which is used to derive cali-

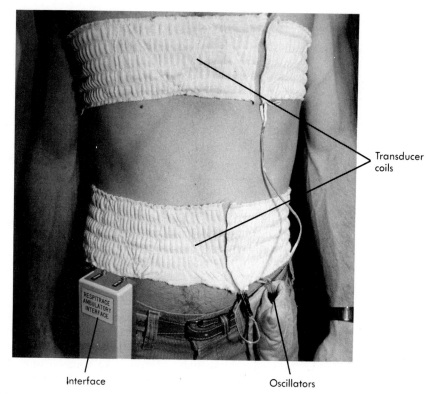

Transducer coils

Interface   Oscillators

FIG 9–32.
Respiratory inductive plethysmograph. A typical application of the respiratory inductive plethysmograph—two elastic bands with Teflon-coated coils sewn in are placed around the rib cage and abdomen. Oscillators connected to the coils (shown hanging from the belt) monitor changes in the cross-sectional areas of the two compartments as changes in inductance. By calibration, the changes in cross-sectional areas can be converted to volume changes in the two compartments to record V_T, rate, and timing of inspiration and expiration.

bration factors for each of the transducers. This may be expressed by the equation:

$$\frac{RC}{SP} + \frac{AB}{SP} = 1$$

where:

RC = the rib cage contribution to the tidal volume

AB = the abdominal contribution to the tidal volume

SP = the volume as measured by spirometry

The calibration "factors" thus obtained are applied to the output of the two channels as gains. Once calibrated, the RIP may be used to measure V_T and respiratory rate. The timing of inspiration (T_I), expiration (T_E), and total respiratory cycle time (T_{tot}) respectively are also easily determined. Various indices relating the extent of paradoxical or asynchronous movement of the rib cage and abdomen also may be quantified.

Because calibration is crucial to accurate measurement of volume change, a microprocessor or small dedicated computer is often used to derive calibration factors once the transducer bands have been placed. The computer also may be used to store and process data derived from the inductive plethysmograph. Graphic representations of the breathing pattern can be rapidly generated via computer.

Changes in body position may affect the calibration factors, so it is important to be able to quickly calibrate the inductive plethysmograph. Once calibration is complete, volume changes can be determined without physical connection to the subject's airway, as is the case with standard methods of assessing ventilation. This feature makes the inductive plethysmograph unique among devices for assessing ventilatory function. Respiratory inductive plethysmography is ideally suited to the study of breathing patterns in a variety of disorders. For subjects in whom connection of a spirometer to the airway is impractical, such as infants or mechanically ventilated patients, it may be the instrument of choice.

RECORDERS AND RELATED DEVICES

An integral part of pulmonary function testing is the recording of volume-time and flow-volume curves, distribution and ventilation tests, lung volumes, and DL_{CO} maneuvers. Many agencies recommend, and some require, inclusion of spirograms as part of the subject's medical record. The ATS has published specific guidelines for the presentation of spirometric waveforms according to the various test categories (see Chapter 11). Graphic representations of MEFV curves are useful for displaying a large amount of information in a succinct manner. Quality control of many instrument functions requires recording of analog signals. For example, to check the accuracy of a computerized method of measuring the FEV_1, the volume signal may be recorded using a device with a known timing accuracy. The FEV_1 then can be compared between the manual method with the software-derived value.

The kymograph is a rotating drum that carries chart paper. Kymographs have been used for recording various physiologic signals including respiratory movements (see Fig. 9–1). A kymograph is a mechanical recorder in the strictest sense. The displacement of the bell or bellows of the spirometer is transferred to a pen as the paper moves beneath it. The accuracy of the kymograph for timed measurements depends almost entirely on the accuracy of the drive motor, which may be easily verified. The kymograph is set rotating and a signal recorded. By introducing inflections in the signal at precise intervals, the time between inflections can be checked against the expected time. If the kymograph motor sticks or is irregular, timed measurements such as the FEV_1 will be in error.

Corrections of gas volumes to BTPS must be made because volume changes in the bell or bellows represent ATPS values. Some recording systems use calibrated chart paper to allow BTPS values to be read directly from the graph. These systems assume that the subject is at 37°C and that the spirometer is at 25°C. These conditions may not always be precise. In such instances, the volume or flow read directly from the graph may be incorrect. Several volume-displacement spirometers incorporate the kymograph recording systems.

A second type of device that uses mechanical recording has a constant-speed motor to provide paper movement along the time axis (X), while the spirometer provides the volume (Y) input. These recorders are referred to as strip chart recorders. This principle is used in many bellows types of spirometers and in some rolling-seal spirometers. For both kymographs and strip chart recorders, the accuracy of the timing motor that drives the graph paper is essential for valid measurements of flow. The paper speed should be at least 1 cm/sec for diagnostic purposes. Speeds of 2 to 3 cm/sec are preferable if timed volumes are to be calculated manually. The volume axis of the graph should have a scale of at least 5 mm/L, but 10 mm/L is preferable if manual calculations are to be done. In order to accurately reproduce the "start-of-test," the paper should be moving at a constant speed before recording the volume deflection; not all recorders fulfill this requirement. The recorder should be able to show at least 10 seconds of volume accumulation after recording begins. It is preferable to use a little more paper than to prematurely terminate the maneuver.

A second type of device for graphing respiratory maneuvers is the electronic X-Y recorder or plotter. This type of recorder has two axes that receive electrical input in the form of analog (DC voltage) signals. The signals drive small servo-controlled motors that regulate pen movement (Fig. 9–33). The X-axis pen can be driven either by an input voltage or by a built-in timer. The Y-axis can be driven by a volume signal, or any other analog signal.

The advantage of this instrument is that signals can be plotted against one another or against time. The same recorder can be used to plot flow-volume or volume-time curves. The signal generated by a pneumotachometer or other flow-sensing device can be recorded in spirographic form. Gas analyzers coupled to such an instrument allow recording of tests such as the SBN_2 and multiple-breath N_2 washout.

The electronic recorder is easy to calibrate. A known voltage can be applied and the recorder gains adjusted to produce an equivalent deflection. For example, 1 volt may equal 1 cm. Volume transducers that produce analog outputs then can be calibrated against the recorder so that a given volume change in the spirometer causes a proportional deflection on the recorder. Many

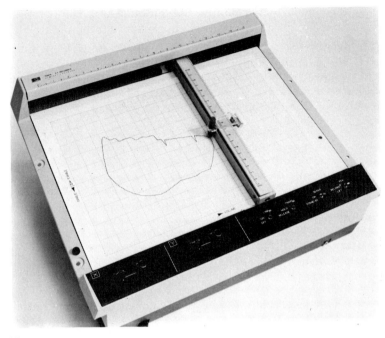

FIG 9–33.
X-Y recorder. An X-Y type of recording device capable of accepting analog inputs for flow, volume, gas concentration, or other typical DC signals, and graphing either against a time base, or plotting one input against another (loops). (Courtesy of Hewlett-Packard, San Diego.)

recorders feature a third dimension (i.e., X-Y-T) for recording superimposed time measurements. This feature is used when the time is not graphed on the X axis. A flow-volume loop typically plots flow on the vertical axis and volume on the horizontal axis. An X-Y-T recorder can interpose time marks or "tics" on the flow-volume tracing. These tic marks allow timed volumes to be obtained from a flow-volume tracing. Most electronic X-Y recorders have variable sensitivity on both axes. These adjustments permit greater flexibility than simple mechanical tracings. X-Y recorders, or plotters, offer a rapid means of graphing complex maneuvers. Most X-Y recorders are unable to faithfully reproduce the wide range of flows generated during a forced expiration in a healthy subject. For this reason, most automated systems that incorporate X-Y recorders store the signals in memory. The signals can then be relayed to the recording device at a slow speed so that rapidly changing flows are accurately represented.

Most pulmonary function systems display graphs and record spirograms or related tracings by computer (see Chapter 10). Computerized systems typically print graphics using thermal, ink jet, dot matrix, or laser techniques. Many automated pulmonary function systems provide for both computer-generated graphics and an alternate form of recording to allow manual measurements for comparison and quality control. A primary advantage of computer-generated graphics is that the data can be manipulated by the computer to provide corrections or linearization before being transformed into a printed tracing. In addition, computer-generated images can be displayed in formats not available with conventional recording devices, such as superimposed flow-volume curves. One disadvantage of computer-generated graphics is that if the stored data are incorrect, the graph of the data will be incorrect as well.

SELF-ASSESSMENT QUESTIONS

1. In order to record flow-volume curves with a water-sealed spirometer, which of the following is required:
   a. A potentiometer
   b. A kymograph
   c. A CO_2 absorber
   d. An He analyzer

2. A bellows-type volume-displacement spirometer is calibrated using a 3-L syringe. Volumes of 2.56 L, 2.57 L, and 2.54 L are measured. Which of the following is the most likely explanation:
   a. A worn potentiometer
   b. Sticking bellows
   c. Nonlaminar flow
   d. An exhausted water absorber

3. Resistance to flow through one-way and two-way valves is mainly determined by:
   a. The size of the valve leaflets
   b. The dead space volume of the valve body
   c. The number and types of pressure taps
   d. The tubing connected to the valve

4. Electronic integration is used to measure volume in which of the following spirometers:
   a. Pressure differential pneumotachometer
   b. Turbine spirometers
   c. Dry-rolling seal spirometers
   d. Ultrasonic flow sensors

5. A pressure-differential pneumotachometer is heated in order to:
   a. Correct the results from ATPS to BTPS
   b. Ensure development of laminar flow in the flow tube

   c. Prevent condensation on the resistive element
   d. Detect slight changes in gas flow

6. Which of the following devices are affected by the composition of the gas
   measured:
      I. Dry rolling-seal spirometers
     II. Pressure-differential pneumotachometers
    III. Respiratory inductive plethysmographs
    IV. Heated-wire pneumotachometers
   a. I, II, III, IV
   b. I, III, IV
   c. II, III
   d. II, IV

7. Which of the following analyzers requires an electrode to be heated to
   700°C:
   a. Zirconium fuel-cell O_2 analyzer
   b. Polarographic O_2 analyzer
   c. Mass spectrometer
   d. Thermal conductivity He analyzer

8. The purpose of the "chopper" motor in conventional infrared analyzers
   is to:
   a. Interrupt the flow of gas through the connecting bridge
   b. Create a slight vacuum to allow ionization
   c. Alternate the radiation to the reference and sample cells
   d. Protect the infrared detector from excessive exposure

9. The thermal conductivity principle is used in which of the following:
      I. Gas chromatographs
     II. He analyzers
    III. CO_2 analyzers
    IV. Emission spectroscopy
   a. I, II, III
   b. I, II
   c. II, IV
   d. III, IV

10. Po_2 electrodes are often polished using a coarse material such as pumice
    in order to:
    a. Remove blood or protein debris
    b. Remove metal ions plated out on the platinum wire
    c. Refresh the sensitive quartz glass membrane
    d. Reduce the actual amount of O_2 reaching the electrode tip

11. Which of the following devices utilizes the principle of luminesence quenching for measuring blood gas values:
    a. Co-oximeter
    b. Optode
    c. Transcutaneous Po_2 electrode
    d. Reflective spectrophotometer

12. The polarographic (Clark) electrode measures partial pressure of O_2 by:
    a. Detecting the presence of polarized light
    b. Measuring pH changes in an electrolyte exposed to O_2
    c. Chemically binding O_2 molecules to a heated wire
    d. Reducing O_2 molecules with a platinum cathode

13. Which of the following devices can be used to measure MetHb:
    a. Spectrophotometric oximeter
    b. Pulse oximeter
    c. Automated blood gas analyzer
    d. Reflective spectrophotometer

14. Which of the following conditions should a recorder meet in order for the FEV_1 to be accurately measured by a manual technique:
    I. The paper must be moving when recording starts
    II. The volume sensitivity must be 10 mm/L
    III. The paper speed must be 2 cm/sec
    IV. Expiratory flow must cause an upward deflection
    a. I, II, III, IV
    b. I, II, III
    c. I, IV only
    d. II, III only

15. Pulse oximeters are capable of measuring which of the following forms of Hb:
    a. O_2Hb, COHb
    b. COHb, MetHb
    c. RHb, total Hb
    d. RHb, O_2Hb

16. Motion artifact, such as shivering, affects the reading of a typical pulse oximeter by:
    a. Forcing the saturation toward a value of 85%
    b. Triggering the low pulse alarm
    c. Causing the saturation to be displayed as 100%
    d. Making the heart rate display (if present) inaccurate

17. The flow-type plethysmograph measures changes in box volume by:
    a. Measuring pressure changes at the subject's mouth
    b. Integrating flow through a sensor in the box wall
    c. Having the subject breathe through a pneumotachometer
    d. Connecting a respirometer to the box

18. Portable peak flow meters measure PEF by means of:
    a. A resistor with a moving scale indicator
    b. Pressure-differential flow sensor
    c. Volume-displacement flow sensor
    d. A flow-sensing thermistor

SELECTED BIBLIOGRAPHY

SPIROMETERS

American Thoracic Society: Standardization of spirometry—1987 update. *Am Rev Respir Dis* 136:1285, 1987.

Eichenhorn MS, Beauchamp RK, Harper PA, et al: An assessment of three portable peak flow meters. *Chest* 82:306, 1982.

Finucane KE, Egan BA, Dawson SV: Linearity and frequency response of pneumotachographs. *J Appl Physiol* 32:121, 1972.

Fitzgerald MX, Smith AA, Gaensler EA: Evaluation of 'electronic' spirometers. *N Engl J Med* 289:1283, 1973.

Gardner RM, Hankinson JL, West BJ: Evaluating commercially available spirometers. *Am Rev Respir Dis* 121:73, 1980.

Glindmeyer HW, Anderson ST, Diem JF, et al: A comparison of the Jones and Stead-Wells spirometers. *Chest* 73:596, 1978.

Hankinson JL: Pulmonary function testing in the screening of workers: guidelines for instrumentation, performance, and interpretation. *J Occup Med* 28:1081, 1986.

Nelson SB, Gardner RM, Crapo RO, et al: Performance evaluation of contemporary spirometers. *Chest* 97:288, 1990.

Permutt S (chairman): Office spirometry in clinical practice. *Chest* 74:298, 1978.

Sullivan WJ, Peters GM, Enright PL: Pneumotachographs: theory and clinical applications. *Respir Care* 29:736, 1984.

Wells HS, Stead WW, Rossing TD, et al: Accuracy of an improved spirometer for recording fast breathing. *J Appl Physiol* 14:451, 1959.

GAS ANALYZERS

Fowler KT: The respiratory mass spectrometer. *Phys Med Biol* 14:185, 1969.

Norton AC: Accuracy in pulmonary measurements. *Respir Care* 24:131, 1979.

Rebuck AS, Chapman KR: Measurement and monitoring of exhaled carbon dioxide. In Nochomovitz ML, Cherniack NS, editors: *Non-invasive respiratory monitoring*. New York, 1986, Churchill-Livingstone.

Sodal IE, Bowman RR, Filley GF: A fast response oxygen analyzer with high accuracy for respiratory gas measurement. *J Appl Physiol* 25:181, 1968.

Wilson RS, Laver MB: Oxygen analysis: advances in methodology. *Anesthesiology* 37:112, 1972.

BLOOD GAS ELECTRODES, OXIMETERS, AND RELATED DEVICES

Barker SJ, Tremper KK: Pulse oximetry: applications and limitations. In Tremper KK, Barker SJ, editors: *International Anesthesiology Clinics*. Boston, 1987, Little, Brown and Co.

Brown LJ: A new instrument for the simultaneous measurement of total hemoglobin, % oxyhemoglobin, % carboxyhemoglobin, % methemoglobin, and O_2 content. *IEEE Trans Biomed Engr* 27:132, 1980.

Divertie MB, McMichan JC: Continuous monitoring of mixed venous saturation. *Chest* 85:423, 1984.

Fahey PJ, Gruber S, Siska D, et al: Clinical evaluation of a new ear oximeter. *Am Rev Respir Dis* 127(suppl):129, 1983.

Huch A, Huch R: Transcutaneous, noninvasive monitoring of pO_2. *Hosp Pract* 11:43, 1976.

Opitz N, Lubbers DW: Theory and development of fluorescence based optical sensors: oxygen optodes. *Int Anesthesiol Clin* 25:177, 1987.

Pologue JA: Pulse oximetry: technical aspects of machine design. In Tremper KK, Barker SJ, editors: *International Anesthesiology Clinics*. Boston, 1987, Little, Brown and Co.

Rebuck AS, Chapman KR, D'urzo A: The accuracy and response characteristics of a simplified ear oximeter. *Chest* 80:860, 1983.

Severinghaus JW, Astrup PB: History of blood gas analysis. V: oxygen measurement. *J Clin Monit* 2:174, 1986.

Severinghaus JW, Bradley AF: Electrodes for blood Po_2 and Pco_2 determination. *J Appl Physiol* 13:515, 1958.

Shapiro BA, Cane RD, Chomka CM, et al: Preliminary evaluation of an intra-arterial blood gas system in dogs and humans. *Crit Care Med* 17:455, 1989.

Shapiro BA, Cane RD: Blood gas monitoring: yesterday, today, and tomorrow. *Crit Care Med* 17:573, 1989.

Taylor MB, Whitman JG: The current status of pulse oximetry: clinical value of continuous noninvasive oxygen saturation monitoring. *Anaesthesia* 41:943, 1986.

Tremper KK, Waxman KS: Transcutaneous monitoring of respiratory gases. In Nochomovitz ML, Cherniack NS, editors: *Non-invasive respiratory monitoring*. New York, 1986, Churchill-Livingstone.

Wiedemann HP, McCarthy K: Noninvasive monitoring of oxygen and carbon dioxide. *Clin Chest Med* 10:239, 1989.

PLETHYSMOGRAPHS

Bargeton D, Barres G: Time characteristics and frequency response of body plethysmographs: International Symposium on Body Plethysmography, Nijmegen. *Prog Respir Res* 4:2, 1969.

DuBois AB, Bothello SY, Bedell GN, et al: A rapid plethysmographic method for measuring thoracic gas volume: a comparison with nitrogen washout method for measuring functional residual capacity in normal subjects. *J Clin Invest* 35:322, 1956.

DuBois AB, Bothello SY, Comroe JH: A new method for measuring airway resistance in man using a body plethysmograph: values in normal subjects and in patients with respiratory disease. *J Clin Invest* 35:327, 1956.

Leith DE, Mead J: Principles of body plethysmography. National Heart, Lung, and Blood Institute-Division of Lung Diseases, 1974.

Lourenco RV, Chung SYK: Calibration of a body plethysmograph for measurement of lung volume. *Am Rev Respir Dis* 95:687, 1967.

RESPIRATORY INDUCTIVE PLETHYSMOGRAPHY

Chadhat TS, Watson H, Birch S, et al: Validation of respiratory inductive plethysmography using different calibration procedures. *Am Rev Respir Dis* 125:644, 1982.

Dolfin T, Duffy P, Wilkes DL, et al: Calibration of respiratory inductive plethysmography (Respitrace) in infants. *Am Rev Respir Dis* 126:577, 1982.

Konno K, Mead J: Measurement of the separate volume changes of rib cage and abdomen during breathing. *J Appl Physiol* 22:407, 1972.

Sackner MA: Monitoring of ventilation without physical connection to the airway: a review. In Scott FD, Raferty CV, Goulding L, editors: *ISAM Proceedings of the Third International Symposium on Ambulatory Monitoring.* London, 1982, Academic Press.

Tobin MJ: Noninvasive evaluation of respiratory movement. In Nochomovitz ML, Cherniack NS, editors: *Noninvasive Respiratory Monitoring.* New York, 1986, Churchill Livingstone.

RECORDERS

Gardner RM, Crapo RO, Billings RG, et al: Spirometry—what paper speed? (abstract). *Am Rev Respir Dis* 125:89, 1982.

Pulmonary Function Standards For Cotton Dust. 29 Code of Federal Regulations; 1910.1043 Cotton Dust, Appendix D. Occupational Safety and Health Administration, 1980.

10

Computers in the Pulmonary Function Laboratory

Computers have become an integral part of almost every pulmonary function testing system because they can efficiently perform the tasks typically involved in the reduction of pulmonary function data. These tasks include the solution of repetitive calculations, data storage and retrieval, printing of reports and graphs, processing of signals from various transducers, and automated control of the instruments themselves. The advantages of computerization of pulmonary function testing are that fewer errors occur in calculations, calibrations can be performed more consistently, and the variability of repeated measurements is reduced. Testing time is often dramatically reduced for both the subject and the technologist, allowing a wider variety of procedures to be performed. Repetition of effort-dependent tests or tests with questionable results is practical because computerization allows immediate inspection of the measurements.

The disadvantages of computerization of pulmonary function testing include decreased understanding and interaction on the part of the technologist. This problem may lead to invalid data being reported if computer-generated results are never questioned. Many computerized systems increase the complexity of the test. Not only must the technologist understand the physiology involved in the measurement technique, but the operation of the computer as well.

This chapter examines some of the general components and terminology used with small computer systems, automated data acquisition, important qualities in a pulmonary laboratory system, languages and programming, and some additional practical applications.

Classification of Computers

Several different levels of computerization are typically found in conjunction with pulmonary function testing systems.

Dedicated microprocessors.   Numerous small, portable spirometers utilize microprocessors to perform calculations and control various instrument functions such as digital display of data. Many flow-sensing spirometers and some volume-displacement devices use a dedicated microprocessor in conjunction with software stored on ROM chips (see Memory section, this chapter) to perform flow and volume measurements (Fig. 10–1). Other devices, such as pulse oximeters and capnographs, also employ dedicated microprocessors to perform unique sets of instructions. Dedicated microprocessors automate measurements, but typically allow only minimal changes (i.e., programming) by the user. Memory chips capable of retaining a large amount of data permit

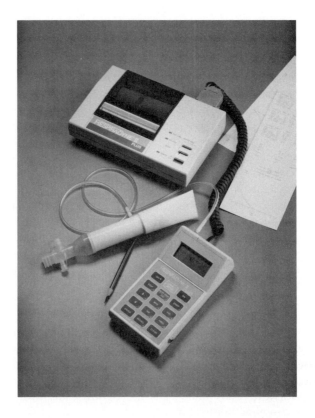

FIG 10–1.
Spirometer with dedicated microprocessor. A flow-based spirometer that uses a pressure differential pneumotachometer interfaced with a dedicated microprocessor. The computer executes instructions stored in read-only memory (ROM). Data for multiple patients may be stored in battery-powered random-access memory (RAM). The stored data may be "dumped" to another computer or directly to the small portable printer pictured. The entire unit is small enough to be easily transported to the bedside. (Courtesy of Sherwood Medical, St. Louis.)

sophisticated functions such as storage of multiple tests, error checking for reproducibility, and user selection of predicted values.

Microcomputers. The next higher level of computerization is the microcomputer, also referred to as a desktop or personal computer. Micro-computers may be incorporated directly into the pulmonary function system, or as stand-alone instruments interfaced to the spirometer and gas analyzers. The microcomputer-based system usually includes disk storage for programs and data, a high resolution video display, and an external printer. Most pulmonary function laboratory systems are now based on the microcomputer (Fig. 10–2). Laptop or notebook-size microcomputers have become widely used with flow-sensing devices for use as portable spirometry systems (see Chapter 9).

Microcomputers are also widely used in conjunction with blood gas analyzers or other laboratory instruments for which management of large amounts of data is necessary. Very fast microcomputers can be used in a network for multiple users. The performance of such a network depends on the speed of the computer, the operating system, and the type of user programs being run.

Minicomputers. Although the microcomputer has largely replaced the minicomputer, some laboratories interface several instruments or workstations to a central minicomputer. Minicomputers have historically been utilized to allow multiple users to access data and programs simultaneously. Pulmonary function equipment, exercise testing equipment, and blood gas analyzers can all be interfaced as part of a multiuser system. The selection of a minicomputer vs. a mainframe depends on the number of users and the types of tasks to be performed. Minicomputers commonly have been employed in laboratory information systems. Multiuser operating systems (see Operating Systems, this Chapter) allow blood gas instrument automation and availability of test results to multiple terminals. Recent advances in microcomputer technology have made networked computers practical on microcomputer as well as mini-computer.

Mainframe computers. Mainframe computers are employed primarily for hospital information systems. As such they are supported by terminals and by networked microcomputers. Pulmonary function testing typically requires a smaller computer system. However, transferring data from the microcomputer used with pulmonary function equipment to the hospital information system requires integration of both types of computers. The need to deliver pulmonary function or blood gas data to referring physicians quickly and accurately has fueled the growth of micro-to-mainframe systems.

A great deal of overlap exists between the various levels of computerization commonly found in the laboratory setting. Dedicated microprocessors can be

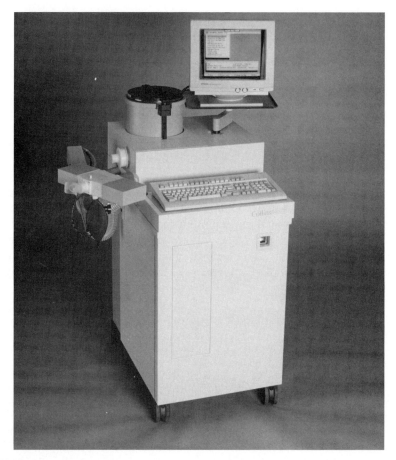

FIG 10–2.
Computerized pulmonary function system. An automated pulmonary function system including Stead-Wells spirometer, gas analyzers, and computer-controlled breathing circuit. This system for performing spirometry, lung volumes and $D_{L_{CO}}$ is interfaced to an MS-DOS microcomputer. The microcomputer allows rapid processing of data, including calculation of test parameters, BTPS and STPD corrections, and display of graphs. Data may be stored on either a floppy diskette or hard disk. The computer also allows trends in patient data to be recalled and displayed. (Courtesy of Warren E. Collins, Inc., Braintree, Mass.)

used to collect data, such as spirometry, at the bedside. The data can then be brought to the laboratory and "dumped" to a microcomputer for permanent storage or printing of results. Microcomputers can be utilized as intelligent terminals, capable of communicating with minicomputers or mainframe computers as well as performing specific functions such as pulmonary function tests.

Selecting a Computer System

The selection of a computerized pulmonary function system should be based on a careful evaluation of the number and complexity of the tests to be performed. Of equal importance is the volume of data to be stored, and the type of reports to be generated. Many applications, such as bedside spirometry, may require only minimal computerization. In some instances, the best computer may be none at all. It may be cost effective to use a system requiring manual measurement of spirograms, particularly if the volume of tests performed is low. However, when choosing a computerized pulmonary function system, the following guidelines may be helpful:

1. Define the *tasks* or types of tests that the system will be expected to perform. Important questions are:

- What tests are required (spirometry, lung volumes, plethysmography, $D_{L_{CO}}$)?
- How many patients will be tested per day, or per month?
- How much data will be stored, and for how long?
- What types of reports are to be generated?
- Will the system be used for other purposes in addition to pulmonary function studies?
- Will the data be transferred to other computer systems or be available to other users?

It is important to rank these characteristics in order of importance.

2. Once the tasks have been clearly defined, the *software* best able to perform the tests should be selected. Each of the tasks identified in step 1 should be compared with the software being evaluated. For example, if only screening spirometry is to be performed, the software will probably not be required to maintain multiple data files on an individual patient for a long time.

3. The actual computer *hardware* that supports the pulmonary function testing software should be the final element in the selection process. In some instances, the manufacturer may offer only one hardware configuration. Many manufacturers now design software that operates on a range of compatible systems. This allows the user to select a computer that meets the present needs (i.e., the tasks identified in step 1) and permits future expansion. Compatibility of the testing software is an important aspect of hardware selection. This is especially true as computer technology has tended to advance more rapidly than that of spirometers or gas analyzers. Software written with future compatibility in mind allows the user to upgrade the computer hardware to take advantage of faster processors and increased storage capabilities while maintaining consistency in testing methods. Ideally, the computer selected should allow

software upgrades as well, rather than require a new computer to implement more sophisticated programs. Modular design of the computer system is advantageous in that it permits the user to change part of the system, such as a printer, while retaining the remainder of the hardware. If more than one hardware option is available, the system chosen should maximize functions offered by the software.

Choosing a laboratory computer for purposes other than pulmonary function testing, such storage of blood gas data or text processing, may differ slightly from the scheme outlined here, but the general approach of defining the tasks to be performed before deciding on software or hardware is useful.

Computer Systems

Most microcomputer and minicomputer systems can be divided into component parts similar to those depicted in Figure 10–3. These components are typical of small computer systems in general, but many have functions specific to pulmonary function testing.

Microprocessor or Central Processing Unit (CPU)

The *microprocessor,* or *CPU,* refers to the "brain" of the computer. Microprocessors are sometimes referred to as the central processing unit, or CPU. The microprocessor performs most, if not all, of the instructions provided by the software. These instructions typically include calculations and storing and retrieving of data from memory. The CPU also controls peripheral devices such as video displays, printers, and disk drives. Microprocessors are classified by the number of "bits" of information that can be handled at one time. A bit is a 0 or 1 in the binary number system. Commonly used in laboratory computer systems are 8-bit, 16-bit, and 32-bit CPUs. Early microcomputers were based on 8-bit processors, capable of addressing 65,536 memory locations. Newer processors (i.e., 16- and 32-bit) are capable of addressing 16 million or more memory addresses. In general, 16-bit and 32-bit processors can perform calculations more rapidly than smaller microprocessors. Their size allows manipulation of large numbers without breaking the number into smaller parts. They also can address more memory directly and are capable of operating at faster clock speeds.

Clock speed refers to the rate at which the microprocessor operates and is usually quantified in terms of megahertz (millions of cycles per second, or MHz). The fastest microcomputer processors operate at speeds in excess of 60 MHz. The actual speed with which the computer is capable of carrying out a task, such as writing a file to disk or retrieving information from memory, depends on the speed of the other computer components as well as the CPU. Fast micropro-

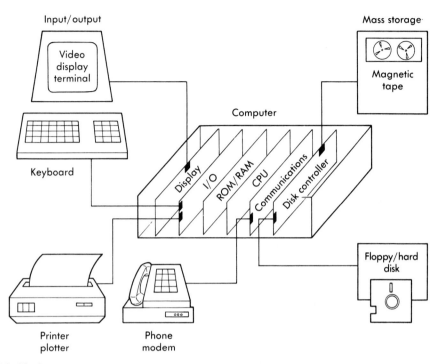

FIG 10–3.
Components of a small computer system. The computer itself includes a central processing unit (CPU or microprocessor) connected to various divisions of memory (ROM/RAM), input/output processors (I/O boards), and controllers for the video display, disk drives, and communication devices. Typical input/output devices include the video display, the keyboard, and printers or plotters. Communications usually include a serial port and modem for transmission of data over conventional telephone lines. Mass storage devices include magnetic tape drives, floppy and hard disk drives, optical (laser) drives, and CD-ROM drives. Many small computer systems allow for addition of various components simply by plugging in different "cards." Not shown is an interface such as might be used to connect the computer to a spirometer or gas analyzers (see Fig. 10–4).

cessors require equally fast input/output devices (see Input/Output section, this chapter).

In order to use very fast microprocessors, most systems rely on special techniques to compensate for slower components. A common technique is "caching." Caching places information into a special memory area, or cache. The cache usually consists of very fast memory. Caching speeds up storage and retrieval from slower devices such as disk drives or regular memory. For example, data being read into the computer from a disk drive is stored in a cache. Then if the same data are needed again, they can be retrieved from the cache rather than accessing the slower disk drive. Caching can dramatically improve the performance of most computers.

Special microprocessors, called co-processors, work in conjunction with the main microprocessor to speed up certain operations. Math co-processors perform arithmetic-intensive calculations. Computers with math co-processors typically perform tasks involving calculations much faster than systems without co-processors. Some advanced microprocessors have math co-processor and memory caching capabilities designed into the CPU itself. Co-processors also may be used for highly specific tasks such as controlling high resolution video displays or managing large blocks of memory.

In addition to faster clock speeds, 16-bit and 32-bit processors are capable of multi-tasking, or running multiple programs simultaneously. Multi-tasking requires a special operating system (see "Operating Systems," this chapter). Multi-tasking permits the user to perform one task in the foreground, while the computer performs other tasks in the background. For example, a multi-tasking testing system could allow spirometry to be performed on one patient while the report from another patient is being printed.

The same types of processors, when used with an appropriate operating system, also allow multiple users to share the computer and peripheral devices such as printers or disk storage. This arrangement is referred to as a network. The network typically consists of a primary powerful computer. This computer is called the server. Other microcomputers are then linked by one of several types of networks. Data can be transferred between any two computers linked by the system. The server usually maintains programs and data that all of the networked users need.

The combination of multi-tasking and multiuser capabilities offers numerous possibilities to enhance laboratory data management. Some multi-tasking systems permit the user to perform diagnostic testing in real time while the computer prints reports or transmits data to another system in the background. A network allows pulmonary function testing to be performed at one terminal while blood gas data is entered at a second terminal, physicians review test results at a third station, and clerical staff print final reports at a fourth work station.

Most commercially available computerized pulmonary function testing systems utilize microcomputers. The typical system is based on either 16-bit or 32-bit CPU architecture. While many laboratories do not require multi-tasking or networking, the availability of microprocessors and software that support these functions permits expansion of the system as utilization increases.

Memory

Memory may be classified as read-only memory (ROM) or random access memory (RAM). The computer's *ROM* usually contains the BIOS (i.e., basic input/output system). The BIOS provides often used instructions such as those for controlling the video display or checking random access memory when the computer is powered on. Incompatibility between certain programs and computers sometimes results from differences in the BIOS. The ROM cannot be changed by a user program, but can be altered if the chip containing the instructions is replaced.

PROMs (programmable ROM chips) or EPROMS (erasable programmable ROM chips) are often used in pulmonary function testing systems. By placing instructions to communicate with a particular piece of equipment on a PROM, it is easy to change to different equipment — just install a new PROM. PROMs and EPROMS are often included in the interface between the computer and the pulmonary function testing hardware (see Data Acquisition and Instrument Control, this chapter).

The *RAM* available in a computer refers to the amount of memory available for user programs. The RAM is normally occupied by the computer's operating system (see Operating Systems, this chapter) and the user's application programs. Both the operating system software and application programs are loaded from an external source such as a disk or tape. Many microcomputers maximize their use of available memory by breaking the application program into modules. Only those segments required for a certain test are loaded. This technique conserves RAM but may slow down overall program execution if many modules are loaded and unloaded. Advances in chip technology have made large amounts of RAM relatively inexpensive, so even microcomputers can manage extremely large and complicated programs.

Both RAM and ROM are quantified in terms of memory units, or *bytes.* Each byte contains 8 bits (either 0 or 1). A byte can take on 256 distinct values. Two bytes taken together form a *word* which contains a 16-bit number. Each memory byte or word can be used to store either data or instructions. A kilobyte, or Kb, is the equivalent of 1024 bytes; 1024 Kb of memory is also referred to as a megabyte or Mb. Most small computer systems use from 640 Kb up to 4 Mb. An 8-bit microprocessor can only address 64 Kb of memory without special adaptations. Early 16-bit CPUs were able to address up to 1024 Kb by combining two 16-bit numbers to derive a 20-bit address. Newer 16-bit and 32-bit microprocessors have address spaces of 16 Mb. Although these microprocessors can physically address 16 Mb or more, most systems utilize a more manageable 2 to 8 Mb. In addition to the ability to accommodate large amounts of real working memory (RAM), many advanced microprocessors, such as the Intel* 80386 and 80486, also can provide as much as 1024 Mb (i.e., a gigabyte) of virtual memory. Virtual memory is mapped into the computer's physical memory. When more memory is needed, the contents of the physical memory are swapped out to a disk drive or other storage device. The computer's operating

---

* Intel is a registered trademark of Intel Corporation.

system has to manage the swapping of actual and virtual memory contents.

Another means of increasing the amount of memory available in the microcomputer is by using bank-switched memory. A special memory board that contains banks of RAM chips is typically added to the computer. Bank-switching (also referred to as expanded memory) allows more memory to be installed in the computer than can actually be addressed by the microprocessor. A special memory manager program then interacts with the user application program to utilize the extra memory banks. Bank-switched memory is very fast, but in some operating systems, the added RAM can only be used for program data, not for the program itself.

Most pulmonary function application programs do not require large amounts of memory in order to run, but more data can be held in memory at one time and sophisticated calculations performed with more available RAM. Storage and high-resolution display of the data from multiple spirometry efforts such as flow-volume curves, may require considerable amounts of RAM. In addition, the amount of RAM available may determine how many different applications can run in a multi-tasking system.

The storage capacity of devices such as tapes, diskettes, and hard disks (see Mass Storage Devices, this chapter) is often classified in terms of either kilobytes or megabytes.

Input/Output Devices

Input/output (I/O) devices are components of the computer system through which data are either entered or displayed. These include the monitor or CRT, the keyboard, pointing devices such as a mouse, mass storage devices like disk or tape drives, printers, modems for communications over telephone lines, and special interfaces between the computer and analog output instruments. Some I/O devices, such as disk drives, modems, and special interfaces perform both input and output. Other I/O devices are for input only, such as the keyboard or mouse. Monitors and printers are examples of output-only devices.

Most of these peripheral devices are quite complex, often using highly specialized integrated circuits (i.e., chips), or even their own microprocessor, to carry out various tasks. Many small computer systems are modular (see Fig. 10–3), utilizing a main circuit board (i.e., mother board) into which various I/O cards may be plugged. This open architecture design is quite flexible and allows systems to be tailored to very specific needs, such as those found in the pulmonary function laboratory. The ability to upgrade a computer system, such as adding a larger disk drive or more memory, is enhanced by being able to replace individual components rather than the entire system. Advanced chip technologies now allow many of the functions previously assigned to specific I/O cards to be placed directly on the mother board. While this limits the flexibility of the system somewhat, the overall size of the computer can be reduced dramatically.

Mass Storage Devices

Mass storage devices include magnetic tape systems, "floppy" and "hard" disks, and optical disks. *Magnetic tape systems* are usually employed on large multiuser systems, such as mainframe computers, where a large amount of data must be maintained. Small tape drive units are sometimes used for data storage where a large volume of data is recorded but does not require rapid or random retrieval. Some tape units are employed as inexpensive backups to floppy or hard disk systems.

On microcomputer-based pulmonary function testing systems, *floppy disk drives,* or a combination of floppy disk and hard drive, are most commonly used. Several different sizes of floppy disk drives are widely available. Common diskette sizes include 5¼ inches and 3½ inches. The volume of data that can be stored on a diskette is described by the number of tracks available and the density with which the data is recorded. The 5¼-inch diskettes hold either 360 Kb or, in the high-density version, 1.2 Mb of data. The smaller 3½-inch diskettes also come in two capacities, 720 Kb and 1.44 Mb. New diskette technology has doubled the capacity on 3½-inch diskettes so that they can be formatted to hold up to 2.88 Mb. Many microcomputers are supplied with one or the other sizes of floppy drives, but some systems utilize both to facilitate transfer of data between computers. The chief advantages of floppy disks for program and data storage are that they are inexpensive, lightweight, and portable. The primary disadvantages of diskettes are that they can be damaged rather easily, are very slow compared with hard disks, and eventually wear out.

The *hard disk,* or *fixed drive,* uses a technology similar to that of the floppy disk, except that instead of a flexible plastic disk, a solid metal platter is employed. The hard drive allows a much greater amount of data to be stored in approximately the same space as a floppy drive. Data on a hard disk can be accessed much more quickly. Hard disks are commonly described by the total storage space provided. Hard disks of 80 to 200 Mb are commonly used for small laboratory systems. Three hundred- to 600-Mb disks are employed in some high volume systems. The advantages of the fixed disk over floppy drives are the large amount of data contained on a single device and the speed with which the data can be accessed. Disadvantages of the hard disk include the necessity of backing up large amounts of information (on floppy disks or tape) and keeping track of hundreds or even thousands of files on a single drive. Advances in hard disk technology have reduced the rate of mechanical failures as well as the cost to store a megabyte of information. Sophisticated software tools are available, and usually required, to manage hard disks. Most of these programs feature file management, diagnostics, and backup features. Several manufacturers offer removable hard disks that allow large amounts of information to be physically moved from one computer to another, or to be removed for security purposes.

The *optical drive,* or laser drive, is a high-capacity storage device that uses a laser to write information on a plastic disk. The simplest type of optical disk is not erasable. Data can only be written to the disk once. These types of devices are commonly referred to as "WORM" drives (i.e., Write Once Read Many). A more sophisticated type of optical drive uses a combination of laser and magnetic pulses to write data on the plastic disk. The data then may be erased or modified by altering the state of the magnetic pulses. Either type of optical disk is ideally suited for storage of large amounts of data such as flow-volume or other physiologic waveforms. Optical drives are very useful for storage of reference information, or for archiving data that must be retained for later retrieval, such as ECG or pulmonary function data. Nonerasable optical disks are capable of holding approximately 900 Mb of data, so that several thousands of routine pulmonary function tests can be archived on a single volume. Erasable optical disks can hold slightly less, approximately 600 Mb. The drive itself is approximately the size of a conventional hard drive and the laser disk about the size of a 5¼-inch floppy.

In addition to optical drives used for data storage, a read-only version, *CD-ROM,* is widely available. CD-ROMs are most commonly used to store reference material. The capacity of the CD-ROM is similar to the erasable optical drive. The hardware for the drive is less complex, as data are read from the disk but never written. CD-ROMs that provide access to large medical databases such as Index Medicus are available.

A related type of pseudo-storage device is the electronic disk or RAM disk. The RAM disk is a disk drive defined in the RAM memory of the computer. It has no physical parts, but acts like a very fast disk drive. RAM disks are ideal for programs that access the disk often for data manipulation or creation of temporary files because they are fast. However, because the RAM disk is not a permanent storage device, any data contained on it must be transferred to a floppy or hard disk before powering down the computer.

Software

Software refers to all of the instructions contained in the memory, both ROM and RAM, of the computer. These sets of instructions are referred to as *programs.* Most microcomputer-based systems utilize an operating system that controls the computer's various functions, and application programs that perform the specific tasks which the user selects, such as pulmonary function testing, word processing, or database management. Most application programs are loaded into the computer from disk, but many basic functions are contained on ROM chips. This is particularly true of many portable spirometry units that feature a dedicated microprocessor (see Fig. 10–1). In these devices, all software is contained on chips (PROMs or EPROMs) and is immediately available when the unit is powered on.

Data Acquisition and Instrument Control

The primary advantages of computerized pulmonary function systems is the ability to process analog signals from various transducers, such as spirometers, pneumotachometers, and gas analyzers, to automatically acquire data. Equally important is the computer's capacity to control instrument functions, such as valve switching and recording, to allow the technologist to manage complex test maneuvers. Both data acquisition and instrument control are implemented by means of an interface (Fig. 10–4) between the computer and various types of pulmonary function equipment.

One of the primary devices used to interface pulmonary function equipment to a computer is the analog-to-digital (A/D) converter. The A/D converter accepts

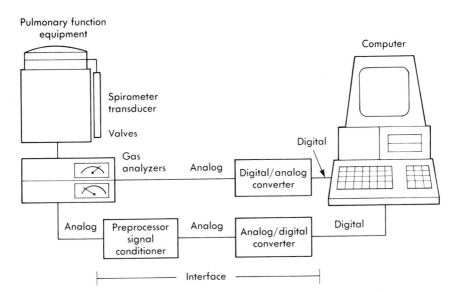

FIG 10–4.
Computer interface for pulmonary function testing. Components of a typical interface between a spirometer, gas analyzers, and a small computer are represented. Analog signals from the pulmonary function equipment are preprocessed so that the analog-to-digital (A/D) converter can manage them. The A/D converter then transforms a voltage, usually DC, into digital data in the form of a binary or hexadecimal number. The digital data is then processed by the computer for calculations, display, and storage. In order for the computer to control various instrument functions, a digital-to-analog (D/A) converter transforms digital data into appropriate analog signals to control system functions such as opening valves or adding gas to the breathing circuit.

an analog signal and transforms the signal into a digital value. The analog signal is usually a DC voltage in the range of either 0 to 10 volts, or -5 to $+5$ volts. Analog-to-digital converters are classified by the number of bits (binary digits) into which they convert the signal. The greater the number of bits, the greater the resolution of the input signal in the resulting digital value. A 12-bit converter can transform a voltage into a number represented by 000000000000 to 111111111111 as a binary number. In the decimal numbering system, this corresponds to a range of 0 to 4096, or 2^{12}. For example, a 10-L spirometer might produce an analog signal ranging from 0 to 10 volts, with 1 volt equal to 1 L. If this spirometer is connected to a 12-bit converter, the signal can be divided into 4096 parts. This arrangement provides a resolution of about 0.0024 volts or 2.4 mL over the 10-L volume range. The smallest volume change that could be detected by the computer would be 2.4 mL for this spirometer system. Some transducers, such as a flow sensor that measures bidirectional flow, have a voltage range of ± 5 volts. A 12-bit converter connected to this transducer would have a similar resolution of 0.0024 volts, because the full scale input range is still 10 volts. However, the actual flow resolution would depend on the sensitivity of the transducer, or the range of flows that produce a -5 to $+5$ voltage. Twelve-bit converters are recommended for most volume- and flow-sampling applications. Eight-bit and 10-bit converters are sometimes used for functions that do not require high resolution.

In addition to the resolution of the A/D converter, the rate at which data are sampled affects the accuracy of the data gathered. Most A/D converter systems have from 8 to 16 distinct channels. Each channel is capable of accepting a separate analog input. The highest sampling rates are usually attained when conversions are done on only one or two channels. For tests in which a great deal of accuracy is required and in which the signal changes very rapidly, such as a forced expiration, conversions may be performed on a single channel. The Nyquist sampling theorem indicates that the sampling rate (i.e., the number of samples taken per second) should be at least twice the frequency of the sampled waveform. The highest frequency components of a typical peak flow signal are within 0 to 12 Hz (cycles per second). The high-frequency components of an FVC maneuver are somewhat less. High-speed converters can perform more than 20,000 conversions per second on a single channel. As more channels are included in the conversion, the rate for each channel is typically reduced. Most computerized pulmonary function systems sample data on multiple channels at rates of 100 Hz or greater. These high rates usually exceed the frequency bandwidth of breathing maneuvers by more than a factor of 2. The maximum accuracy is attained by matching the output of a particular transducer, such as a spirometer, to an A/D converter with the appropriate sampling rate and voltage resolution.

High sampling rates and high-resolution conversion require very fast microprocessors. Increased memory for storing large amounts of raw data are also needed. The lowest sampling rate that will allow acceptable resolution of the signal also allows the greatest flexibility in terms of processing times and computations. Another approach to sampling for volumes or flow signals is to measure the time required for a predetermined volume or flow change. For example, the number of clock ticks that occur for a volume change of 100 mL can be measured, and flow calculated. This technique typically requires a spirometer that includes a position encoder or that generates pulses for each volume increment. The accuracy of an encoder system depends on the resolution of the clock during rapid flow and the size of the volume increment.

Some analog signals require special handling before A/D conversion. Computations on the digital data also may be included in the conversion. These signal-conditioning functions are often included in the interface between the test instrument and the computer. Signal conditioning is also referred to as "preprocessing." Most transducers include amplifiers that allow setting of offsets and gains. These are forms of signal preprocessing. A common example of signal preprocessing involves transforming a resistance into a voltage so that A/D conversion is possible. Other preprocessing functions of an interface include peak signal detection, counters, and timers. Many analog-to-digital converter systems have the capacity to process and store data in their own memory (RAM) until the computer requests it. This on-board storage allows high-speed data acquisition by the interface and provides flexibility in programming the computer. The "smart" interface performs data acquisition and holds the information so that the computer can retrieve the data at a slower rate. In addition, the interface may make computations and corrections before the computer retrieves the data. Smart interfaces permit data to be transmitted in any one of several formats, such as ASCII codes.* Standardized formats allow modification of the software which reads the data. This arrangement permits the computer or software to be upgraded without replacing the entire testing system.

Many instruments such as pulse oximeters and capnographs utilize their own microprocessor and A/D board to display data. Such instruments typically have a communication port so that an external computer or printer can be interfaced. The RS-232 serial port is typically used, but other faster types (i.e., RS-422, RS-485) are becoming commonplace. A "serial" port transmits data 1 bit at a time, usually in a fixed pattern. The speed at which the transmission occurs is called the baud rate (i.e., bits/second). The baud rate may vary from 300 to more than 19,000, depending on the type of connection and equipment involved. The pattern of bits needed to transmit a byte of data may range from 8 to 10. Along with the data bits are extra bits to signal the beginning or end of a byte. Most computers that have a serial port can be interfaced to the instrument using a standardized protocol. Some laboratory instruments support parallel ports. Parallel ports transmit entire bytes of data at one time rather than in bits

---

* American Standard Code for Interchange of Information.

(i.e., serially). Parallel ports are typically used for interconnection with printers.

Another function of the interface between the computer and the test instrument is the conversion of digital information from the computer into analog signals. This is accomplished by a digital-to-analog (D/A) converter that can be viewed as the complement to the A/D converter described above. In this case, a digital input results in an analog output voltage proportional to the value of the input byte. In its simplest form, the D/A converter acts as a relay switch between the computer and an instrument. For this reason, it is commonly referred to as digital I/O or digital expansion. A nonzero value sent from the computer can be used to activate an electrically operated valve or solenoid. The converter, on receiving the digital input, generates the required voltage (typically 5 volts DC). Digital-to-analog conversion allows the computer to control functions such as activating kymographs or recorders, switching valves in automated circuits, and opening solenoids to add oxygen, helium, or other gases. Digital-to-analog signal conversion allows the user to check various instrument functions that are normally under software control or to perform automatic calibration. This is accomplished by diagnostic procedures built into the application software. Diagnostic software helps in tracking down equipment problems by isolating those attributable to the transducers (i.e., spirometer, gas analyzers) from those which may result from failure of the computer hardware or software.

Manual pulmonary function systems provide alternate means of controlling various functions that are normally computer controlled. Manual controls allow use of the spirometer, gas analyzers, and associated equipment, even if the computer becomes unavailable.

Computerized Pulmonary Function Testing Systems

The interdependence of pulmonary function equipment and computers makes the capabilities of the computer system especially important. The technology of small computers and their peripherals advances very rapidly. For this reason, most users cannot anticipate all the possible applications that the computer may have in the future. An important consideration is whether the hardware and software is both "upward" and "downward" compatible. Upwardly compatible hardware means that the computer itself can be enhanced and still perform tests with the same spirometer or gas analyzers. This type of compatibility is often determined by the interface used as described earlier in this chapter. A related concern may be whether the computer system can accommodate enhancements to the testing system, such as the addition of equipment to perform $D_{L_{CO}}$ tests, body plethysmography, or exercise/metabolic studies.

Upward and downward compatibility in software means that a new version of a program (i.e., "upward" changes) does not invalidate or render unusable previously generated data. If a program enhancement allows new or more accurate data to be generated while allowing previously stored data to be used, the program is "downward" compatible. This type of compatibility is especially important for longitudinal studies in which subjects may be tested over a period of years. Most vendors of pulmonary function systems continually enhance both hardware and software. Conversion programs are often used to update previously generated data files so that they can be used with the upgraded hardware or software.

Accuracy and Dependability

The most important quality of a computerized pulmonary function system is its ability to dependably perform accurate measurements. In addition to accuracy of the transducers (i.e., spirometer, gas analyzers), the computer hardware and software must be designed so that overall accuracy is not compromised by the automated acquisition of data. Careful selection and implementation of data acquisition hardware (see Data Acquisition and Instrument Control, this chapter), appropriate sampling rates, and controlling software is typically the responsibility of the manufacturer. The simplest means for users to assess the accuracy of a computerized system is to compare computer-generated results with those obtained by manual calculation. A means of recording raw signals from spirometers and gas analyzers, as well as documentation of all equations used by the software, is required for this type of comparison. Testing normal subjects, such as lab personnel, is typically easier than using a test simulator. Devices that furnish reproducible flow signals (see Chapter 11) provide controlled inputs for repeated testing. Digitized spirometry waveforms may be used to simulate the FVC maneuver using a computer-controlled syringe, or simply to check the accuracy of the software that reduces the data obtained. Although not practical for most laboratories, the use of standardized waveforms is recommended by the ATS for the validation of spirometers and spirometry software. If the accuracy of any test cannot be easily verified, the system may be difficult to maintain day to day.

The software required for data acquisition in spirometry, lung volume determinations, $D_{L_{CO}}$, and plethysmography is complex. It is relatively rare that a program is completely free of errors. This high level of complexity requires that the program developer offer continuing program upgrades and support. A system for documentation of hardware or program modifications and validation of measurements should be maintained.

Computerized pulmonary function testing can enhance the quality of the data obtained. Most pulmonary function software checks for errors during data acquisition and after results have been calculated. Examples of this include calculation of the back-extrapolated volume during spirometry and analysis of the reproducibility of the FVC and FEV_1 (see Chapter 11).

Computerized and Manual Testing

A second important quality of any automated system is its ability to perform nonautomated tests. As noted previously, manual calculation of component tests is the best means of assessing the accuracy of the measurements. Small computers and peripherals such as disk drives, printers, and interfaces are typically complex. Failure of a single component can often disable a computer-dependent pulmonary function testing system. In a high-volume laboratory, a computer failure may cause cancellation of many procedures.

A serious shortcoming of some computerized systems is that all graphic and tabular data are computer generated. No analog recording system may be available. A computer malfunction under these circumstances often means that no data can be recorded. In some circumstances, the technologist may need to alter the exact method or sequence that the automated system normally requires. A valuable asset is a computer system that allows user intervention for data verification or modification of the test maneuver sequence.

Software Design

The ease of use of a computerized pulmonary function system is one of the most desirable qualities of an automated testing system. The computer should speed up the test routine while enhancing the quality and accuracy of the data obtained. The software should allow the necessary repetition of maneuvers required for obtaining valid data. The program should be able to hold at least three FVC maneuvers in memory for comparison and selection. The ability to store more than three FVC maneuvers may be important in some applications. The software should accommodate two to four slow VC maneuvers, two to four MVV efforts, one or more lung volume determinations, two to four $D_{L_{CO}}$ tests, and multiple panting maneuvers if plethysmography is implemented. The software should not constrict the user in choosing which data will be reported. Some software designs do not allow the technologist to "override" the computer. For example, a computerized spirometry system may select the largest FVC recorded to be reported. If the largest FVC measurement is in error because of a leak or similar problem, the user should be able to select an alternate data set.

Carefully designed software makes allowances for the degree of cooperation of the subject tested. The software must be able to handle unusual occurrences, such as the subject interrupting the sequence of the test. Sequence breaks should not result in loss of data or system lockup. Computerization of spirometry requires pattern recognition algorithms for determining the start and end of test. These algorithms should be implemented so that various breathing patterns can be accommodated. Lung volume determinations or $D_{L_{CO}}$ measurements require computer control of breathing circuits, valves, and gas analyzers. Automated testing should be able to handle unusual occurrences, such as coughing.

The capacity for user modification is an important aspect of well-designed software. The simplest means of customizing software is to build modifiable parameters into the program. The user may then select the desired options and save them in a configuration file. User-selected program options allow the software to meet a wide variety of laboratory needs. Important areas that should be user modifiable include report formats, reference values, and test sequences. Standards, such as those set forth by the ATS for spirometry and $D_{L_{CO}}$, should be user selectable when appropriate. This is an important asset when a standard permits different methods of calculating or reporting results.

Many systems employ a *turnkey* approach in software design. The program is written so that the operator may perform tests with little or no knowledge of what the computer is doing. Turnkey systems are best for simple maneuvers that only require minimal intervention. This software method allows the technologist to concentrate on eliciting the maximal effort from the subject. The turnkey approach, however, does not completely eliminate the need for the technologist to perform some computer-related procedures, such as backing up patient data. Another drawback of turnkey systems is lack of flexibility in the choice of options the technologist may have.

Most pulmonary function software uses *menu-driven* programs. Menu-driven programs prompt the user by using a list of choices. The choices are typically displayed somewhere on the video display. The list may be numbered or arranged alphabetically. Each choice usually can be selected by a single keyboard entry. A well designed menu-driven program allows the user to select tasks quickly. Menu-driven programs can be learned without prolonged orientation. Many menu-driven applications provide a means of pointing at specific menu items. This may be accomplished using the directional keys on a keyboard or by using a pointing device such as a mouse. A popular implementation of the menu-driven approach incorporates the use of window-based applications. As the user navigates among different menu options, a series of windows open on the video display, either side by side or overlaying one another. Each window contains a related set of options. The window technique helps the user decide what input is required.

Hardware and Software Documentation

Documentation provided by the manufacturer or programmer is as important as any of the previously described attributes for computerized pulmonary function systems. The complexity of data acquisition programs and of the computer's operating system necessitates thorough documentation. Appropriate documentation includes all the information necessary to install the system and make it operational. The documentation should be suitable even for the novice pulmonary function computer user. Information should be included that describes the interconnection of all peripheral devices. Initialization or installation programs that must be executed should be fully described. If the system is provided in several different configurations (i.e., different computers or printers), each should be clearly described, and separate instructions should be provided for each component.

Every segment of the pulmonary function application software should be carefully outlined. Diagrams of screen displays and printouts should be included. Step-by-step instructions related to user input are required. Examples, either in text format or as sample data from the computer itself, are invaluable for training new users on complicated systems. Most commercially available pulmonary function systems use generic operating systems such as MS-DOS,* OS/2,† or UNIX.‡ Some manufacturers support their own proprietary operating systems. The functions of the operating system, such as file handling and backup of data, should be fully documented along with the pulmonary function application programs. A useful adjunct is "on-line" or context-sensitive help messages. Context-sensitive help usually consists of one or more screens of text that the operator can access from within the pulmonary function testing program. Some application programs display the appropriate help screen when an error occurs. On-line help functions facilitate orientation to a new system. It is also useful for functions that may not be performed on a routine basis. A glossary of computer terms is helpful, particularly if the applications program redefines keys on the computer keyboard. An explanation of error messages is important in tracking down software problems and user errors.

Computational errors may occur in the software. The potential for these errors dictates that there should be documentation of how the automated testing system arrives at the reported results. Manufacturer-supplied operation manuals should include detailed descriptions of all equations that the software uses in its calculations, both for tests and for predicted values. All formulas should be adequately referenced to the scientific literature. Software source codes may be furnished by the programmer. The actual program code may be as useful as detailed descriptions of software functions, depending on the programming expertise of the user. The user should be able to manually calculate all values for comparison with the software-generated results. Manual calculations require that the testing equipment provide all necessary raw data (as described previously). Tracings, such as spirograms or flow-volume curves, should be standardized to allow manual measurement of flows and volumes. Changes in computational methods, pattern-recognition algorithms, or in equations themselves that are made when software is upgraded should be detailed by the programmer. Test results may change significantly following a software upgrade. This is particularly important when the upgrade corrects a software problem. Modification of previously stored data may be necessary.

---

* MS-DOS is a registered trademark of Microsoft, Inc.
† OS/2 is a registered trademark of IBM.
‡ UNIX is a registered trademark of AT&T.

capacity of the hard disk system is increased. Some computer systems support moderately sized storage devices (i.e., 10 Mb to 20 Mb) that have removable media. These devices may be cost effective in maintaining large amounts of data.

Individual laboratories must carefully decide on the most appropriate means of maintaining subject data files. Laboratory protocols should include scheduled backups, archiving of records, and security of computer-stored information. Another important attribute of a computerized data system for pulmonary function studies is means for editing stored data and transferring the data to other computers for use with other programs. Most commercially available pulmonary function software allows selection of the actual data to be saved. Data selection may be assisted by computer-based algorithms. The final choice of valid data should be left to the user. A file editor is useful for correcting erroneous user input. An editor also may be helpful if data obtained by an independent means must be included.

Printers and Plotters

Computerized pulmonary function testing supports the generation of high-quality, high-resolution graphic representations of volume-time spirograms, flow-volume curves, and plethysmograph tangents. Tabular data can be printed rapidly as well. Peripherals utilized for printing graphic images and reports include dot matrix printers, ink-jet printers, thermal printers, laser printers, and digital plotters.

Dot matrix printers.   These printers utilize from 9 to 24 pins to generate both alphanumeric characters and graphics. The fastest dot matrix printers can print more than 200 characters per second. Fast dot matrix printers use fewer pins in order to achieve high speed, but text characters are not fully formed. Many dot matrix printers can produce either near letter-quality or draft characters. Near letter-quality characters can be generated at lower speeds. When a quick report is needed, draft characters can be produced. Dot matrix printers have the ability to generate high-resolution graphic images, but usually at rates slower than when printing text characters. Some dot matrix printers, especially high-speed models, may be noisy in the testing area. Color graphics and text can be printed by dot matrix printers that utilize multicolor ribbons.

Thermal transfer printers.   Thermal printers are extremely quiet but require heat-sensitive paper that may discolor with time. Thermal printers are utilized on some portable spirometers to generate text and graphic reports. Their small size (paper widths may vary from 2 to 8 inches) makes them transportable. Text characters resemble those produced by dot matrix printers. The speed of thermal printers is typically slower than fast dot matrix printers.

Ink-jet printers.   These printers apply a small jet of ink directly to the paper to form both characters and graphic images. Ink-jet printers are very quiet. Their speed equals that of thermal and standard dot matrix printers. Text quality equals most 24-pin dot matrix printers, and is close to the high-quality characters produced by laser printers. Color ink-jet printers allow text and graphics to be printed in a wide range of colors.

Laser printers.   These printers offer the highest quality in text and graphics. Resolution on printers is gauged in dots per inch. Laser printers typically have resolutions of 300 to 600 dots per inch. This is approximately double the resolution of most dot matrix printers. Only the ink-jet printer has similar resolution. Laser printers use a laser beam to form the images of letters or graphs. This image is formed on a drum which then transfers toner to paper, printing an entire page at one time. The speed of laser printers is described by the number of pages of text that can be printed per minute. Typical laser printers can print from 6 to 10 text pages per minute. Graphic images are more complex and take longer to format and print. The speed of laser printers often exceeds that of dot matrix printers. Laser printers are quiet and relatively easy to maintain. The high-quality text and graphic images that laser printers produce are not inexpensive. A laser printer can cost two to three times as much as a good quality dot matrix printer. The cost per printed page is also higher for laser printers than for the other types discussed. Laser printers are large and heavy, often occupying more space than the microcomputer itself. Laser printers contain their own microprocessor and memory (RAM). More than 1 Mb of memory or special interface cards are usually required if full graphic pages are to be printed. Standard laser printers cannot print in multiple colors.

Combination-type printers may be useful in some laboratory settings. These printers typically employ laser imaging, but can double as copiers, scanners, or facsimile (i.e., FAX) devices. Combination printers can accept output from computer software in the standard mode. In the copier mode, they can reproduce pages of text or graphics. In the scanner mode, the image is translated into one of several formats for storage in the computer. In the facsimile mode, page images can be transferred via modem (see Communications, this section).

Digital plotters.   Plotters interface directly to many computers. With appropriate software drivers, plotters can produce high-quality, multicolor representations of any figures generated on the video display. Plotters are usually slower than dot matrix printers when producing alphanumeric characters, but produce graphs rapidly. Plotters are quiet—this may be an important consideration in a busy laboratory.

Printing text reports or graphic images may take considerable time (i.e., minutes). In order for the computer to be used while the printer is working, many systems use a printer buffer or a software spooling program. A printer buffer is a device that contains memory (RAM). The buffer is placed between the computer and the printer. The printer buffer can accept data much faster than the printer itself. Data are stored and then fed to the printer at a slower rate, making the computer available to perform other tasks. Many printers have built-in memory to provide a buffer.

A spooler is a special program that resides in memory along with the pulmonary function application program. The spooler functions much like the hardware buffer. The spooler accepts data then "spools" them to the printer at an appropriate rate. Dumping graphic images, even with a buffer or spooler, may be slow because of the number of bytes required for high-resolution graphics. Spoolers are somewhat less efficient than hardware buffers. The computer's microprocessor must control the spooler while the hardware buffer has its own processor. Operating systems that support multi-tasking can perform printing as a background process with little or no loss of speed.

Hardware and Software Compatibility

One of the benefits of a computerized pulmonary function laboratory is that the computer may be used for tasks other than automated testing. This perhaps explains the trend many manufacturers are following of interfacing pulmonary function equipment with generic microcomputers and peripherals (see Figs. 10–1 and 10–2). There are two important considerations if the computer will be used for programs other than pulmonary function testing. The first of these is whether the system is compatible with commercial (off-the-shelf) software. The second consideration is how easily the pulmonary function software can be used in conjunction with other programs.

Compatibility with commercial software depends largely on the micropro-cessor and operating system the computer employs. Because of the variety of microcomputers available, determining software compatibility may require testing on the system in question. In addition, the user may need to become familiar with a specific program to ascertain if the computer incorporated in the pulmonary function system supports that program (see Additional Applications, this chapter). For example, if a pulmonary function testing system uses an ink-jet printer, a word processing program that does not support the ink-jet printer would be limited in its usefulness.

Use of commercial programs as adjuncts to the pulmonary function software may be easy, or may require high-level programming. A common example would be the export of pulmonary function data to a spreadsheet or database program (see Additional Applications, this chapter). The pulmonary function application often can be enhanced by using an operating system shell, memory resident utilities such as calculators or help files, print spoolers, or RAM disks.

Compatibility with these types of programs requires testing. Compatibility may depend on whether the pulmonary function software was designed to operate with other programs in memory.

Transfer of data among the pulmonary function software and other applications may be extremely useful. For example, if the pulmonary function program creates standard text files (i.e. ASCII files), then a simple word processor can be used to modify the file or generate customized reports. Most database and spreadsheet programs have functions that allow them to import data, if that data is in a common format. If the pulmonary function software is well documented or the source code is available, custom programs can interface to the application. These programs are usually developed in a high-level language such as BASIC, C, or PASCAL (see Languages and Programming, this section). Interfacing programs are usually developed to access data generated by the pulmonary function software. Some manufacturers provide this type of customization with the purchase of the system. Other vendors provide source code and documentation so that customization can be provided by the user.

Communications

An application of pulmonary function testing that is becoming more common is *outreach* testing. Outreach testing consists of pulmonary function equipment located at a remote site that communicates with a central computer using standard telephone lines. The satellite laboratory may be miles away or within the same building. The telecommunications supporting this type of system is implemented by means of modems. A modem translates digital data from the computer into tones that can be transmitted over a telephone line. The tones are decoded back into digital data by a modem in the receiving computer. Many computers have a built-in RS232C serial communication port. The serial port allows data to be transmitted one bit at a time very rapidly. The serial data can be sent either to a modem, for remote transmission, or to a local device such as another computer. The modem allows a small computer at a remote site to transmit and receive data from a centrally located host computer. Many portable computers such as laptop and notebook types, have a built-in modem. The host computer supports software that allows communications with one or more remote computers. Pulmonary function tests may be performed at the remote site, and a copy of the data transmitted to the host system, where it can be evaluated and interpreted.

Most microcomputers can use internal *FAX* (i.e., facsimile) boards. FAX boards allow the computer to send and receive text and graphic images, one page at a time. FAX transmission requires simple telephone-line connections. The data transmitted via FAX is in graphic format. In order to manipulate this type of data, the graphic images of characters must be translated back into ASCII characters. This can be accomplished using optical character recognition (OCR) software. This translation process may be required if the data transmitted by FAX must be edited or otherwise altered. If simple transmission of data is all that is required, a FAX board alone is sufficient.

A related type of system is the multiuser computer, in which a centrally located computer communicates with other computers or simple terminals to share programs and data. This arrangement is referred to as a *local area network*. Although multiuser systems previously required a mainframe or minicomputer, faster and more powerful microcomputers can support multiple users. Local area networks require one computer to function as the server. The server maintains the network operating system, and usually provides disk storage. Local area networks may be ideal in large laboratories that perform pulmonary function testing, exercise testing, and blood gas analysis. A multiuser computer permits stations to be dedicated to particular tasks. Programs that are needed in several areas can be accessed from the server. Transferring data from one location to another can be done quickly and easily. Local area networks are complex and somewhat difficult to implement. A properly designed network may save time and money in a high-volume pulmonary function laboratory.

System Maintenance

A large, automated pulmonary function testing system may include various interfaces as well as monitors, disk drives, printers, plotters, and modems. System maintenance of this type of automated system is usually complex. In addition to the service to spirometers and gas analyzers, the computer and its peripherals also require preventive or corrective maintenance.

A common source of problems is the software itself. Programs may load improperly or fail while accessing data from a storage device or other peripheral. Most operating systems and languages provide error messages to help track down software problems. Well-designed programs report full error messages. Some programs report only error codes, which must then be looked up in a manual. Careful evaluation of error codes or messages often indicates the source of the error.

Programs often fail when attempting to communicate with a peripheral device that is not ready, or that is operating incorrectly. For example, if the program expects data from the A/D converter but the converter malfunctions, the program may process incorrect data. Well-designed software contains error traps to handle most types of input or communication errors. Not every problem can be anticipated. A trouble-shooting guide is invaluable in tracking down computer problems. The guide should be keyed to the error messages that the program displays. Many systems contain diagnostic programs that allow checks of memory, disk drives, and related hardware. These diagnostics may help to determine if a particular error is software or hardware based. Many utility programs are available for microcomputers and peripherals that allow testing of disk drives, file integrity, and system performance.

Most programs utilize disk drives to store data and programs. Errors related to disks or disk drives are common. Because hard drives are capable of holding large amounts of data, a device failure may mean the loss of significant information. The most direct solution to these errors is to maintain adequate backups of all programs and data, and to rotate backup disks or tapes at regular intervals (Fig. 10–5). A simple protocol for backing up data is to use an alternate-day scheme. Two backup disks or tapes are employed, one designated *even day,* and the other *odd day.* Files are copied to each backup on alternate days. This system prevents loss of all data if the hard drive fails during the backup process. Data backup may be full or incremental. A full backup copies all files. An incremental backup copies only those files that have been added or modified since the previous backup. The type of backup used may depend on the method of data storage (see Data Management, this section). The alternate-day scheme usually also includes a weekly backup. The weekly backup should be a full backup and should include file verification. File verification checks each file as it is copied to assure its integrity. File verification may not be used during some backup routines in order to speed up the process.

For hardware malfunctions, such as printer breakdowns or disk drive failures, the usual action is to replace the suspected component. Many systems utilize components that are easy, though not always inexpensive, to replace. Dirt, dust, smoke, and humidity quite often interfere with sensitive electronics, but can be managed with a minimum of preventive care. Cabling and connectors between components are another source of hardware errors that should be evaluated whenever a peripheral begins functioning erratically or stops functioning suddenly.

Because of the variety of computerized systems available, not every capability can be completely described. Those discussed in this section include many of the important aspects related to automated data handling in the pulmonary

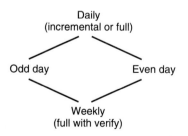

FIG 10–5.
Typical data backup protocol.

function laboratory. These features may be considerations in the selection of a computerized testing system.

Languages and Programming

The pulmonary function technologist may utilize computerized pulmonary function testing systems without programming expertise. To fully understand data acquisition and processing, a background in programming concepts may be helpful. Understanding how the computer controls various peripheral devices is useful for investigating hardware or software malfunctions. Programming skill may allow the development of utilities to supplement a full-scale testing package. Many application programs, such as databases, utilize their own "command" languages. These command languages allow programming of often-used functions. Understanding the operating system that controls most computer functions is a valuable tool for the technologist. Familiarity with operating system commands allows the technologist to manage not only the pulmonary function software, but various utility programs as well.

Computer Languages

Each microprocessor recognizes a set of instructions that are referred to as *"machine language."* These instructions are usually in binary format (i.e., 0 or 1) and represent the lowest-level language for controlling the computer. Because it is difficult to program using binary numbers, "assembly" language is utilized. Assembly language applies mnemonics to each low-level command. An assembly language program may be written using a simple text editor. The program code is then processed by an assembler that converts the mnemonics into machine language instructions. The resulting low-level program is usually stored in the form of hexadecimal bytes. Hexadecimal notation refers to the number system with a base equal to 16 in the decimal system. Assembly language programs are extremely fast, and usually do not require a large amount of RAM. Writing large programs in assembly language is a task that requires programming expertise. The programmer must understand the machine language instructions and be familiar with the specific hardware that the microprocessor will address. Many commercially available programs, such as word processors and spreadsheets, as well as some pulmonary function programs, are written in assembly language.

BASIC (Beginner's All-purpose Symbolic Instructional Code) has been used since the 1960s. BASIC is popular with the scientific and technical community because it can be learned easily. High-level mathematic and text-handling functions as well as file management are all possible in BASIC. BASIC programs may be too slow for applications that communicate with fast devices such as A/D converters. Two solutions to the slow execution problem with BASIC programs are widely applied. The first is to use a combination of machine language subroutines with BASIC to speed up critical portions of the program. A machine language routine might be used to access the A/D converter, and then pass the numeric values back to the BASIC program that called the subroutine. The second solution is to "compile" the BASIC program code. Compiled BASIC instructions are similar to native machine language. With careful programming, a speed increase of tenfold or more is often possible using compiled BASIC. Some BASIC commands cannot be compiled easily, particularly those that allow BASIC to function through the computer's operating system. Compiled BASIC programs cannot be easily modified without recompiling the source code. Nonetheless, some pulmonary function software packages use one or more of these techniques and support BASIC as the primary program language. For relatively short programs, especially when execution time is not critical, BASIC functions well. BASIC is easy to learn and allows programs to be modified quickly. Sophisticated versions of BASIC are available that support graphical user interfaces (see Operating Systems, this section).

FORTRAN (FORmula TRANslation) is the high-level language implemented for most scientific and technical applications on minicomputers. FORTRAN is a compiled language. The source program is coded according to a structured format and then compiled before the program is actually run. In general, compiled programs execute very quickly, as error checking is carried out during the compilation phase. FORTRAN supports calls to machine language subroutines so that it can be used as high-level language and still manage tasks such as reading data from A/D converters or other instruments. FORTRAN was designed primarily for numeric manipulations, and does not allow for easy handling of text characters. A large number of programs and subroutines are already written for FORTRAN. Because FORTRAN is available for most microprocessors it may be attractive for laboratories developing their own software.

A third high-level language with increased implementations in pulmonary function laboratories is *PASCAL*. PASCAL is a compiled language that requires a highly structured source program. The source program is compiled into an intermediate form called p-code, which is then interpreted at the time the program is run. PASCAL supports a number of functions that allow complex programs to be written easily. Because it is highly structured, PASCAL programs can be written in modules. The modules are then linked together or used repeatedly as necessary. Another advantage of the highly structured nature of PASCAL is its ability to create libraries of routines that can be incorporated into programs.

The high-level language that has assumed a leading place in the development of many commercial software packages is C. C has a block structure similar to PASCAL, but is more concise and efficient. By design, C is a simple language. It is often categorized as the lowest of the high-level languages. The flexibility of

C allows it to duplicate many assembly language functions. Its simplicity allows programs to be written in more understandable and easily maintained code. Because C is capable of relatively low level operations, C programs can achieve levels of speed and efficiency comparable to assembly language programs. C programs are built around functions, with one main function as the entry point into the program. Functions can call other functions, including themselves, and retrieve values from the called routine. C has been widely used for development of operating systems as well as application programs. UNIX,* the popular multiuser, multi-tasking operating system, is written almost entirely in C. C is also well suited for applications running under the MS-DOS,† Windows, or OS/2‡ operating systems. The simplicity and flexibility of C allows C programs to be highly transportable. As long as the program does not use hardware-specific features, applications developed for one microprocessor can be easily adapted to run on other microprocessors.

Many language systems support interaction between languages. This allows one high-level language to call subroutines or functions written in another language, either high or low level. New high-level languages provide facilities to define new and complex data structures, called objects. Programs written using these structures are called *object-oriented programs* (OOPs). Object-oriented programming adds more structure to languages like PASCAL, BASIC, and C by binding data together with routines that act on it. Special implementations of these languages, such as C++, are designed around the concept of objects. Object-oriented programs are highly modular, making it easy to replace or enhance parts of a program without affecting the rest of it.

Operating Systems

The language most often used in pulmonary function laboratories is the operating system (OS) or disk operating system (DOS). The OS is primarily responsible for supervising input and output functions of the computer. These functions include file management, controlling information sent to the video display, and accepting input from the keyboard or other devices. The OS also coordinates functions from the application programs running on the computer. The technologist may use the OS for several important functions: copying files or programs, backing up data files, viewing a directory of files on a particular device, sorting files, and running specific application programs.

Most operating systems support an automatic mode of control. A file-based control mode allows the user to perform multiple procedures by executing a single program. Commands normally entered from the keyboard are stored in a special file called a *"batch"* or *"job control"* file. By calling the batch file, the

---

* UNIX is a registered trademark of AT&T.
† MS-DOS and Windows are registered trademarks of Microsoft, Inc.
‡ OS/2 is a registered trademark of IBM.

same steps can be repeated as often as needed. Batch files are extremely helpful for initializing small computer systems. Programs for controlling printers, screen displays, and other devices can be loaded automatically so that the main program functions correctly. Batch files also can be used for tedious tasks such as backing up selected data files on a routine basis. Other OS utilities include programs for formatting storage media (i.e., diskettes), editing files, protecting files with passwords, deleting files, and setting parameters for the operation of the video display and the printer.

Many OS functions are initiated by entering commands at the keyboard. "Shell" programs provide an alternate interface so that the user does not have to remember the system's commands or type them. Shell interfaces allow the user to indicate the desired function with a special pointing device, such as a mouse or touch screen. A series of menus or windows on the display provide the user with choices. These graphical user interfaces provide an intuitive approach to operating the computer. Rather than learning and entering long lists of commands, the user simply points to the desired option. Programs that conform to the standards set forth in the graphical interface tend to be similar. This similarity allows the user to quickly learn new programs.

Many different OSs are in use on minicomputers and microcomputers. A few of these are quite common: MS-DOS, Windows, OS/2, and UNIX. Some pulmonary function systems support a proprietary OS. Most, however, utilize one or more of the "off-the-shelf" systems to provide compatibility with other commercially available software. MS-DOS has a large base of application programs, but is limited to providing single-user microcomputer functions. OS/2, UNIX, and Windows all have versions that support both multi-tasking and multiple users. Many hybrid OSs are available that allow programs designed to run under one OS to be used in different operating environments, or to enhance program capabilities by allowing access to more sophisticated OS functions.

While most pulmonary function laboratories utilize computers for performing tests, relatively few do extensive programming. Development of a comprehensive pulmonary function testing package, complete with interfacing to all necessary laboratory instruments, is an involved task. Most laboratories developing their own software find it useful to engage professional programmers and consultants. The cost, in time and money, of producing a custom testing program is usually prohibitive, unless special computer resources, such as programming facilities, are available. Programming skills using languages such as C, PASCAL, BASIC, FORTRAN, or ASSEMBLY can allow in-house development of utilities and supplementary programs to enhance or extend commercially available software. A working knowledge of the OS used by a particular computer can greatly enhance day-to-day functions of the laboratory. Skill in using other application programs, such as spreadsheets or word processors, can increase the productivity of a system designed primarily for pulmonary function testing.

Additional Applications

Several types of application programs lend themselves to use in the pulmonary function laboratory. These include interpretation programs for pulmonary function tests, blood gas data and quality control programs, spreadsheets, database managers, word processing programs, and educational applications.

Pulmonary Function Interpretation Programs

Many pulmonary function software packages include an interpretation program. Interpretation programs use one or more sets of algorithms for defining obstructive, restrictive, combined, or normal patterns based on spirometry, lung volumes and $D_{L_{CO}}$. These interpretive programs analyze the results from testing, comparing the values to reference values. The algorithms are based on the same logic that a clinical interpreter might use. The computerized interpreter, however, does not have the benefit of including the subject's clinical history or other laboratory findings in the interpretation process. Depending on the sophistication of the program, computerized interpreters can detect the presence of obstruction or restriction reasonably well. An incorrect computerized interpretation may occur if test results are invalid because of inadequate effort or nonreproducible data. Computerized interpretation in no way substitutes for evaluation by a qualified interpreter. It may be helpful in situations when an immediate report of abnormalities is necessary, such as in a screening program. Computerized interpretation also can be used in an educational setting. If a computerized interpretation is included in the medical record, it should be clearly labelled as such. Computerized interpretations should never be used as the only interpretation, but should always be reviewed by a qualified reader.

Blood Gas Programs

Blood gas interpretation by computer is implemented by applying algorithms to evaluate acid-base and oxygenation status. Computerized blood gas interpretation can be useful in situations in which an immediate interpretation to rule out gross abnormalities is required. Because the computer can routinely evaluate all the measured and calculated blood gas parameters, it often may suggest abnormalities that the casual interpreter might overlook. As with computerized pulmonary function interpretation, blood gas interpretations should always be held as preliminary until verified by a qualified interpreter.

Another context in which computerization is useful in the blood gas laboratory is quality control and data reporting. Because evaluation of multiple levels of controls requires statistical manipulation of large amounts of data (see Chapter 11), the computer is ideally suited to maintaining a quality assurance program. Most quality control programs require the calculation of means and standard deviations (see Appendix) for each level of pH, Pco_2, and Po_2. Because controls are usually run daily or more often, many times on multiple instruments, computerization of data files greatly reduces the record keeping in a busy laboratory. A second advantage is that the computer can be utilized to interpret the results of quality control runs in real time. This allows the technologist to immediately determine the status of each individual blood gas electrode (see also Chapter 11). Quality assurance programs that are compatible with a variety of microcomputers are available from several professional organizations.

Result reporting lends itself to computerization, as many patients receive multiple blood gas analyses. Most automated or semiautomated analyzers can be interfaced via the standard serial port so that blood gas data can be stored on disk or tape, with reports generated as required. Interfacing a blood gas analyzer directly to a hospital information system allows blood gas results to be available wherever a terminal is located. Automated result reporting tends to reduce transcription errors and lost results. Blood gas instruments that are interfaced to a hospital information system should permit results to be reviewed and edited before final posting.

Databases

Database programs are available for almost every microcomputer or minicomputer. Most allow the user to design what information will be stored and how it will be arranged. Computer databases permit the user to save information in much the same manner as a conventional file might be used. The computer can rapidly sort the information, search for records meeting specific criteria, and generate reports as required. A common application in the pulmonary function laboratory is maintaining records of tests performed, patient demographics, diagnoses, and referral sources. Many pulmonary function software packages support the export of test data from patient files using popular database formats. Other uses include records of departmental inventory, expenditures, and quality assurance programs.

Some pulmonary function software packages utilize a relational database for storing test results from pulmonary function or blood gas studies. The combination of a relational database and a large-capacity hard disk makes it possible to maintain a large number of patient studies that can be retrieved using typical database queries. Reference lists and bibliographies can be maintained as a database. A number of free-form databases are available in which all disparate types of data such as memos, reports, references, and test results can be accessed in a manner similar to the records in a conventional database. Many commercially available database programs can be integrated so that information from spreadsheets, word processing programs, or even pulmonary function data can be easily exchanged.

Spreadsheets

Electronic spreadsheets were originally designed as financial planning tools, replacing the ledger book. However, their ability to organize numeric data and perform repetitive calculations make them ideal for many scientific and technical purposes. Spreadsheets utilize matrix arithmetic. Numbers or formulas are placed in the cells of a matrix. A value or the result of an equation then can be accessed by referring to its row and column location in the spreadsheet. By adding mathematic and logic functions, rows or columns can be added, subtracted, averaged, or otherwise evaluated. Spreadsheets are quite useful for statistical calculations, such as computation of means and standard deviations for blood gas quality control. Many spreadsheets have built-in statistical functions.

Reducing data from procedures such as exercise tests, in which the same calculations are performed at each exercise work load, can be quickly performed using a spreadsheet. An equation can be entered in one cell and then replicated to additional cells. The variables in the replicated equations are adjusted relative to the position of the cell in the spreadsheet. If a formula sums the two cells immediately above it, a copy of that formula will always add the two cells above it. Any data that are normally reduced using a calculator can be managed by a spreadsheet.

Most spreadsheets support functions used for storing and editing numeric data, and for generating customized reports. Typical spreadsheet applications include conventional database functions, as well as importing data from and exporting data to other applications and generating graphic representations of numeric data.

Word Processing

Word processing is a frequent application for small computers. Using an appropriate printer, word processing software can be used to generate any document that normally would require typing or printing. The document is saved, allowing revisions or copies as needed. In the laboratory environment, word processing software is ideal for maintaining documents that require continual updates, such as procedure manuals. Word processing software can be used to generate customized reports. In many instances, data can be transferred directly from a spreadsheet or database, and incorporated into the document. Multi-tasking operating systems allow text or graphics to be cut from one program and "pasted" into another.

Pulmonary function software that stores data in text files often can be interfaced to a word processing program for custom report generation. Some pulmonary function application programs include an editor for inserting comments or adding an interpretation to the final report. Although simple text editors do not support many word processing functions, they permit text to be stored and retrieved along with tabular data.

Educational Programs

Computer-assisted instructional software has several applications in the pulmonary function laboratory. Information that is usually taught by repetitive drill can often be administered by computer. Many programs are available to allow multiple choice and other types of questions to be administered by computer. The computer can easily score the results of a test taken. For training, the computer can be an educational and evaluation tool. Computerized simulations can be adapted for laboratory personnel. Simulations can be used to review interpretation of pulmonary function studies or blood gas analyses.

Libraries of reference material covering a variety of subjects are available on CD-ROM disks. These devices allow huge amounts of reference data to be available via the computer, and may replace conventional reference texts for information that does not change often.

SELF-ASSESSMENT QUESTIONS

1. One megabyte of random access memory (RAM) is equal to:
   a. 1,000,000 bytes
   b. 4096 Kb
   c. 1024 Kb
   d. 1000 bytes

2. Which of the following are used to increase the speed of data storage:
   a. ROM
   b. CD-ROM
   c. Virtual memory
   d. Cache memory

3. In order for a volume-displacement spirometer to be interfaced to a computer, which of the following are necessary:
   I. Hard drive
   II. A/D converter
   III. Potentiometer
   IV. Parallel port
   a. I, II, III, IV
   b. II, III, IV
   c. I, IV only
   d. II, III only

4. The most important quality of a computerized pulmonary function system is:
   a. Microprocessor speed
   b. Hard disk storage capacity

   c. The number of megabytes of RAM

   d. Accuracy of the interface hardware and software

5. Software for performing spirometry should allow _____ FVC efforts to be held in memory for comparison:

   a. 2

   b. 3

   c. 8

   d. 12

6. In order to check the accuracy of a computerized pulmonary function system, the manufacturer's documentation should include:

   a. The sampling rate of the A/D converter

   b. All equations used in the software

   c. Source code for the command menu

   d. An example of a patient data file

7. The factor that limits the volume of pulmonary function data that can be stored by computer is:

   a. The type of database utilized

   b. The storage media (hard or floppy disk)

   c. The amount of RAM available (in megabytes)

   d. The computer language used in the application program

8. In addition to the pulmonary function equipment, which of the following would be required to implement a remote-site (outreach) testing facility:

   I. Host computer

   II. Modems

   III. Local-area network (LAN)

   IV. Communications software

   a. I, II, III, IV

   b. I, II, IV

   c. I, II

   d. III, IV

9. Which of the following is an operating system:

   a. FORTRAN

   b. MS-DOS

   c. Pascal

   d. C++

10. In order to interface an automated blood gas analyzer to a hospital information system, which of the following is required:

   a. A serial port on the analyzer

   b. A text editor

    c. A graphic user interface

    d. A D/A converter

SELECTED BIBLIOGRAPHY

COMPUTERIZED PULMONARY FUNCTION TESTING

American Thoracic Society. Committee on Proficiency Standards for Clinical Pulmonary Laboratories: Computer guidelines for pulmonary laboratories. *Am Rev Respir Dis* 134:628, 1986.

Black KH, Petusevsky ML, Gaensler EA: A general purpose microprocessor for spirometry. *Chest* 78:605, 1980.

Crapo RO, Gardner RM, Berlin SL, et al: Automation of pulmonary function equipment—user beware! (editorial). *Chest* 90:1, 1986.

Dickman ML, Schmidt CD, Gardner RM, et al: On-line computerized spirometry in 738 normal adults. *Am Rev Respir Dis* 100:780, 1969.

Gardner RM, Crapo RO, Morris AH, et al: Computerized decision-making in the pulmonary function laboratory. *Respir Care* 27(7):799, 1982.

Jones NL: *Clinical exercise testing,* ed 3. Philadelphia, 1988, WB Saunders.

COMPUTER DATA ACQUISITION

Engleman B, Abraham M: Personal computer signal processing. *Byte* April:94, 1984.

Mellichamp D, editor: *Real-time computing—with applications to data acquisition and control.* New York, 1983, Van Nostrand Reinhold.

Tompkins WJ, Webster JG, editors: *Design of microcomputer-based medical instrumentation.* New Jersey, 1981, Prentice-Hall.

Wyss CR: Planning a computerized measurement system. *Byte* April:114, 1985.

COMPUTER APPLICATIONS

Byers RA: *Everyman's database primer.* Culver City, Calif, 1984, Ashton-Tate.

Cohn JD, Engler RC, DelGuercio RL: The automated physiologic profile. *Crit Care Med* 3:51, 1975.

Ellis JH, Perera SP, Levin DC: A computer program for the interpretation of pulmonary function studies. *Chest* 68:209, 1975.

Gardner RM, Cannon GH, Morris AH, et al: Computerized blood gas interpretation and reporting system. *Computer* 8(1):39, 1975.

Miller H: Introduction to spreadsheets. *PC World* 2:66, 1984.

Silage DA, Maxwell C: A spirometry/interpretation program for hand-held computers. *Respir Care* 28:62, 1983.

LANGUAGES AND PROGRAMMING

Duncan R: *Advanced OS/2*. Bellevue, Wash, 1988, Microsoft Press.

Kernighan BW, Ritchie DM: *The C programming language*, ed 2. Englewood Cliffs, NJ, 1988, Prentice-Hall.

Norton P: *Inside the IBM-PC*. New York, 1986, Brady Books.

Waite M, Martin D, Prata S: *Unix primer plus*. Indianapolis, 1983, Howard W. Sams and Co.

Wolverton V: *Running MS-DOS*, ed 2. Bellevue, Wash, 1988, Microsoft Press.

11

Quality Assurance in the Pulmonary Function Laboratory

ELEMENTS OF LABORATORY QUALITY CONTROL

Quality control is essential to the operation of the pulmonary function laboratory in order to obtain valid and reproducible data. There are four primary elements to consider in regard to a quality assurance program.

1. *Methodology.* The type of equipment used (i.e., spirometer, gas analyzer, recorder) largely determines the procedures that are required for calibration and quality control. The methods used also determine how often quality control procedures must be performed. The methods used for spirometry, lung volumes, $D_{L_{CO}}$, blood gases, and exercise testing are usually determined by the needs of referring physicians. The number and complexity of the tests performed also may dictate which equipment and methods are employed. Methods and equipment that have been validated in the scientific literature should be used whenever possible. Quality control is usually easier to perform when standardized techniques or equipment are employed.

2. *Instrument Maintenance.* The type and complexity of the instrumentation for a specific test will determine the long-term and short-term maintenance that will be required. *Preventive maintenance* is that which is scheduled in anticipation of equipment malfunction, in order to reduce the possibility of equipment failure. *Corrective maintenance* or *repair* is unscheduled service that is required to correct equipment failure. The failure is often signaled by quality control procedures or extreme results during testing. Familiarity with the

TABLE 11–1.

Pulmonary Function Procedure Manual

Items to be included in a typical procedure manual for a pulmonary function laboratory. For each procedure performed, the following should be present:

1. *Description* of the test, and its purpose.
2. *Indications* for ordering the test and contraindications, if any.
3. Description of the *general method(s)* and any specific equipment required.
4. *Calibration* of equipment required prior to testing (manufacturer's documentation may be referenced).
5. *Patient preparation* for the test, if any (withholding medication, etc.).
6. Step-by-step procedure for both computerized and manual *measurement/calculation* of results.

7. *Quality control* guidelines with acceptable limits of performance and corrective actions to be taken.
8. *Safety precautions* related to the procedure (infection control, hazards, etc.), and alert values that require physician notification.
9. *References* for all equations used for calculating results and for predicted normals, including a bibliography.
10. Documentation of *computer protocols* for calculations and data storage; guidelines for computer downtime.
11. Dated *signatures* of the medical and technical directors.

operating characteristics of spirometers, gas analyzers, plethysmographs, and computers is best accomplished by manufacturer support and thorough documentation. A procedure manual (Table 11–1) and accurate records are essential to a comprehensive maintenance program. Documentation of procedures and repairs are required by most accrediting organizations.

3. *Control Methods.* Appropriate test signals for each instrument are necessary to determine accuracy and precision of the data reported. Control signals or materials must be available for spirometers, gas analyzers, blood gas analyzers, and other instruments. Because many laboratories utilize computerized pulmonary function or blood gas analyzers, control signals are required to assure that both software and hardware are functioning within acceptable limits. Control methods may vary from mechanical flow generators for spirometers to tonometered blood for blood gas analyzers.

4. *Testing and/or Sampling Technique.* A primary means of assuring quality data is to rigidly control the methods and procedures by which data is obtained. In the case of pulmonary function testing, "sampling technique" refers to the ability of the technician to perform the test procedure, and to elicit the subject's cooperation in the test maneuvers. Technician and subject performance, as well as proper equipment function, must be evaluated on a test-by-test basis. This may be accomplished by applying appropriate criteria to determine the acceptability of the results.

This chapter deals primarily with the appropriate control signals for instrument maintenance and calibration. Also discussed in the chapter are criteria for acceptability of pulmonary function tests, such as spirometry, lung volumes, and $D_{L_{CO}}$. The operating characteristics (methodologies) of various types of pulmonary function testing equipment was discussed in Chapter 9.

Each laboratory should have a written quality assurance program which includes:

- The methods employed for specific tests
- The limitations of the procedure (if any)
- Indications or schedules for maintenance
- Quality control materials or signals to be used
- Action to be taken if controls exceed specified limits
- Specific guidelines as to how tests are to be performed

The quality assurance program should be included as part of the laboratory procedure manual.

Two concepts that are central to quality assurance are the definitions of *accuracy* and *precision*. Accuracy may be defined as the extent to which measurement of a known quantity results in a value approximating that quantity. For most laboratory tests, this is accomplished by taking repeated measurements and calculating the mean, or average, of the data. If the mean value approximates the "known," the instrument is considered accurate. Precision may be defined as the extent to which repeated measurements of the same quantity can be reproduced. If the same parameter is measured repeatedly and the resulting values are similar, the instrument may be considered precise.

Accuracy and precision may not always be present concurrently in the same instrument. For example, a spirometer that consistently measures a 3-L test volume as 2.5 L is precise, but not very accurate. A spirometer that evaluates a 3-L test volume as 2.5, 3.0, and 3.5 L on repeated maneuvers, shows an accurate mean of 3.0 L, but the individual measurements are not precise. Determination of the accuracy *and* precision of instruments such as spirometers is particularly important because many common pulmonary function tests are "effort dependent." The largest value observed, rather than the mean, is often reported as the "best test" (see Criteria for Acceptability of Spirometry, this chapter). Reporting the largest result observed is based on the rationale that the subject cannot overshoot on a test that is effort dependent.

CALIBRATION AND QUALITY CONTROL OF SPIROMETERS

Calibration is the process in which the signal from a spirometer is adjusted to produce a known output. This may be accomplished by one or more of several methods:

1. Adjustment of the analog output signal from the primary transducer (i.e., bell, bellows, flow sensor).
2. Adjustment of the sensitivity of the recording device.
3. Software correction or compensation.

Spirometers that produce a voltage signal by means of a potentiometer (see Chapter 9) normally allow some form of *"gain" adjustment* so that the analog output can be matched to a known input of either volume or flow. For example, a 10-L volume-displacement spirometer may be equipped with a 10-volt potentiometer. This potentiometer amplifier would be adjusted so that 0 volts equals 0 L, and 10 volts equals 10 L. The calibration could be checked by setting the spirometer at a specific volume and noting the analog signal (i.e., 5 L should equal 5 volts).

A related technique is the adjustment of the sensitivity of the *recording device*. This technique is used with an X-Y plotter or strip chart recorder. In this technique, a known volume is injected into the spirometer and the deflection of the recording device adjusted to match the volume. For example, a strip chart recorder is turned on and has the recording pen adjusted to read 0 L when the spirometer is empty. A volume of 3 L is then injected. The gain of the recorder is adjusted so that the tracing deflects 3 L on the graph paper. This method is appropriate when the recorded tracing is to be measured manually. In computerized systems, the signal produced by the spirometer is often corrected by applying a *software calibration factor*. A known volume, or flow, is injected into the spirometer using a large-volume syringe, usually 3 L. A correction factor is calculated based on the measured vs. expected values:

$$\text{Correction factor} = \frac{\text{Expected volume}}{\text{Measured volume}}$$

The correction factor derived by this method is then stored, usually in memory and on disk. The correction is then applied to all subsequent volume measurements. For example, if a syringe with a volume of 3 L is injected into a spirometer, and a volume of 2.97 L is recorded, the correction factor would be:

$$1.010 = \frac{3.00 \text{ L}}{2.97 \text{ L}}$$

The correction factor 1.010 would then be used to adjust subsequent volume measurements. This method assumes that the spirometer output is linear, so that the correction factor would be correct for any volume, large or small. Many computerized systems allow the correction factor to be verified by reinjecting a known volume, not necessarily 3 L, and checking the input against the output. Care should be taken that the gas in the syringe, which is at ambient temperature (ATPS), is not "temperature corrected" by the software. Inappropriate temper-

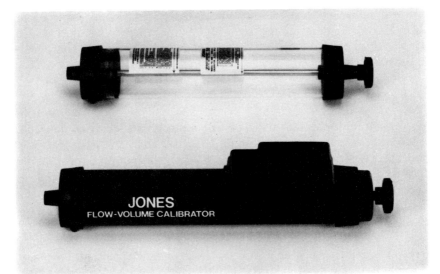

FIG 11–1.
Equipment for spirometer calibration. **Top,** 3-L syringe used for volume calibrations or for connection to FRC and $D_{L_{CO}}$ calibration setups. A 3-L syringe is recommended for both calibration and quality control. **Bottom,** computerized FVC simulator that uses a microprocessor to measure FEV_1 and other flows during injection of a 3-L volume. The volumes and flows delivered can be compared with those reported by the spirometer. (Courtesy of Jones Medical Instrument Co., Oakbrook, Ill).

ature correction would produce an erroneously high measured value, and a low correction factor.

Other factors that might influence establishment of the software correction value include the accuracy of the large-volume syringe and the speed with which the injection is performed. An inaccurate syringe or leaks in the connection to the spirometer will produce erroneous software corrections. Some systems, particularly flow-based spirometers, may require that the syringe volume be injected within certain flow limits so that the software can generate correction factors based on a series of injections. Flow-based spirometers that measure both inspiratory and expiratory volumes usually require the syringe volume to be injected and withdrawn. This allows corrections for both inspired and expired gas to be generated.

Quality control of spirometers is closely related to calibration, and the two are sometimes confused. An important distinction is that calibration (i.e., adjustment) may or may not be needed, but quality control must be applied on a routine basis. Calibration, whether it includes the output of the spirometer, recorder sensitivity, or generation of a software correction factor, involves *adjusting* of the device to perform within certain limits. Quality control is a *test* performed to determine the accuracy and/or precision of the device using a known standard or signal. Various control methods (i.e., signal generators) are available for spirometers:

1. *Simple large-volume syringe.* A syringe of at least 3-L volume (Fig. 11–1, top) should be used to generate a control signal for checking the volume deflection of volume-displacement spirometers and the associated deflection of the recording device. A large-volume syringe also may be used to check the volume accuracy of flow-sensing devices. Spirometer quality control should be performed at least each day that the device is to be used. For field studies, such as industrial applications or epidemiologic research, in which the spirometer is moved or used for a large number of tests, accuracy should be checked several times daily to prevent reporting of erroneous values. Different volumes should be used to assess the accuracy of the spirometer across its volume range. The spirometer should record 1, 3, and 5 L with equal accuracy. For volume-displacement spirometers, accuracy should be checked across the volume range at least quarterly. A 3-L syringe injection performed when the spirometer is nearly empty or nearly full should yield comparable results. The volume accuracy of a spirometer should be tested over a range of flows. Different flows can be generated by varying the speed at which the syringe is emptied, but it is impossible to reproduce those flows to check the precision of the spirometer. Applying different flows and measuring the resulting volumes may provide insight as to whether the device and its software are accurate at low and high flows. For example, three different injection times, 0.5 to 1.0 seconds, 1.0 to 1.5 seconds, and 5.0 to 5.5 seconds, may be used with a 3-L syringe to simulate a wide range of flows.

Computerized syringes (see Fig. 11–1, bottom) are available for assessing the accuracy of commonly measured parameters such as FEV_1 and $FEF_{25\%-75\%}$. These syringes utilize a built-in microprocessor that times the volume injection and calculates the flow parameters. The microprocessor displays its volume and flows for comparison with those recorded by the instrument being tested. The computerized syringe offers the advantage of being able to deliver a 3-L volume for calibration or volume checks, and test the accuracy for commonly reported flows.

Volume accuracy checks should be applied as if a subject were being tested, with a few exceptions. For volume-displacement spirometers, a check for leaks should be performed daily before assessing volume accuracy. Fill the device with air to approximately half of its volume range and apply a constant pressure, by means of a weight or spring. No change in the volume tracing should be noted while the pressure is applied. The spirometer should return to its original volume baseline when the pressure is removed. The large-volume syringe should be connected to the subject port with whatever circuitry is employed for the actual test. In order to prevent automatic correction to BTPS, the spirometer temperature correction should be set to 37°C. Most computerized spirometers provide a specific routine for volume checks or calibration that overrides temperature corrections. In some systems, temperature correction cannot be overridden. In these instances, injection of a 3-L volume at ATPS results in a reading greater than 3 L because the system attempts to "correct" the volume to body temperature (BTPS). For water-seal spirometers, the syringe should be filled and emptied several times to allow equilibration with the humidified air of the device. For some flow-sensing spirometers, a length of tubing must be connected between the flow sensor and syringe. This avoids artifact caused by the turbulent flow generated by the syringe.

The accuracy of any spirometer can be calculated as follows:

$$\% \text{ Error} = \frac{\text{Expected volume} - \text{Measured volume}}{\text{Expected volume}} \times 100$$

where:

$$\text{expected volume} = \text{the actual volume of the syringe}$$

$$\text{measured volume} = \text{the result recorded for the test}$$

The maximum acceptable error, according to the ATS recommendations (Table 11–2), is ±3% or ±50 mL, whichever is larger. If the percent of error exceeds ±3%, a careful examination of the spirometer, recording device, software, most recent calibration, and the testing technique should be carried out.

2. *Sine-Wave Rotary Pumps.* A second method of checking volume accuracy of spirometers involves a syringe or piston driven by a rotary motor. This type of device produces a biphasic volume signal. A biphasic signal may be useful for checking volume and flow accuracy for both inspiration and expiration. This type of device has limited use for assessing the accuracy of spirometers for most flow measurements. A rotary-drive syringe is ideal for checking the frequency response of a spirometer, particularly at high flow rates. A sine-wave signal is necessary to evaluate a spirometer's ability to adequately record tests such as the MVV. The ATS recommends that spirometers that measure MVV record a 2-L sine wave within ±5% from 0 to 250 L/min. Although tests such as this are impractical for most clinical laboratories, they should be available from manufacturers where necessary. Sine-wave pumps are also commonly used in the calibration of body plethysmographs.

3. *Automated Syringes.* These devices are similar to large-volume syringes that are used manually, but have some combination of computer-controlled motor drive or digital output. Computerized syringes are usually employed only by equipment manufacturers or for research applications concerned with testing available clinical equipment. Other commercially available devices utilize

TABLE 11–2.
Minimal Spirometry Standards*

Test	Range/Accuracy BTPS (L)	Flow Range (L/sec)	Time (sec)	Resistance/Back pressure	Test Signals
VC	7 L ± 3% or 50 mL, whichever is greater	0–12	30		3-L calibrated syringe
FVC	7 L ± 3% or 50 mL, whichever is greater	0–12	15		24 standard waveforms
FEV_T	7 L ± 3% or 50 mL, whichever is greater	0–12	T	Less than 1.5 cm H_2O/L/sec at 12 L/sec flow	24 standard waveforms
Time zero	Time point from which all FEV_T measurements are taken			Determined by back-extrapolation	
$FEF_{25\%-75\%}$	7 L ± 5% or 0.2 L/sec, whichever is greater	0–12	15	Same as FEV_T	24 standard waveforms
$\dot{V}$	12 L/sec ± 5% or 0.2 L/sec, whichever is greater	0–12	15	Same as FEV_T	Manufacturer proof
MVV	Sine wave 250 L/min at 2-L tidal volume to ± 5% of reading	0–12 ± 5%	12–15 ± 3%	Less than ± 10 cm H_2O at 2-L tidal volume at 2.0 Hz	Sine-wave pump 0.4 Hz ± 10% at 12 L/sec

*Summarized from Standardization of spirometry—1987 update. *Am Rev Respir Dis* 136:1285, 1987.

sensors coupled to microprocessors to calculate various flows such as FEV_1 and $FEF_{25\%-75\%}$ as described previously (see Fig. 11–1, bottom).

4. *Explosive Decompression Devices.* Explosive decompression simulates the exponential flow pattern of a forced expiratory maneuver. Such devices use a known volume of gas compressed to a fixed pressure, which is released through an orifice. Some devices use air while others utilize CO_2 as the compressed gas. The primary advantage of this type of device is that it allows flow and volume signals to be reproduced. Reproducible flows permit quality assurance checks of most spirometric parameters, and evaluates both hardware and software. Because the test signal can be reproduced as often as necessary, both accuracy and precision can be measured. Explosive decompression devices may be limited in automated systems that require a particular pattern of respiration in order to trigger recording, such as inspiration-expiration-inspiration. Another potential limitation is the use of CO_2 as the compressed gas. Flow-sensing spirometers that are affected by gas density may yield unacceptable values if 100% CO_2 is used (see Chapter 9).

5. *Biologic controls.* A semi-quantitative means of assessing accuracy and precision of a spirometer uses repeated measurements of known subjects. Routine spirometric measurements may be performed on subjects who will be available for future comparison, such as laboratory personnel. Although individual signals for FVC, FEV_1, and $FEF_{25\%-75\%}$ show day-to-day variability when test subjects are used, all aspects of the testing protocol are evaluated. This method includes hardware, software, and the testing procedure itself. Biologic controls are a readily available check of the overall function of the spirometer. They do not, however, replace accuracy checks by means of a known-volume syringe. The mean and standard deviation (see Appendix) of 5 to 10 spirometric measurements for each reported parameter should be recorded for at least three known subjects. These subjects should have repeat tests at least quarterly, or whenever questionable test results are observed. The control subjects should reflect the patient population routinely tested (i.e., adults, children). Interlaboratory testing of biologic controls in two or more laboratories allows a form of proficiency testing, so that the accuracy of an individual laboratory can be assessed. Testing of healthy subjects, usually 10 or more, can be useful in assessing the appropriateness of the reference value equations used for predicting normals (see Using Normal Values, Appendix).

In addition to checking the volume and flow accuracy of spirometers, there are several other important aspects of quality control that require routine evaluation:

1. *Flow resistance.* The "back pressure" from a spirometer should be less than 1.5 cm H_2O at a flow of 12 L/sec. Resistance to flow is measured by placing an accurate manometer or pressure transducer at the subject connection and

applying a known flow. This is easily accomplished with flow-sensing devices but somewhat difficult with volume-displacement devices. Measurement of flow resistance is normally performed only when there is some reason to suspect that the spirometer is causing undue resistance.

2. *Frequency response.* Frequency response refers to the spirometer's ability to produce accurate volume and flow measurements across a wide range of frequencies. Frequency response is most critical in the MVV maneuver. Frequency response is usually evaluated by means of a sine-wave pump. It should be measured as part of the manufacturer's validation, and rechecked only if the spirometer is suspect.

3. *Flow.* Flow-sensing spirometers directly measure flow and indirectly calculate volume by integration or counting volume pulses. It is sometimes necessary to assess the flow accuracy of such devices. Inaccurate measurement of flow almost always results in inaccurate volume determinations. A rotameter may be used in conjunction with an adjustable compressed gas source to supply gas at a known flow to the device. A weighted volume-displacement spirometer, such as a water-seal, also can be used to generate a known flow. Many flow-sensing spirometers use a volume signal to perform software calibration as described previously. It may be useful to check the flow signal from the spirometer at different known flows if the volume accuracy is observed to vary with flow.

4. *Recorders.* Recording devices are perhaps as important as the volume/flow transducers themselves in providing accurate spirometric tracings. The ATS recommends that a recording device be included with all spirometers. Slightly different recorder standards are recommended, depending on the intended application of the spirometer. For *diagnostic* functions such as recognition of disease patterns or unacceptable maneuvers, the recorder must have a sensitivity on the volume axis of at least 5 mm/L (BTPS) and a time base of at least 1 cm/second. For *manual measurements* and for instrument validation, a volume sensitivity of at least 10 mm/L (BTPS), and a time base of at least 2 cm/second is required. Hard-copy recordings of volume-time or flow-volume tracings should be made as part of all spirometric measurements. Flow-volume curves should be plotted with expired flow upwards on the vertical axis and expired volume from left to right on the horizontal axis. A 2-to-1 ratio of the flow-to-volume scales should be maintained. For diagnostic purposes, the flow sensitivity of the flow-volume display should be at least 2.5 mm/L/sec, while for manual measurements or validation the flow sensitivity should be at least 5 mm/L/sec. Sensitivity on the volume axis of flow-volume displays should be the same as for volume-time curves. A standard flow-volume curve for manual measurement would then have a flow sensitivity of 2 L/sec equal to 10 mm, and a volume sensitivity of 1 L equal to 10 mm. Accurate recorder speed and volume sensitivity are particularly important when the results to be reported are obtained by manual calculation. Recorder accuracy should be checked at least

quarterly. Paper speed of strip chart recorders can be easily checked with a stopwatch. With the paper or recording pen moving, a volume signal is applied at regular intervals so that deflections are placed on the tracing. The intervals between the deflections are then measured and compared with the speed of the recorder. Electronic plotters or strip chart recorders can usually have their speed adjusted. Kymographs and similar mechanical recording devices may require repair or replacement of drive motors if paper speed is determined to be inaccurate.

Common Problems

Some of the common problems detected by routine quality control of spirometers include:

- Cracks or leaks (in volume-displacement spirometers)
- Low water level (in water-seal spirometers)
- Sticking or worn bellows
- Inaccurate or erratic potentiometers
- Obstructed or dirty flow tubes (flow sensors)
- Mechanical resistance (in volume-displacement spirometers)
- Leaks in tubes and connectors
- Faulty recorder timing
- Inappropriate signal correction (BTPS)
- Improper software calibration (corrections)
- Defective software or computer interface

Calibration and Quality Control of Gas Analyzers

Accurate analysis of inspired and expired gases is required for measurement of lung volumes, $D_{L_{CO}}$, and gas exchange during exercise or metabolic testing. The accuracy of these tests depends on the accuracy of the volume transducer and the gas analyzers used. Various types of gas analyzers are commonly used in pulmonary function testing (see Chapter 9). Some general principles apply when considering their calibration and quality control. Calibration refers to the process of adjusting the output of the instrument to meet certain specifications. Quality control refers to a method of routine checking of the accuracy and precision of the device. Calibration techniques for gas analyzers include the following:

1. *Physiologic range.* Some analyzers are not linear or exhibit poor accuracy over a wide range. Many analyzers are calibrated to match the physiologic range over which measurements are to be performed. Oxygen analyzers may be used to measure fractional concentrations from 0.21 to 1.00, representing a wide

physiologic range. If the O_2 analyzer is to be used for exercise tests in subjects breathing room air, it should be calibrated over the range of 0.12 to 0.21. This narrow interval represents the physiologic range of expired O_2 likely to be encountered during an exercise test. Reducing the physiologic range of an analyzer generally allows greater accuracy and precision. Some types of analyzers provide range adjustments or user-selected amplification just for this purpose. Test gases used for calibration should represent the extremes of the physiologic range.

2. *Sampling conditions.* Gas analyzers must be calibrated under the same conditions that will be encountered during the test procedure. Analyzers that are sensitive to partial pressure of the test gas (see Chapter 9) may be affected by the sample flow rate. For certain tests, gas is sampled continuously from the breathing circuit using a pump. The sampling flow rate of the pump must be adjusted *before* calibration, then left unchanged during sampling. If gas flow is stopped before the measurement is actually performed, the sampling flow rate is not critical. This type of analyzer must be calibrated under conditions of no flow. Measurement errors may occur when the analyzer is calibrated and then the configuration of the sampling circuit is changed. This typically happens with the addition of tubing, valves, or stopcocks. Any absorber circuits such as those used for CO_2, H_2O, or dust should be in place during calibration as well.

3. *Two-point calibration.* The most common technique for analyzer calibration involves introducing two known gases. If the test involves a gas that is not normally present in expired gas, such as He, CO, or Ne, room air may be used to zero the analyzer. A calibration gas representing the upper end of the physiologic range may be used to *span* the analyzer. The He dilution FRC and $D_{L_{CO}}SB$ are examples of such tests. The He and CO analyzers are zeroed by drawing room air into the measuring chambers. Helium and CO are assumed to be absent from the atmosphere. Test gas containing a known concentration of the gas to be analyzed is then introduced. The analyzer gain is adjusted to match the known concentration. The test gas approximates the concentration to be analyzed during the test. The analyzer then may be re-zeroed, and the entire process is repeated to verify the calibration. A similar technique may be employed using two gases of known concentration if the expirate normally contains varying concentrations of the gas. For example, room air and 12% O_2 might be used to perform a two-point calibration for an O_2 analyzer for exercise testing. Depending on the stability of the analyzer, calibration may have to be repeated before each test or measurement. Regardless of the methodology employed, gas analyzers should be calibrated before each patient for lung volume determinations, $D_{L_{CO}}$, exercise tests, and metabolic studies. Gas analyzers used for monitoring, such as capnographs, should be calibrated on a schedule appropriate for the extent of use. All calibration procedures should be performed in accordance with the manufacturer's recommendations. The accuracy of the calibration gas should reflect the necessary accuracy of the

measurements involved. For exercise or metabolic studies, calibration gases should be accurate to at least two decimal places (i.e., one hundredth of a percent). Calibration gases may require verification by an independent method.

4. *Multiple-point (linearity) calibration.* An assumption made by the two-point technique is that analyzer output is linear between the points used for calibration. In order to verify linearity or to determine the pattern of nonlinearity, three or more calibration points must be determined (Fig. 11–2). A multiple-point calibration is performed in a manner similar to the two-point calibration except that the concentrations of known gases across the range to be analyzed are checked and plotted. If multiple points are determined, linear regression may be used to determine the slope of the line relating the measured gas concentrations to the expected gas concentrations. Most statistics textbooks describe the calculation of simple linear regression. If the analyzer is linear, the points plotted fall in a straight line. If the analyzer is nonlinear, a calibration curve may be constructed in order to correct analyzed samples. In most instances, an equation describing the nonlinear curve can be generated. This equation then can be used either manually or by software to correct meter readings. Many nonlinear analyzers incorporate electronic circuitry that linearizes the output. Linearity of analyzers used for $D_{L_{CO}}$, lung volumes,

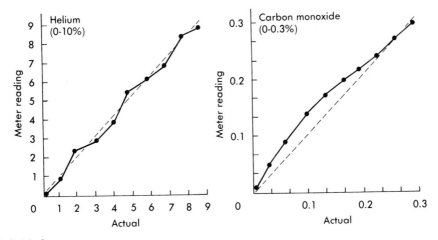

FIG 11–2.
Calibration and linearity check of gas analyzers. Typical plots of varying gas concentrations in relation to the meter readings of the analyzers for two gases (He and CO). Different dilutions of each gas are prepared and submitted to the analyzer. The meter reading is then compared with the calculated value. In the example, the He analyzer shows good linearity in the comparison of measured (meter reading) vs. expected (actual) concentrations. The CO analyzer shows a nonlinear pattern, as might be expected for an infrared CO analyzer. If enough points are determined a "calibration" curve can be generated for correction of the meter readings. By mathematically fitting the curve, an equation can be generated for subsequent correction of meter readings. Computerized systems often use a table of points representing a calibration curve.

exercise, and metabolic studies should be re-evaluated at least every 6 months. Some analyzers may require more frequent checks, depending on the extent of use.

Quality control of gas analyzers can be performed by submitting known concentrations of gases to the analyzer by testing a lung analog or biologic control. Multiple gases with concentrations spanning the range of the analyzer can be maintained. This may be a rather complex means of quality control for most clinical laboratories. A simpler technique is to prepare serial dilutions of a known gas using a large-volume syringe. The syringe may be the type used for volume calibration. For example, 100 mL of He and 900 mL of air may be mixed in a 1-L syringe to produce a 10% He gas mixture, then injected into the analyzer. Subsequently, 100 mL of He might be diluted in 1000 mL, then 1100 mL, and so on, with the expected concentrations calculated as follows:

$$\text{Expected \% test gas} = \frac{\text{Volume of test gas}}{\text{Total volume of gas}} \times 100$$

where:

$$\text{total volume of gas} = \text{test gas} + \text{added air} + \text{syringe dead space}$$

As each dilution is analyzed, the meter reading is recorded and plotted against the expected percentage (see Fig. 11–2). This method is simple and available to most laboratories. When preparing samples in this way, care must be taken that air does not leak into the syringe and further dilute the test gas. The volume of air in the syringe connectors (i.e., dead space) must be included when calculating the dilution of the test gas. Some calibrated syringes account for the connector volume.

A second method of verifying analyzer performance involves simulating either lung volume or $D_{L_{CO}}$ maneuvers. This may be accomplished using a fixed or variable volume lung analog. A lung analog is simply an airtight container of known volume (Fig. 11–3). The lung volume simulator is attached at the subject connection with the system prepared for lung volume or $D_{L_{CO}}$ determination. A large-volume syringe is used to "ventilate" the lung analog, mimicking a subject's breathing. At the end of the test the resulting lung volume (i.e., FRC) is compared with the known volume of the analog system. A calibrated syringe alone also may be used to simulate the maneuver. Starting with a known volume of air in the syringe, the test is performed by filling and emptying the syringe to the starting volume.

Simulation of the $D_{L_{CO}}SB$ maneuver using either technique should produce values very near zero. Both He and CO are diluted equally in the lung analog, and their relative concentrations should be identical. If the two analyzers are not linear in relation to one another, the ratio of He to CO will not equal 1.0. The

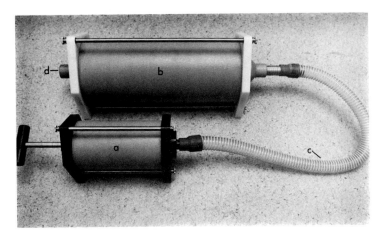

FIG 11–3.
FRC/DL_CO test system. A typical setup for quality control of either an open- or closed-circuit FRC system, or a DL_COSB system. **A,** large-volume syringe. **B,** variable-volume closed container. The volume may be varied by setting an internal piston. **C,** connective tubing used so that the syringe can be used to "ventilate" the closed container. **D,** system connection for attachment to the subject port. The system volume is determined by adding the volume set on B plus the volume of C (determined by filling with water and measuring) plus any dead space contained in the connections. The large-volume syringe is then used to simulate breathing. A 3-L syringe alone can be used to simulate a lung by starting the test with the syringe partially filled with air.

calculated $D_{L_{CO}}SB$ will be either above or below zero. This method tests not only the gas analyzers but the volume transducer, breathing circuit, and software as well. Temperature or gas corrections should be overridden or not performed. By varying the volume of the lung analog, a linearity check at different dilutions can be performed.

Some computerized systems do not allow lung simulators to be used. The software may be designed to make all necessary corrections for human subjects and may produce erroneous results when a simulator is used. However, if the software reports gas analyzer values directly, the accuracy and linearity of various dilutions can be checked.

Testing biologic controls (i.e., known subjects) is a third means of quality checking gas analyzers. This method may not detect small changes in analyzer performance because the entire lung volume, $D_{L_{CO}}$, or exercise system is used. Despite a variability of as much as 10% in $D_{L_{CO}}$ or exercise parameters that occurs in known subjects, malfunctions of systems involving gas analyzers can be detected. Tests on at least 3 subjects should be performed quarterly and results recorded in a database. The mean and standard deviation of these repeated measurements provide an index of the precision of the system. The biologic controls may be retested whenever questionable values are obtained. The known subject method may be the easiest means of checking automated exercise testing and metabolic measurement systems. Abnormal results of biologic controls can then be followed with more specific tests of suspect components.

Common Problems

Some of the common problems occurring with gas analyzers which may be detected by routine quality control checks include:

- Leaks in sampling lines or connectors
- Blockage of sampling lines
- Exhausted water vapor or CO_2 absorbers
- Contamination of photocells or electrodes
- Improper mechanical zeroing (taut band display)
- Inadequate warm-up time
- Deterioration or contamination of column packing material (gas chromatographs)
- Poor vacuum pump performance (mass spectrometer or emission spectroscopy analyzers)
- Chopper motor malfunction (infrared analyzers)
- Electrolyte or fuel cell exhaustion (O_2 analyzers)
- Aging of detector cells (infrared analyzers)
- Poor optical balance (infrared analyzers)

CALIBRATION AND QUALITY CONTROL OF PLETHYSMOGRAPHS

The calibration techniques described here apply primarily to a variable-pressure, constant-volume plethysmograph. Users of flow-based plethysmographs should perform the calibration procedure for the box transducer according to the manufacturers instructions. The mouth pressure and pneumotachometer calibration are similar for both types of plethysmographs.

Calibration

1. *Mouth pressure transducer.* Physical calibration can be done by directly connecting the pressure transducer to a water or mercury manometer. The manometer is a U-shaped tube with a calibration scale. The range of the transducer should include pressures usually measured, approximately ±25 cm H_2O. Care should be taken in using a mercury-filled manometer because of the high toxicity of mercury. Air is injected into one port of the manometer. For example, a small volume of air may be introduced to cause a deflection of 5 cm. This, in effect, creates a difference of 10 cm between the two columns of the

manometer. The gain of the mouth pressure amplifier is then adjusted so that the signal appearing on the display deflects by an amount equivalent to 10 cm H_2O per centimeter. The display device may be an oscilloscope, a plotter, or most commonly a computer terminal. This deflection then becomes the calibration factor for the mouth pressure transducer. In the previous example, each pressure change of 10 cm H_2O would result in a 1-cm deflection on the display. In computerized systems the analog output of the transducers is measured and a software correction factor determined. The correction factor is calculated in a manner similar to that used for spirometer output (see Calibration and Quality Control of Spirometers, this chapter). The correction factor is then applied by the software as the signals are acquired.

2. *Box pressure transducer.* Physical calibration of the box pressure transducer is accomplished by sealing the plethysmograph and applying a volume signal comparable to that which occurs during subject testing. In a 500-L plethysmograph, a volume signal of 25 to 50 mL is typical. A sine-wave pump connected to a small syringe is ideal for box calibration. The same volume can be alternately added and removed from the box at varying frequencies. With the pump operating, the gain of the box pressure transducer is adjusted so that the volume change in the box causes a specific deflection on the display device. For example, the pressure signal generated by a 30-mL volume might be adjusted to cause a 2-cm deflection on the display. The box pressure calibration factor would then become 15 mL per cm. This procedure may be repeated at varying frequencies from 0.5 to 5.0 cycles per second (i.e., Hz). Varying the frequency allows the frequency response of the box and transducer to be checked. The volume deflection should not change at different frequencies. Flow-based plethysmographs may be calibrated similarly. The output of the box flow transducer is adjusted rather than that of a pressure transducer. The plethysmograph is normally calibrated empty. A volume correction for the subject is then applied in the calculation of results (see the Appendix).

3. *Flow transducer.* The pneumotachometer is physically calibrated by applying a known flow of gas. An exact flow is generated using a rotameter or other calibrated flow device. The type of pneumotachometer usually employed is the pressure-differential type (see Chapter 9). A pressure transducer connected to the pneumotachometer is adjusted in a manner similar to that used for the mouth and box pressure transducers. The gain is adjusted so that a known flow causes a specific deflection on the display. For example, a flow of 2 L per second may be set to cause a 2-cm deflection. This results in a flow calibration factor of 1 L/sec/cm. If an adjustable rotameter is used, the linearity of the pneumotachometer can be verified by checking the deflections at various flows. A weighted spirometer also may be used to generate a known flow. Many computerized plethysmographs avoid the need for a flow generator by using a simple calibrated syringe. A 3-L volume can be injected through the pneumo-tachometer. The flow is integrated, and the gain of the flow signal is then

adjusted until the output of the integrator produces the known volume. In practice, a software correction factor, or table of factors, may be used rather than a physical adjustment of the flow signal.

As described previously, many computerized plethysmographs provide for electronic or software adjustment of the transducers. Known physical signals are applied, but gain adjustments are done electronically, or by generating a software correction factor. Another check provided by some systems is a calibrated voltage signal applied to the display device. For example, a microswitch may be depressed to send a 1-millivolt signal to a recorder. This reference signal might cause a recorder deflection of 1 cm. A procedure such as this is useful if the recorder will then be used to check the output of a transducer. This type of signal should not be confused with the actual physical calibration described above, but may be used to check an oscilloscope or recorder.

Quality Control

Quality control of a body plethysmograph may be accomplished by use of an isothermal lung analog, a biologic control, or comparison with gas dilution or radiologic lung volumes.

An *isothermal volume analog* can be constructed from a 4- or 5-L glass bottle that has been filled with metal wool, usually copper or steel. The metal wool acts as a heat sink (Fig. 11–4). The mouth of the bottle is fitted with two connectors. One fitting is attached to the subject connection of the mouth shutter. The other is attached to a rubber bulb of 50- to 100-mL volume. The actual volume of the lung analog can be determined by subtracting the volume of the metal wool from the volume of the bottle. The volume occupied by metal wool is calculated by its weight times its density. Alternately, the gas volume of the bottle may be measured by filling it with water from a volumetric source. The dead space of the connectors and rubber bulb also should be added to the total volume.

The accuracy check is performed with an assistant seated in the sealed plethysmograph. The isothermal volume device is connected to the mouthpiece. The mouth shutter is then closed. While breatholding, the assistant squeezes the bulb. A P_{mouth}/P_{box} tangent is recorded just as would be done in testing a subject. The volume (V_{TG}) is calculated as usual, except that the P_{H_2O} is not subtracted (see Appendix). The volume calculated should equal the volume of the isothermal lung analog (as measured previously) within ±5%. The correction for the subject volume, normally based on the subject's body weight, should include the subject plus the known volume of the isothermal lung analog. The procedure may be repeated at frequencies from 0.5 to 5.0 cycles per second to check the frequency response of the box. If the frequency response is "flat," the tangents or angles should not change as the bulb is compressed at different rates. The lung analog must contain a sufficient volume of metal wool to act as a heat sink. The metal

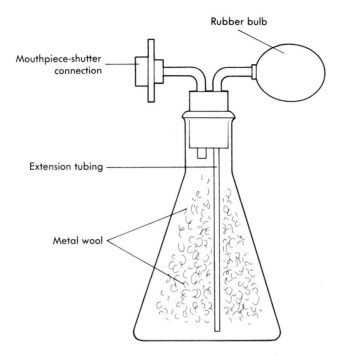

FIG 11–4.
Isothermal lung analog. A schematic of an isothermal lung analog for quality control of the body plethysmograph. A 3- to 4-L jar is fitted with a stopper with two openings. One opening connects to the mouthpiece shutter apparatus of the plethysmograph. The other opening is connected to a rubber hand bulb with an extension to the bottom of the jar. Copper or steel wool is used to fill the container. The metal wool acts as a heat sink so that pressure changes in the bottle cause only minimal changes in gas temperature. By having a subject in the plethysmograph hold their breath and squeeze the bulb, a V_{TG} maneuver can be simulated. A P_{mouth}/P_{box} angle may be recorded and the volume of the container calculated. The calculated volume should compare within 5% of the volume of the device. The true volume may be determined by filling the container with water and subtracting the volume of the metal wool. The volumes of the connectors and rubber bulb should be considered as well.

wool "absorbs" changes in temperature that result from the compression and decompression of gas in the box. Inadequate metal wool allows small temperature changes to affect the volume determination.

The accuracy of the pneumotachometer can be assessed by the use of known resistances. Resistors can be made using orifices with fixed diameters. Alternately, resistances of different magnitudes can be constructed by placing capillary tubes lengthwise in a flow tube. In either case, the pressure drop across the resistor is measured at a known flow rate. The resistor then may be added in front of the pneumotachometer while a subject breathes, or a known flow is applied. The increase in measured resistance should equal that of the resistor.

A second means of checking the plethysmograph's accuracy is to measure V_{TG} and/or Raw from a biologic control. A series of 10 measurements provides an adequate mean value for comparison with subsequent results. Day-to-day variability in trained subjects is usually less than 10%. This method allows checking the box itself, the transducers, the recording devices, and the software. Unfortunately, discrepancies between the mean of previous measurements and an individual quality control trial often do not indicate which section of the equipment may be causing the problem. Routine application of biologic controls, in conjunction with checks of the calibrations performed, may demonstrate which transducer or component is responsible for a problem.

A third method of checking the accuracy of the plethysmograph is to compare the V_{TG} with lung volumes determined by gas dilution or radiologic techniques. Correlations greater than 0.90 have been demonstrated between gas dilution, radiologic, and plethysmographically determined lung volumes in healthy subjects. Differences greater than 10% in volumes measured by plethysmograph and one of the other methods are nonspecific, but may indicate equipment malfunction. Because this method and the biologic control technique previously described are based on measurements of individuals, it is important that the subject performs the breathing maneuvers correctly (see "Criteria for Acceptability of Plethysmographic Measurements").

Common problems that may be identified by routine quality control of body plethysmographs include:

- Leaks in door seals or connectors (pressure boxes)
- Improperly calibrated pressure transducers
- Obstructed or perforated pneumotachometers
- Excessive thermal drift
- Poor frequency response
- Excessive vibration (poorly mounted transducers)

CALIBRATION AND QUALITY CONTROL OF BLOOD GAS ANALYZERS

Blood gas analyzers may be divided into two categories based on the type of calibration used—manual or automatic. Although both automatic and manual calibrations are similar, some important differences exist, particularly in the technologist's role in instrument maintenance.

Manual calibration of the blood gas electrodes involves exposing the gas electrodes (i.e., Po_2, Pco_2) to two or more gases with known partial pressures of O_2 and CO_2. Two or more known buffers are used to calibrate the pH electrode. Calibration gases spanning the physiologic ranges of the Po_2 and Pco_2 electrodes are used just as for gas analyzers described above. Typical combinations would include one calibration gas with a fractional O_2 concentration of 0.20 (20%), and a fractional CO_2 concentration of 0.05 (5%). The second calibration gas would have a CO_2 concentration of 0.10 (10%) with an O_2 concentration close to zero. If blood specimens with very high or very low partial pressures of oxygen are to be analyzed, the analyzer can be calibrated with a gas of similar fractional concentration. For shunt studies in which the subject breathes 100% oxygen, the analyzer may be calibrated with 80% to 100% O_2.

Calibration gases are bubbled through water at 37°C to saturate them with water vapor. Then the gas is allowed to flow into the measuring chamber. The partial pressures of the calibration gases depend on the barometric pressure. For each gas, the partial pressure is calculated as follows:

$$P_{gas} = F_{gas} \times (P_B - 47)$$

where:

P_{gas} = partial pressure of calibration gas

F_{gas} = fractional concentration of the same gas

P_B = ambient barometric pressure

47 = partial pressure of water vapor at 37°C

Each calibration gas is kept in the measuring chamber until equilibrium is reached. Once the partial pressure reading has stabilized, the appropriate control is adjusted to match the electrode to the calculated pressure. As with expired gas analyzers, a "low" gas is used to zero (sometimes referred to as "balancing") the electrode. A "high" gas is used to adjust the gain (also called the "slope") of the electrode. Zeroing the electrode does not necessarily require a gas with a partial pressure of zero, but simply setting the low range of the electrode. Two-point calibrations are commonly used to calibrate gas analysis devices. More than two calibration gases, however, must be used to prove the linearity of a blood gas electrode. Most blood gas analyzers utilize a combination of calibration gases. The P_{O_2} electrode is usually calibrated over a range of 0 to 150 mm Hg. The P_{CO_2} electrode is typically calibrated for the range of 40 to 80 mm Hg.

Some blood gas analyzers use precision gases to calibrate the gas electrodes, while gas tensions are measured in a liquid (i.e., blood). Some difference may exist between analysis of the same partial pressure in gas or liquid, especially for O_2. The reduction of O_2 at the tip of the polarographic electrode occurs more rapidly in a gaseous medium than in a liquid. If the electrode is calibrated with a gas, its response when measuring a liquid will be to read slightly lower. This difference is called the gas-liquid factor. A correction factor can be derived by calibrating the electrode using a liquid that has been tonometered (see discussion of tonometry in this section). The calibration gas and tonometered liquid are analyzed, and a ratio based on the difference between the two is computed. Gas-liquid corrections may be clinically important when measuring high partial pressures of oxygen, particularly above 400 mm Hg. Some blood gas analyzers use tonometered solutions for routine calibration of the gas electrodes. This technique avoids the necessity of determining the gas-liquid ratio.

Manual calibration of the pH electrode is performed by exposing the electrode to two or more known buffers. The "low" buffer typically has a pH of 6.840. This value is similar to the sealed-in buffer used in the pH electrode. A "high" buffer in the range of 7.38 is used to adjust the gain. This value is close to normal adult blood pH. The zero and gain of the pH voltmeter are adjusted to match these known points.

Automatic calibration of blood gas analyzers differs slightly from manual calibration. The gases and reagents involved are similar. The role of the technologist in assuring that the procedure achieves the desired outcome is different. The gas electrodes are balanced and sloped by a microprocessor using gases of known fractional concentrations or tonometered solutions. Adjustment of the output of each electrode's amplifier is also performed by the microprocessor. The computer brings the calibration gases or buffers into contact with the electrodes. The measured values are then stored. The microprocessor compares the measured values with expected calibration values. The microprocessor then adjusts the zero and gain (for a two-point calibration) to correct for the observed differences between the measured and expected values. Most computerized blood gas analyzers store the calibration results for comparison with the subsequent calibration. The amount of drift that occurs between calibrations can then be used to check an electrode's stability. Automatic calibration of the pH system is performed similarly. The microprocessor adjusts the electrode output to match two or more known buffers.

Most automated systems include checks of various other conditions that are fundamental to accurate blood gas analysis, such as the temperature of the measuring chamber. Some computerized systems tonometer solutions for calibration of the gas and pH electrodes. The microprocessor calculates the partial pressures of the calibration gases based on its reading of an internal barometer. Once the P_{CO_2} of the tonometered solution is calculated, the pH can be determined. This is relatively simple because the buffers are usually a bicarbonate-based solution. The built-in tonometer allows expected values for all three electrodes to be determined.

Automatic calibrations can be programmed to occur at predetermined intervals. Adjustments are performed automatically, based on the response of the electrodes. Because of this, all conditions for an acceptable calibration must be met before the procedure actually begins. During an automatic calibration, inadequate buffer or the wrong calibration gas may cause the microprocessor to adjust an electrode incorrectly. A similar problem can arise when blood or protein contaminates the tip of an electrode, altering its sensitivity. If an automatic calibration occurs, the microprocessor adjusts the electrode's output in an attempt to bring it into range. This process may work well for minor changes in electrode sensitivity, but the electrode cannot be properly calibrated if the debris at the measuring surface is excessive. The technologist must maintain the buffers, gases, and electrodes themselves so that automatic calibration can occur successfully. Inappropriate adjustments that occur may be detected easily by routine checking of calibration results. Although automated analyzers may seem easier to maintain, they require greater understanding and diligence by the technologist.

Manual and automatic calibration of blood gas analyzers each has its advantages and disadvantages. Manual instruments allow complete control over the analysis, including determination of the end point of the measurement. Manual calibration with gases of high or low partial pressures permits adjustment of the measuring range of the instrument to accommodate special tests. This may be important if the laboratory does a large number of shunt determinations. Manually calibrated instruments tend to be less precise than automated analyzers. This increased variability may result from different techniques of those using the equipment. The chief advantage of instruments that calibrate automatically is increased precision. The microprocessor controls sample size, timing, rinsing, and most other aspects of sample analysis and of calibration. The apparent simplicity of the automated calibration may be misleading. Although less attention may be required on the part of personnel performing analyses, those same technologists must be even more proficient in identifying electrode malfunctions. Most computerized instruments provide error flags or warnings if an automatic calibration senses unacceptable electrode performance. The technologist is responsible for assessing and correcting the problem.

Systematic errors can sometimes be masked by instruments that calibrate themselves. Contamination of the calibrating gases or buffers is a common example. If the microprocessor adjusts electrodes to match a contaminated calibration standard, the calibrations appear normal, but analysis of control samples will show differences. Detection of these types of systematic errors usually requires proficiency testing as described later in this section.

Two general methods of *quality control* for blood gas analysis are in widespread use: 1. tonometry, and 2. commercially prepared controls. The interpretation of blood gas quality control is the same with either of these methods, with a few minor differences.

Tonometry

A tonometer is a device that allows precision gas mixtures to be equilibrated with either whole blood or a buffer solution. One type of tonometer creates a thin film of blood or buffer by spinning the sample in a chamber flooded with the precision gas. A second type bubbles the gas through the sample to create a large surface for gas exchange. In both designs, the tonometer is maintained at 37°C and the gas is humidified. After an equilibration period determined by the gas flow rate and the volume of the control sample being prepared, a portion of the sample is transferred to the blood gas analyzer. The expected gas tensions are calculated from the fractional concentrations of the precision gas, just as described for manual calibrations in this section. If whole blood is used as the control material, then Po_2 and Pco_2, but not pH, can be checked. Blood is ideal for quality control of the gas electrodes because its viscosity and gas exchange properties are the same as patient samples. No other control material provides the oxygen carrying capacity of whole blood. For the most precise control of the Po_2 electrode, tonometry is the method of choice. Unless the buffering capacity of tonometered blood is known, however, the pH cannot be accurately calculated. Tonometry of a bicarbonate-based buffer using a known fractional concentration of CO_2 allows both gas and pH electrodes to be quality controlled. However, the gas exchange characteristics of buffers differ from those of whole blood.

Tonometry can be performed inexpensively using pooled waste blood and small amounts of precision gas. Using pooled blood requires special care. All blood specimens must be handled using Universal Precautions (see "Infection Control and Safety," this chapter). Quality control of the pH electrode must be accomplished by tonometry of a buffer. Three levels of control materials are typically used to provide checks over the physiologic range of the electrodes. Three precision gas mixtures are therefore required.

Accuracy of tonometry is highly dependent on a standardized technique. Sampling syringes must be lubricated and then flushed with the precision gas. Careful attention to the preparation and sampling from the tonometer is required to obtain reliable results. The values obtained using tonometry may depend on individual technique. Problems that occur with tonometry include contamination of the precision gas resulting from leaky connections, improper temperature control of the chamber, or inadequate gas flow to reach equilibrium.

Commercially Prepared Controls

Commercially prepared controls fall into three general categories: blood based, aqueous, or fluorocarbon based. The blood-based matrix consists of a solution containing buffered human red cells. The aqueous material is usually a bicarbonate buffer. The fluorocarbon-based control material is a perfluorinated compound that has enhanced oxygen-dissolving characteristics. These control materials are packaged in sealed glass ampules of 2- to 3-mL volume. They require minimum preparation for use. The blood-based material must be refrigerated. Incubation at 37°C for several minutes and agitation is required before use. The aqueous- and fluorocarbon-based controls can be stored in refrigeration for long periods, or at room temperature for day-to-day use. Most aqueous- and fluorocarbon-based controls have shelf lives of 1 year. Each of these require agitation for 10 to 15 seconds before use. Multiple levels of these materials are used to provide control over the range of values clinically seen. Commercially prepared controls may be considerably more expensive than tonometered samples. They are convenient to use, and may be less susceptible to handling errors than tonometered materials. One difficulty associated with aqueous controls (and to a lesser extent with fluorocarbon solutions) is poor precision of the P_{O_2}. This deficiency is especially bothersome at low partial pressures of O_2. Aqueous or fluorocarbon controls may produce such a wide range of "expected" values that the control may be of limited clinical usefulness. Some of these difficulties may be overcome by careful statistical handling of the P_{O_2} control data as described in this section.

A sound method of interpretation of the results of "control runs" is necessary to assist the technologist in detecting and repairing a malfunctioning electrode. A common method for detecting "out-of-control" situations is to calculate the control mean ± 2 standard deviation (SD). A series of runs of the same control material are performed. Twenty to 30 runs provide an adequate base for calculation of the mean and SD (see Appendix for a sample calculation). One SD on either side of the mean in a normal distribution includes about 67% of the data points. Two standard deviations include 95% of the data points in a normal distribution. Ninety-nine percent of the data points in a normal series fall within 3 SDs of the mean. A quality control value that falls within ± 2 SDs of the mean can be considered "in control." If the control value falls between 2 and 3 SDs from the mean, there is only a 5% chance that the run is in control. This normal variability which occurs when multiple measurements are performed is called "random error." One of 20 control runs (i.e. 5%) can be expected to produce a result in the 2-SD to 3-SD range and still be acceptable.

In order to distinguish true out-of-control situations from random errors, more complex sets of rules have been developed. The most widely used rules are those proposed by Westgard (see the Selected Bibliography). These rules are a subset of many statistical models. The rules are selected to provide the greatest probability for detecting real errors and rejecting false errors. This approach to quality control is called the multiple-rule method. The multiple-rule method usually requires that two or more control levels be evaluated on the same measurement device (electrode). The multiple-rule method may be applied as follows:

1. When one control observation exceeds the mean $\pm$ 2 SDs, a "warning" condition exists.
2. When one control observation exceeds the mean $\pm$ 3 SDs, an out-of-control condition exists.
3. When two consecutive control observations exceed the mean + 2 SDs or the mean − 2 SDs, an out-of-control condition exists.

4. When the range of differences between consecutive control runs exceeds 4 SDs, an out-of-control condition exists.
5. When four consecutive control observations exceed the mean + 1 SD or the mean − 1 SD, an out-of-control condition exists.
6. When 10 consecutive control observations fall on the same side of the mean ($\pm$), an out-of-control condition exists.

The multiple rule method attempts to detect marked changes in electrode performance, sometimes referred to as a "shift" by examining how far from the mean a single control value falls (rules 1 and 2). "Trends" in the performance of the electrode are detected by examining the recent history of control runs (rules 3–6). Similar rules may be applied to more than one level of control material by linking. For example, if three different levels of Po_2 controls are all between 2 SDs and 3 SDs higher than their respective means, it is unlikely that the Po_2 electrode is in control.

One problem with using a strict statistical approach is that when outliers (i.e., values more than 2 SDs from the mean) are repeatedly rejected, the standard deviation tends to become smaller, so eventually good data may be rejected. This situation can be managed by including data into the database that are clinically acceptable. With the multiple-rule approach, it is necessary to evaluate not only the mean and standard deviation of the current control run, but to keep a control history as well. This is usually accomplished by means of a control chart (Fig. 11–5).

In order to provide adequate quality control of a blood-gas analyzer, three levels of control materials are normally used. Three levels of control for each of the three electrodes (i.e., pH, Pco_2 and Po_2) require that 9 means and 9 SDs must be calculated for each instrument. When controls are run several times daily, tracking consecutive control runs can become quite cumbersome. In order to automate this procedure, computerized quality control programs are commonly employed. Such programs are available from professional organizations as well as commercial vendors. Many computerized laboratory information systems also support statistical databases for evaluation of control data. The chief advantages of such programs are simplified data storage and maintenance of necessary statistics. Rules such as those outlined can be applied easily to each new control run to detect errors. These types of records for quality control and instrument maintenance are required by many accrediting agencies (see the Appendix for a list of some regulatory agencies).

Quality control of blood gas analyzers should be performed on a schedule commensurate with the number of specimens analyzed. For most laboratories, controls must be performed daily or more often. In busy laboratories, multiple levels of controls may be required on each shift or whenever electrode maintenance is performed. Quality control runs establish the *precision* of the electrodes. Instrument precision must be known so that blood gas interpretation

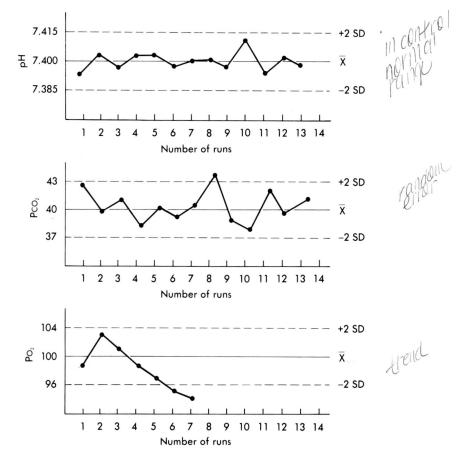

FIG 11–5.
Blood gas quality control charts. Three examples of Shewhart/Levey-Jennings charts for pH, P_{CO_2} and P_{O_2}. The mean for a specific control material is plotted as a *solid line* and the ± 2 standard deviation (SD) lines are dotted. The *left axis* on each graph is labelled with the actual mean and 2 SD values. Consecutive control "runs" are plotted along the *horizontal axis*. On the pH control chart, all of the values vary about the mean in a regular fashion — the electrode appears "in control" for the 13 measurements plotted. The P_{CO_2} chart shows a slightly different pattern. Control run 8 shows a value outside of the +2 SD range. This value is probably a "random" error, as it is the only control value outside the ± 2 SD limits. Subsequent controls show normal variability about the mean also suggesting that run 8 was a random error. The P_{O_2} chart shows a "trend" of decreasing control values. Runs 6 and 7 both produce values more than -2 SDs below the mean. This pattern suggests that the electrode is malfunctioning and needs to be serviced. By applying multiple rules to the interpretation of consecutive control runs, with or without charts, most "out-of-control" situations can be detected.

can be related to a range of values. For example, the variability of a P_{O_2} electrode may be determined to be $\pm$ 6 mm Hg (2 SDs). Each P_{O_2} result then can be interpreted within a range of 6 mm Hg above or below the reported value.

Several other techniques related to quality control of blood gas analyzers are commonly employed. *Interlaboratory proficiency testing* consists of the comparison of unknown control specimens from a single source by multiple laboratories. This allows an individual laboratory to compare its results with those of other laboratories. Results using different methodologies (i.e., analyzers) also may be compared. Results of proficiency tests are also reported as means and SDs for each type of instrument participating in the program. Proficiency testing does not establish the level of precision as does day-to-day quality control. It does, however, provide a measure of the absolute *accuracy* of the individual laboratory. A laboratory may have an acceptable level of precision as determined by daily control runs, but be inaccurate when compared with other laboratories. Proficiency testing often detects systematic errors that result from improper calibration techniques, contaminated buffers, or procedural errors. Multiple levels of unknowns are usually provided to check the typical ranges of values seen in clinical practice. Proficiency testing programs are available from professional organizations such as the College of American Pathologists as well as from commercial vendors. Satisfactory performance on interlaboratory proficiency testing has been mandated by the U.S. Department of Health and Human Services under the Clinical Laboratory Improvement Amendments of 1988 (see Regulatory Agencies in the Appendix).

Comparison of either controls or random samples on *multiple instruments* provides another means of quality control. Because many blood gas laboratories have two or more instruments, interinstrument comparisons provide a type of proficiency testing that yields immediate information. Monitoring either controls or samples by independent methods may provide a means of checking the accuracy of a particular instrument. For example, measurement of pH by means of an automated blood gas analyzer and a manual pH electrode could be used to verify the accuracy of the automated calibration system.

Some of the common problems encountered in the blood gas laboratory that are detected by quality control and proficiency testing include the following.

Electrode malfunction.   The most common causes of out-of-control situations relates to problems arising from the gas and pH electrodes. Protein and blood product buildup on the membranes covering the electrodes is quite common and can usually be remedied by careful cleaning. Leaks in the membranes themselves and depletion of electrolyte solution also commonly lead to electrode drift.

Temperature control.   Failure of the water or air baths to maintain the measuring chamber at 37°C or thermometer inaccuracy may lead to unacceptable electrode performance. Temperature control systems should be checked routinely against a certified thermometer (National Bureau of Standards traceable).

Improper calibration.   Improper manual calibration, either one or two point, is often related to operator error. Analysis of quality control data may determine if the technologist is performing calibration or sampling incorrectly. Problems arising from automatic calibration almost always relate to the instrument performing a calibration with inadequate buffer, or a poorly functioning electrode.

Reagent contamination or loss.   Contamination of calibration buffers and gases leads to inaccurate calibration and sample analysis. Quality control data that are consistently high or low may indicate a problem with reagents. Analysis of the buffers, reagents, or gases by an independent method may be required to detect deficiencies.

Mechanical problems.   A common source of error is the mechanism responsible for pumping or aspirating the sample into the measuring chamber. Leaks in pump tubing, or poorly functioning pumps, allow calibrating solutions, controls, and patient samples all to be contaminated. If air bubbles are introduced during analysis, gas tensions may be in error while pH determinations may be acceptable, but large changes in Pco_2 can cause alterations in the pH. Inadequate rinsing of the measuring chamber also may occur with pump problems or improperly functioning valves. This usually results in blood clotting in the transport tubing or measuring chamber.

Improper sampling techniques.   Failure to collect arterial specimens anaerobically, failure to properly store the sample in ice water, and bubbles in the specimen all may result in questionable results. Excess heparin typically results in a dilution of the sample with changes in the Po_2 and Pco_2. Improperly iced blood gas specimens exhibit changes in pH, Pco_2 and Po_2; red and white blood cells consume O_2 and produce CO_2 with a reduction in the pH. Air bubbles in the specimen shift the gas tensions in the sample toward room air. Low Po_2 values move toward 150 mm Hg while values above 150 mm Hg are reduced. Another common problem related to sampling is obtaining a venous specimen inadvertently. Adequately functioning electrodes, as demonstrated by good quality control, can detect poor sampling techniques, in distinction to actual clinical abnormalities.

CRITERIA FOR THE ACCEPTABILITY OF PULMONARY FUNCTION STUDIES

Quality assurance in the pulmonary function laboratory focuses not only on instrumentation, calibration, and controls, but on careful attention to the *testing technique.* Testing technique may be compared with "sampling" technique in other laboratory sciences. In pulmonary function testing, sampling may be defined as the procedures used to obtain patient data. These include effort and cooperation by the subject, instruction and encouragement from the technologist, as well as the correct performance of the equipment. Applying objective criteria to determine the validity of data is one means of providing high-quality results.

The criteria described in the sections that follow are arranged by test category. Standards for spirometry and the single-breath $D_{L_{CO}}$ have been set forth by the ATS. Guidelines for other tests are much less standardized. For each test category, a similar method may be used. To apply the criteria, these steps may be followed:

1. *Examine the printed or displayed tracings* whenever available. A direct recording, such as a kymograph tracing for spirometry, is ideal. Computer-generated graphics, either printed or on a video display, may be used as well. Compare the observed tracing with the characteristics of an acceptable curve.

2. *Look at the numerical data.* Are the results reproducible? Are the two highest values of multiple efforts within 5% of one another?

3. Are *key indicators* for a particular test present? Such indicators might include a minimum change in a gas concentration or duration of a maneuver. The key indicators may vary with the methodology used in each test category.

4. Are the *results consistent* among different test categories? Do spirometry, lung volumes, $D_{L_{CO}}$, and blood gas values all suggest a similar interpretation?

These general guidelines form the basis for applying the criteria to individual sets of patient data.

CRITERIA FOR ACCEPTABILITY OF SPIROMETRY

The following criteria may be used to judge the acceptability of tests from the forced expiratory volume (FEV) maneuver:

1. The volume-time tracing should show maximal effort, with a smooth curve. There should be no coughing or hesitation at the beginning of the maneuver. The tracing should show at least 6 seconds of forced effort. An obvious plateau with no volume change for at least 2 seconds should be achieved. Some subjects with severe obstruction may continue exhalation well past 15 seconds, so 6 seconds is simply a minimum. In severe obstruction, very low flows may be observed at the end of expiration, and continuation of the maneuver will not appreciably change the interpretation. The FEV maneuver may be terminated if the subject cannot continue for clinical reasons such as excessive coughing or dizziness.

2. The start-of-test should be abrupt and unhesitating. Any maneuver that displays a "slow" start must have the back-extrapolated volume calculated. The FEV_1 and all other flows must be measured after back-extrapolation (Fig. 11–6). If the volume of back-extrapolation is greater than 5% of the FVC or 100 mL (whichever is greater), the maneuver is not acceptable and should be repeated. The subject should be reinstructed in the correct technique for performing the maneuver. Demonstration by the technologist is often helpful.

3. A minimum of 3 acceptable efforts should be obtained. The two largest FVC and FEV_1 values should be within 5% or 100 mL, whichever is greater. These may be calculated:

$$\frac{2\text{nd largest FVC}}{\text{largest FVC}} \times 100$$

The same calculation is applied for the FEV_1. For the test results to be considered reproducible, this calculation should produce a value of 95% or more. If the two

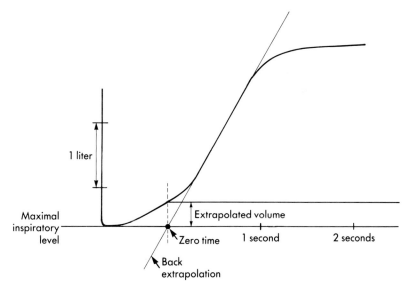

FIG 11–6.
Back-extrapolation of a volume-time spirogram. Back-extrapolation is a means of correcting measurements made from a spirogram that does not show a sharp deflection from the baseline maximal inspiratory level. This occurs when a subject does not begin the forced exhalation rapidly enough. A straight line drawn through the steepest part of a volume-time tracing is extended to cross the volume baseline (maximum inspiration). The point of intersection is the back-extrapolated time zero. Timed intervals, such as 1 second for the FEV_1, are measured from this point rather than from the initial deflection from the baseline or from the point of maximal flow. The perpendicular distance *(dashed line)* from the zero time point to the volume-time tracing defines the back-extrapolated volume. To accurately determine the time zero point, the extrapolated volume should be less than 5% of the FVC or 100 mL, whichever is greater. Tracings with larger extrapolated volumes may be considered unacceptable.

largest FVC or FEV$_1$ values are not within 5% (or 100 mL), the maneuver should be repeated. The test may be repeated any number of times. If reproducible values cannot be obtained after 8 attempts, testing may be discontinued. The reproducibility criteria should be applied only after the maneuver has been deemed acceptable, as described previously. Individual spirometric maneuvers should not be rejected solely because they are not reproducible. Bronchospasm or fatigue may affect reproducibility. The interpretation should include comments regarding the reproducibility (or lack of it) for the test maneuvers. The only criteria for eliminating a test completely is failure to obtain 2 acceptable maneuvers after at least eight attempts.

4. The MEFV tracing, if obtained, should show reproducible flows at similar lung volumes. The PEF (peak flow) should be consistent, and is a good indicator of subject effort. Superimposing MEFV curves, or displaying them side by side, provides a simple means of checking reproducibility. Complete loops should close. Inspiratory and expiratory VC values should be similar.

Data from all acceptable maneuvers should be examined. The largest FVC and the largest FEV$_1$ (BTPS) should be reported, even if the two values do not come from the same test maneuver. Flows that depend on the FVC, such as the FEF$_{25\%-75\%}$ and $\dot{V}_{max50}$, should be taken from the single "best" test maneuver. The "best" test is that maneuver with the largest sum of FVC and FEV$_1$ (Table 11–3).

A common problem may occur when using these criteria to produce a spirometry report. If a single volume-time or flow-volume tracing is included in the final report, it may not contain the FVC or FEV$_1$ that appears in the tabular data. It is advisable to maintain recordings, or raw data, for all acceptable maneuvers. Other methods of selecting the "best" test have been suggested, and are sometimes used. These include using the PEF as an indicator of maximal effort, or combining data from several MEFV loops to create an "envelope" loop.

TABLE 11–3.

Comparison of Spirometry Efforts

Test	Trial 1	Trial 2	Trial 3	"Best" test
FVC	5.20	5.30	5.35*	5.35
FEV$_1$	4.41*	4.35	4.36*	4.41
FEV$_1$/FVC	85	82	82	82
FEF$_{25\%-75\%}$	3.87	3.92	3.94	3.94
$\dot{V}_{max50}$	3.99	3.95	3.41	3.41
$\dot{V}_{max25}$	1.97	1.95	1.89	1.89
PEFR	8.39	9.44	9.89	9.89

*These values are keys to selecting the "best" test results. The FEV$_1$ is taken from Trial 1, even though the largest sum of FVC and FEV$_1$ occurs in Trial 3. All FVC-dependent flows (average and instantaneous flows) come from Trial 3. It should be noted that the FEV$_{1\%}$ (FEV$_1$/FVC) is calculated from the FEV$_1$ of Trial 1 and the FVC of Trial 3. The MEFV curve, if reported, would be the curve from Trial 3 as well.

Using the peak flow may cause errors if the FVC and FEV_1 are not also evaluated. The PEF is highly effort dependent and occurs at the beginning of the forced expiration. Combining loops to generate an envelope will provide the maximal flow achieved at any lung volume.

Spirometry may be performed in either the sitting or standing position for adults or children. There is some evidence that FEVs may be larger in the standing position in adults and in children younger than 12 years. The position used for testing should be indicated on the final report. The use of noseclips is recommended for spirometric measurements that require rebreathing, even if just for a few breaths. Some spirometers record only expiratory flow and require the subject to place the mouthpiece into the mouth after inspiring to TLC. If this is the case, noseclips are usually unnecessary. Care should be taken, however, that the subject places the mouthpiece into the mouth before beginning the forced expiration. Failure to do so may result in an undetectable loss of volume. It may be impossible to accurately calculate the volume of back-extrapolation from a tracing that displays only expiratory flow. In either type of spirometry system, rebreathing or expiratory flow only, a mechanical recorder should have the pen or paper moving at recording speed when the forced expiration begins. Systems that initiate pen or paper movement at the same time as expiration may be unable to adequately record the start-of-test, and may incorrectly record expiratory flow.

CRITERIA FOR ACCEPTABILITY OF THE MVV

The maximum voluntary ventilation (MVV) maneuver may be considered acceptable if the following criteria are met:

1. The volume-time tracing should show a continuous, rhythmic effort for at least 12 seconds. The end-expiratory level should remain relatively constant. If significant air trapping occurs, the end-expiratory volume may increase. On spirometers such as the water-sealed type, a leak at the mouthpiece may cause the spirometer volume to fall. This gives a false appearance of gas being trapped in the lungs. Most subjects show a change in the end-expiratory level during the first few breaths of the MVV. The change occurs as the subject adjusts to a mechanically efficient lung volume. This change may appear on the tracing as a decrease in spirometer volume, as most subjects perform the MVV at a lung volume slightly above FRC. The first three to five breaths may be discarded if the maneuver was continued long enough for a 12-second interval to be measured. Performing the test for 12 to 15 seconds is usually adequate.

2. At least two acceptable maneuvers should be obtained. The results should not differ by more than 10%. If a difference greater than 10% is observed, the test should be repeated until the two best maneuvers are reproducible. Other less

strenuous tests may be performed between MVV efforts to minimize fatigue that may accompany repeated MVV trials. Patients with hyperreactive airways may experience bronchospasm or coughing induced by hyperventilation occurring with the MVV maneuver. A marked decrease in the MVV with repeated efforts may be evidence of hyperreactivity and should be noted in the final report.

3. The MVV should approximate the largest FEV_1 multiplied by 35. Because there is a good correlation between the two tests, subject effort can be judged by comparing the MVV with an acceptable FEV_1 maneuver. If the MVV is much smaller than the $FEV_1 \times 35$, subject effort should be considered, as well as other conditions that might cause a decreased MVV (see Chapter 3). Similarly, if the MVV exceeds the $FEV_1 \times 35$ by a large amount, the validity of the FEV_1 itself may be questionable.

The "best" test should be the largest MVV observed from an acceptable maneuver. If the subject is unable to perform the MVV for 12 seconds because of coughing, fatigue, or shortness of breath, that fact should be noted on the final report.

CRITERIA FOR ACCEPTABILITY OF THE SLOW VITAL CAPACITY (VC)

A slow VC maneuver may be considered acceptable if the following criteria are met:

1. The end-expiratory volume of the three breaths immediately preceding the VC maneuver should not vary by more than 100 mL. Increasing or decreasing end-expiratory levels usually indicates that the subject is not breathing consistently near FRC, or that a leak is present. Even if the end-expiratory level is constant, the V_T usually increases when the subject is asked to breathe through a mouthpiece with a noseclip in place. This increase in V_T may change the inspiratory capacity (IC) or the expiratory reserve volume (ERV), depending on the pattern of breathing that the subject assumes.

2. The subject should expire smoothly to RV and then inspire without interruption to TLC. A volume plateau should occur at both maximal expiration and maximal inspiration. The slow VC may be measured either from maximal inspiration (inspiratory VC) or from maximal expiration (expiratory VC).

3. At least two acceptable VC maneuvers should be obtained. The volumes measured from these trials should be within 5% of one another. If the VC values are not within 5%, the maneuver should be repeated.

4. The VC should be within 5% of the largest FVC. If the slow VC is less than 95% of the FVC, poor subject effort may be the cause. If the VC is much larger than the FVC, dynamic compression of the airways during the FVC maneuver

may be causing air trapping. Insufficient subject effort during the FVC also may cause discrepancies between FVC and VC. Subjects who have obvious signs of airway obstruction are most likely to display an FVC that is smaller than the VC. If the VC is significantly larger than the FVC, the $FEV_{1\%}$ may be overestimated.

Obtaining a valid slow VC is important. The subdivisions of the VC, IC and ERV, are used in the calculation of RV and TLC. An excessively large V_T (i.e., greater than 1 L) or an irregular breathing pattern during the VC maneuver may reduce the ERV or IC. When an artificially reduced ERV is subtracted from the FRC, the RV will be calculated as larger than it actually is. Similarly, if an artificially reduced IC is added to the FRC, the TLC will be underestimated.

The same criteria should be applied to the VC if it is done alone or in conjunction with the lung volume determination by gas dilution or plethysmography. The VC maneuvers performed during the He dilution FRC measurement may show slightly lower ERV values. The ERV appears smaller because the subject exhales through the CO_2 absorber. The IC and ERV may be measured from an FVC maneuver if tidal breathing is also recorded. The end-expiratory level should be well defined as described previously in this section. Measuring lung volume compartments (i.e., IC and ERV) from the FVC maneuver without performing a slow VC may overlook clinically significant differences between the two.

CRITERIA FOR ACCEPTABILITY OF LUNG VOLUMES AND PLETHYSMOGRAPHY

Helium Dilution FRC

The He dilution (closed-circuit) FRC determination may be considered acceptable if the following criteria are met:

1. The "system" baseline should be flat. A tracing or display of the spirometer volume should indicate that no leaks are present. The He concentration should be stable up to the point when subject begins breathing through the system. A stable He concentration also indicates that no system leaks are present.

2. The rebreathing pattern of the subject should be regular. Tidal breathing should be regular, with successive breaths showing a gradually falling end-tidal level as O_2 is consumed. The addition of oxygen should return the system volume to the starting volume. Excessive addition of oxygen to maintain a stable baseline indicates a leak. This pattern may be difficult to detect in computerized systems that automatically add O_2. A pattern of increasing V_T and rate usually indicates inadequate CO_2 absorption. A similar pattern is observed if the addition of O_2 is

inadequate to meet the subject's needs. Both situations are uncomfortable for the subject, and may be dangerous. Both will affect the He analyzer readings and the results of the test.

3. The test should be continued until the He concentration changes by less than 0.02% over a 30-second interval. If the He analyzer is not capable of readings as small as 0.02%, 0.05% in 30 seconds may be used. In some computerized systems, the He concentration is recorded only at 30-second intervals. When using such a system, the test should be continued for at least 3 minutes, even if the equilibration criteria described is met before 3 minutes. This avoids a "false" equilibrium that may occur with irregular breathing patterns or frequent addition of oxygen.

4. The addition of oxygen should be appropriate for a quietly breathing subject (i.e., 200 to 400 mL/min). Some systems estimate O_2 consumption during rebreathing by noting the volume of O_2 added and dividing it by the time of the test. In the stabilized-volume method, the oxygen consumption can be estimated by noting how often and how much oxygen is added. During the oxygen bolus method, the rate of fall of the spirometer volume is proportional to the oxygen consumption rate. High O_2 consumption usually indicates a leak. Very low or no oxygen consumption means that the subject is receiving oxygen from outside the system, also usually a leak.

5. The He equilibration curve, if plotted, should be smooth and regular. The shape of the equilibration curve will depend on the evenness of ventilation. The curve should show gradually decreasing He concentrations. The tracing or display should be flat at equilibrium.

The time to reach equilibrium also should be reported. If the subject fails to achieve equilibrium within 7 minutes, that also should be reported. Extremely large or small FRC values, especially in healthy subjects, should be examined carefully using the criteria described. Comparison of He dilution lung volumes to those obtained by an independent method is helpful. In healthy subjects or those with purely restrictive disease, lung volumes by plethysmography, chest x-ray method, or single-breath dilution (as done with $D_{L_{CO}}SB$) should be similar. In moderate or severely obstructed subjects, He lung volumes are typically smaller than plethysmograph volumes, and greater than the volume determined from a single-breath dilution.

If He dilution is the only available method and a questionable value is obtained, the procedure should be repeated, allowing at least 4 minutes between tests to wash residual He out of the subject's lungs.

Nitrogen Washout FRC

The N_2 washout (closed-circuit) lung volume determination may be considered acceptable if the following criteria are met:

1. The washout should show a regular pattern without increases or abrupt variations in end-tidal N_2. Individual breaths may vary, particularly in subjects with irregular breathing patterns or uneven ventilation. The tracing should show gradually falling N_2 concentrations. Leaks in tubing, the N_2 sampling head, or at the mouthpiece usually allow room air containing N_2 to enter the system. If a Tissot collection system is used, the volume of the spirometer should be constant when the valves are closed to the patient, indicating no leak in the spirometer.

2. Washout times should be appropriate for the type of subject being tested. Healthy subjects should wash out in approximately 3 minutes or less. Washout should be complete. At the end of the test, the end-tidal concentration should be approximately 1% N_2 in subjects without obstruction. Incomplete washout in unobstructed subjects usually indicates a leak or a contaminated oxygen source. An improperly calibrated or poorly functioning N_2 analyzer also may cause the washout to appear prolonged or incomplete. In systems that integrate a flow signal with the N_2 analyzer signal, changes in the lag time between the two signals can cause inaccurate measurement of the breath-by-breath volume of N_2 washed out.

The washout time should be reported. Failure of the subject to wash out within 7 minutes also should be noted. Extremely large or small FRC values in healthy subjects should be questioned in regard to the criteria described. Lung volume determinations by an independent method should compare as described previously for He dilution FRC measurements. If the N_2 washout is the only method available and questionable results are obtained, the test should be repeated after a delay of at least 15 minutes to allow re-establishment of the normal N_2 and O_2 tensions in the lung and body tissues. Longer delays may be necessary if the subject is severely obstructed.

Body Plethysmography (V_TG)

The thoracic gas volume (V_{TG}) determined using the body plethysmograph may be considered acceptable if the following criteria are met:

1. The displayed or recorded tracing should indicate that the subject panted correctly (Fig. 11–7). The P_{mouth}/P_{box} panting loop should be closed or nearly closed. The loop should be contained within the pressure range for which the transducers were calibrated. If full-scale deflection is ± 10 cm H_2O on the mouth pressure axis, then the mouth pressure deflection should not exceed ± 10 cm H_2O. If the oscilloscope or display is calibrated appropriately, pressure signals that exceed the calibration limits will go "off screen" and are easily detected. Open loops may indicate compression of gas in the oropharynx, especially with the cheek muscles, or leaks at the mouth. Panting loops that drift across the

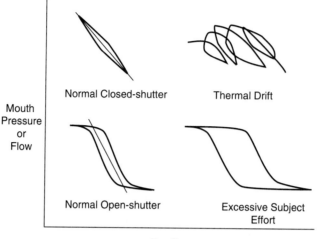

Mouth Pressure or Flow

Normal Closed-shutter

Thermal Drift

Normal Open-shutter

Excessive Subject Effort

Box Pressure

FIG 11–7.

Normal and abnormal plethysmograph recordings. **Top,** a normal closed-shutter maneuver in which mouth pressure is plotted against box pressure. The loop should be closed or nearly closed. If thermal equilibrium has not been reached, the loop tends to be open and to drift across the screen. **Bottom,** a normal open-shutter measurement in which flow is plotted against box pressure. If the subject pants near FRC, the loop takes on a nearly closed S-shaped appearance. If the subject pants too rapidly or too deeply, the tracing becomes open and flattened. Thermal drift also can cause the open-shutter tracing to resemble excessive patient effort.

display usually indicate that thermal equilibrium has not been attained, or that the panting volume is excessive.

2. A minimum of three acceptable panting maneuvers should be obtained. The angles should agree within 10% of the average of the angles measured. This may not always be practical if only three acceptable tangents are obtained and all three vary significantly. In such cases, the average may be used without rejecting individual maneuvers, but the variability of the angles should be considered when interpreting the reported lung volumes. Visual inspection of tracings or displays of the panting maneuvers often allows markedly different efforts to be discarded. Computerized plethysmographs that allow the mouth shutter to be closed at lung volumes other than at FRC may display widely varying angles. For these systems, the calculated FRC values determined from the various panting maneuvers should be compared, and outliers discarded. Most computerized plethysmographs use least-squares regression analysis to determine a best-fit line through the angle generated by the panting maneuver. The technologist may need to override the computer-generated tangent depending on the quality of the data obtained from the panting maneuver.

Similar criteria may be applied to measurements of angles for calculation of airways resistance (Raw), except that the angles for open-shutter and closed-shutter maneuvers are not averaged. Because the $\dot{V}/P_{box}$ angle and P_{mouth}/P_{box} angles are interdependent, airway resistance is derived for each maneuver separately, and the results of the maneuvers averaged. In most instances, the closed-shutter angles measured during airway resistance maneuvers will be less than those measured to derive V_{TG}. This occurs because most subjects pant *above* FRC. Higher lung volumes result in smaller angles.

If the subject cannot perform at least three acceptable maneuvers, it should be noted on the report. The V_{TG} should be determined from the average of three or more acceptable maneuvers. As described for the gas dilution techniques, it is often helpful to compare lung volume determinations by two or more independent methods. In subjects who have obstructive lung disease, lung volumes using a plethysmograph usually exceed those measured by the gas dilution techniques. The V_{TG} also compares favorably with radiologic lung volumes that have been measured reliably (see Chapter 1).

CRITERIA FOR ACCEPTABILITY OF $D_{L_{CO}}SB$

The ATS has published guidelines for the standardization of the $D_{L_{CO}}SB$ test (See Table 11-4: $D_{L_{CO}}SB$ Recommendations). The $D_{L_{CO}}SB$ maneuver may be considered acceptable if the following criteria are met:

1. The volume-time tracing (see Fig. 5–2) should show a smooth, rapid inspiration from RV to TLC. The rate of inspiration should be rapid enough so that 90% of the VC is inspired in 2.5 seconds in healthy subjects, and in less than 4 seconds in patients with obstruction. The breathhold baseline should be flat. The exhalation of dead space gas should be rapid and smooth. The volume of dead space gas expired should be between 0.75 and 1.00 L. If the subject's VC is less than 2 L, the dead space volume may be reduced to 0.5 L. The tracing should indicate the switch-in to alveolar sampling. Alveolar sample volume should be 0.5 to 1.0 L and should be collected in 3 seconds or less.

2. The volume inspired (VC or V_I) should exceed 90% of the largest previously measured VC value, either FVC or VC. If the inspired volume is less than 90% of the known VC, it may be assumed that the subject did not exhale to RV, did not breathhold at TLC, or both. For purposes of standardization, the breathhold should be as close to the true TLC as possible. If the inspired volume exceeds the best previously determined VC, then that VC should be questioned and may need to be repeated.

3. The breathholding time should be between 9 and 11 seconds. Any tests outside these limits should be discarded. Various methods of timing are

TABLE 11–4.

$D_{L_{CO}}SB$ Recommendations*

A. *Equipment*
  1. Volume accuracy same as for spirometry.
  2. Gas concentrations: O_2, CO, He, other gases.

CO	0.3	± 0.05%
He	10.0	± 1.0%
O_2	21.0	± 1.0%

  3. Documented CO and He analyzer linearity.
  4. CO analyzer calibrated at least every 6 months.
  5. Timing mechanism checked quarterly.
  6. Documented instrument dead space (inspiratory/expiratory).
  7. Check for leaks and volume accuracy (3-L calibration) daily.
  8. Validate system by testing healthy, nonsmokers.
B. *Technique*
  1. Subject should refrain from smoking for 24 hours before test.
  2. Subject should be instructed carefully before procedure.
  3. Subject should achieve an inspired volume >90% of VC.
  4. Subject should perform breathhold for 9 to 11 seconds.
  5. Deadspace washout should be 750 to 1000 mL, (unless VC <2 L).
  6. Alveolar sample volume should be 500 to 1000 mL.
  7. Four minutes should elapse between repeat tests.
C. *Calculations*
  1. Average at least two acceptable tests.
  2. Use Ogilvie or Meade-Jones methods of timing breathhold.
  3. Adjust for dead space volumes (instrument and subject).
  4. Determine inspired gas conditions (ATPS or ATPD).
  5. Correct for CO_2 and H_2O absorption.
  6. Report D_L/V_A in ml CO (STPD)/min/mm Hg per L (BTPS)
  7. Correct for Hb concentration (Cotes method).
  8. Adjustment for COHb (recommended).
  9. Adjustment for altitude (recommended).

*Summarized from Single breath carbon monoxide diffusing capacity (transfer factor). *Am Rev Respir Dis* 136:1299–1307, 1987.

employed with the $D_{L_{CO}}SB$ (see Chapter 5). Again, for purposes of standardization, the breathholding time should be kept close to 10 seconds. Rapid inspiration and expiration tends to reduce differences produced by the method of timing employed. In subjects with obstruction, prolonged expiration adds to the time for diffusion to occur and may overestimate diffusing capacity. Reducing the washout volume may shorten the measured breathhold time, but also may lead to inaccuracies. Sampling earlier will add more dead space gas to the alveolar sample, particularly in those subjects who may have increased dead space. The breathhold itself should be relaxed against either a closed glottis or the valve. A sustained inspiratory effort (Mueller maneuver) will increase $D_{L_{CO}}SB$ because of an increase in pulmonary capillary blood volume. Excessive positive pressure during the breathhold (Valsalva maneuver) tends to reduce pulmonary capillary blood volume and $D_{L_{CO}}SB$. The only practical means of detecting excessive pressure during the breathhold is careful observation by the technologist conducting the test.

4. Duplicate determinations should be within 10% or 3 mL CO/min/mm Hg (STPD), whichever is greater. The difference between two tests may be calculated as follows:

$$\frac{\text{Test 1} - \text{Test 2}}{\text{Average}} \times 100$$

The reported value should be the average of two or more acceptable maneuvers. The number of acceptable maneuvers averaged should be included in the report.

If the subject is unable to perform acceptable maneuvers, that fact should be included in the report. If a dead space washout volume other than the "standard" 0.75 − 1.00 L is used, it should be noted. The lung volume calculated from the $D_{L_{CO}}$ maneuver (V_A) may be compared with previously measured lung volumes, but must be expressed in liters (BTPS). In normal and even moderately restricted subjects, the V_A correlates reasonably well with the TLC if the single-breath maneuver is performed acceptably. In obstructed subjects, the single-breath lung volume may be smaller than lung volumes by multiple-breath gas dilution techniques, by radiologic estimation, or by plethysmography. The $D_{L_{CO}}SB$ may be reported using the standard single-breath technique, or by calculating the diffusion capacity using an independently determined lung volume in a similar equation.

Corrections for the subject's hemoglobin, COHb, and the altitude of the laboratory (see Chapter 5) are recommended but not required. If the Hb is corrected, both the adjusted and unadjusted values should be reported. Carboxyhemoglobin and altitude corrections, if made, should be documented on the final report for interpretive purposes.

Several conditions affecting the subject may influence the acceptability of the $D_{L_{CO}}SB$. The subject should be instructed to refrain from smoking for 24 hours before the test. The subject should be relaxed and in a sitting position, and should be carefully instructed in each of the required steps of the procedure. For duplicate determinations, at least 4 minutes should elapse between tests to allow test gas to wash out of the subject's lungs.

Infection Control and Safety

Pulmonary function tests, including blood gas analysis, are used often to test patients with blood-borne or respiratory pathogens. Reasonable precautions applied to testing techniques and equipment handling can prevent cross-contamination between patients. Similar techniques can prevent infection of the technologist performing the tests.

Policies and Procedures

Each laboratory should have written guidelines concerning safety and infection control. The guidelines should be part of a policy and procedures manual (see Table 11–1). Procedures should include, but not be limited to, handwashing techniques, use of protective equipment such as lab coats and gloves, and guidelines for equipment cleaning. The handling of contaminated materials (i.e., waste blood) should be clearly described. Policies and procedures should include education of technologists regarding proper handling of biologic hazards. Most accrediting agencies require written plans for safety, waste management, and chemical hygiene. In the U.S., the Occupational Safety and Health Administration (OSHA) has published strict guidelines regarding the handling of blood and other medical waste (see "Regulatory Agencies" in the Appendix).

Pulmonary Function Tests

Pulmonary function testing does not present a significant risk of infection for either patients or technologists. There are, however, some potential hazards involved. Most respiratory pathogens are spread either by contact with contaminated equipment or by an airborne route. Airborne organisms may be contained in droplet nuclei, on epithelial cells that have been shed, or in dust particles. The following guidelines can help reduce the possibility of cross contamination or infection:

1. Disposable mouthpieces and noseclips should be used for spirometry. Reusable mouthpieces should be disinfected or sterilized after each use.

2. Tubing or valves through which subjects rebreathe should be changed after each test. This is particularly important for maneuvers such as the FVC, where there is a potential for mucus, saliva, or droplet nuclei to contaminate the device. Breathing-circuit components should be stored in sealed plastic bags after disinfection.

3. Spirometers should be cleaned according to the manufacturer's recommendations. The frequency of cleaning should be appropriate for the number of tests performed. Flow-based spirometers in which the flow sensor is located at the subject's mouth may require daily cleaning. Some flow-based systems offer pneumotachometers that can be changed between subjects. These may be advantageous if patients with known respiratory infections must be tested. Pneumotachometers not located proximal to the patient are less likely to be

contaminated by mucus, saliva, or droplet nuclei. Such systems may require disinfection less frequently. Disposable flow sensors should not be reused. Water-sealed spirometers should be drained at least weekly and allowed to dry completely. Only distilled water should be used for filling. Bellows and rolling-seal spirometers may be more difficult to disassemble, but should be disinfected on a routine basis. Most spirometers present little risk of cross contamination to patients. Routine cleaning also helps maintain the spirometer in good working condition.

4. Bacteria filters may be used in some circuits to prevent equipment contamination. Filters may impose increased resistance that will affect maximal flows. Some types of filters show increased resistance after continued use in expired gas. If filters are used for low-flow procedures such as lung volume determinations, their volume must be included in the calculations. Filters may be useful in protecting equipment from contamination when patients with respiratory pathogens must be tested.

5. Small-volume nebulizers, such as those used for bronchodilators or bronchial challenge, offer the greatest potential for cross contamination. These devices, if reused, should be sterilized in order to destroy vegetative micro-organisms, fungal spores, tubercle bacilli, and some viruses. Preferably, disposable single-use nebulizers should be used. Metered-dose devices may be used for bronchodilator studies by utilizing disposable mouthpieces or "spacers" to prevent colonization of the device.

6. Risk of infection for the technologist may be minimized by the use of gloves or other barriers to remove used mouthpieces, tubing, or valves, particularly when dealing with subjects with documented infections. The risk of transmission from subjects with hepatitis B or human immunodeficiency virus (HIV or AIDS) through respiratory secretions is slight. There is a risk of acquiring infections such as tuberculosis or *Pneumocystis carinii* occurring in infected individuals. A mask should be worn by the technologist when testing subjects who have active tuberculosis or other diseases that can be transmitted by coughing. Masks may be required for "reverse isolation" when testing immu-nocompromised patients.

7. If routine pulmonary function testing includes a large number of patients with respiratory pathogens, such as tuberculosis, specially ventilated rooms may be necessary. The risk of cross contamination or infection can be greatly reduced by filtering and increasing the exchange rate of air in the testing room.

8. Surveillance should include routine cultures of reusable components such as mouthpieces, tubing, and valves following disinfection.

Blood Gases

The Centers for Disease Control (CDC) have established *universal precautions* that apply to personnel handling blood or other body fluids containing blood. Universal precautions apply to blood, semen, vaginal secretions, cerebrospinal fluid (CSF), synovial fluid, pleural fluid, pericardial fluid, and amniotic fluid. Some of these fluids are commonly encountered in the blood gas laboratory. These fluids present a significant risk to the health care worker. Hepatitis B, HIV, and other blood-borne pathogens must be assumed to be present in these fluids.

Body fluids to which the universal precautions do not apply include feces, nasal secretions, sputum, sweat, tears, urine, and vomitus, unless they contain visible blood. Some of these fluids may be encountered in the pulmonary function laboratory. These fluids present an extremely low or nonexistent risk for HIV or hepatitis B. They are, however, a potential source for nosocomial infections from other non–blood-borne pathogens. Universal precautions do not apply to saliva, but infection control practices such as use of gloves and handwashing further minimize the risk involved in contact with mucous membranes of the mouth.

These universal precautions should be applied in the pulmonary function or blood gas laboratory:

1. Treat *all* blood and body fluid specimens as potentially contaminated.

2. Exercise care to prevent injuries from needles, scalpels, or other sharp instruments or devices. Do not resheath used needles by hand. If a needle must be resheathed, use a one-handed technique or a device that holds the sheath. Do not remove used needles from disposable syringes by hand. Do not bend, break, or otherwise manipulate used needles by hand. Use a rubber block or cork to obstruct used needles after arterial punctures. Place used syringes and needles, scalpel blades, and other sharp items in puncture-resistant containers. Locate the containers as close as possible to the area of use.

3. Use protective barriers to prevent exposure to blood, body fluids containing visible blood, and other fluids to which the universal precautions apply. Examples of protective barriers include gloves, gowns, lab coats, masks, and protective eye wear. Gloves should be worn for drawing blood samples. Gloves cannot prevent penetrating injuries caused by needles or sharp objects. Gloves are also indicated if the technologist has cuts, scratches or other breaks in the skin. Protective barriers should be used in situations where contamination with blood may occur, such as obtaining blood from an uncooperative patient, when performing finger/heel sticks on infants, or when receiving training in blood drawing. Examination gloves should be worn for procedures involving contact with mucous membranes. Masks, gowns, and protective goggles may be indicated for procedures that present a possibility of blood splashing. Blood splashing may occur during arterial line placement or drawing samples from arterial catheters.

4. Wear gloves while performing blood gas analysis. Lab coats or aprons that are resistant to liquids also should be worn. Protective eye wear may be

necessary if there is risk of blood splashing during specimen handling. Maintenance of blood gas analyzers, such as repair of electrodes and emptying of waste containers, should be performed wearing similar protective gear. Lab coats or aprons should be left in the specimen handling area. Blood waste products, such as blood gas syringes, should be disposed of in clearly marked biohazard containers.

5. Immediately and thoroughly wash hands and other skin surfaces that are contaminated with blood or other fluids to which the universal precautions apply. Hands should be washed after removing gloves. Blood spills should be cleaned up using a solution of 1 part 5% sodium hypochlorite (bleach) in 9 parts of water. Bleach also should be used to rinse sinks used for blood disposal.

SELF-ASSESSMENT QUESTIONS

1. Multiple injections of a 3-L syringe into a flow-based spirometer produce an average of 2.92 L; this value indicates:
   a. The spirometer meets ATS accuracy requirements
   b. There is a system leak
   c. Excessive flows were used for calibration
   d. The spirometer should not be used for children

2. A 3-L syringe is used to calibrate a computerized spirometer; at ATPS, the spirometer reads a volume of 2.94. The software correction factor for this system would be:
   a. 1.02
   b. 1.00
   c. 0.98
   d. 0.95

3. According to ATS recommendations, the acceptable "back pressure" (flow resistance) from a spirometer is less than:
   a. 3.0 cm H_2O at 3 L/sec
   b. 3.0 cm H_2O at 12 L/sec
   c. 1.5 cm H_2O at 7 L/sec
   d. 1.5 cm H_2O at 12 L/sec

4. A spirometer recorder that is used for plotting flow-volume curves has a volume (X-axis) sensitivity of 25 mm/L; the flow (Y-axis) sensitivity should be:
   a. 12.5 mm/L/sec
   b. 25.0 mm/L/sec
   c. 50.0 mm/L/sec
   d. 50.0 mm/L

5. A CO_2 analyzer is calibrated using a 5% CO_2 mixture with the sampling pump set at 500 mL/min; a water vapor absorber is then added to the sample line. Which of the following should be done before using this system:
   a. Increase the sampling pump flow to at least 750 mL/min
   b. Decrease the sampling pump flow to less than 50 mL/min
   c. Recalibrate the analyzer
   d. Calculate the "corrected" CO_2 reading

6. A helium analyzer is checked using a 3-L syringe. 300 mL of He is added to 2.70 L of air in the syringe. If the dead space of the syringe and tubing is 100 mL, what is the expected concentration of He in the syringe:
   a. 11.1%
   b. 10.2%
   c. 9.7%
   d. 8.8%

7. A 50-mL sine-wave pump is used to calibrate a 450-L plethysmograph. While the pump is running, the display is adjusted so that the tracing deflects 2 inches. The box calibration factor for this system would be:
   a. 1.0 L/inch
   b. 100 mL/inch
   c. 25 mL/inch
   d. 12.5 mL/inch

8. An automated blood gas analyzer performs two-point calibrations that match expected values. Subsequent quality control runs show unacceptable values for Pco_2 and Po_2, but pH is acceptable. Which of the following is most likely the cause:
   a. Contaminated buffers
   b. Contaminated calibration gas
   c. Analyzer temperature is not 37°C
   d. Computer error

9. Which of the following control materials would be best suited for quality control of a Po_2 electrode used to measure O_2 tensions less than 50 mm Hg:
   a. Fluorocarbon-based control
   b. Aqueous-based control
   c. Tonometered buffer
   d. Tonometered whole blood

10. Quality control runs on a Pco_2 electrode have produced a mean of 40 mm Hg $\pm$ 2 mm Hg (1 SD); what are the chances of obtaining a value of 45 mm Hg on a control run, even if the electrode is functioning properly:

a. 95%
b. 50%
c. 5%
d. less than 1%

11. A subject performs spirometry and these results are recorded from 3 acceptable trials:

	Trial 1	Trial 2	Trial 3
FVC (L)	4.4	4.4	4.5
FEV_1 (L)	3.7	3.8	3.3
$\dot{V}_{max50}$ (L/sec)	1.7	1.2	1.3

If the flow-volume curve is to be reported with this study:
a. The curve from trial 1 should be used.
b. The curve from trial 2 should be used.
c. Either trial 1 or trial 3 may be used.
d. The peak flow must be known to select the curve.

12. A patient performs spirometry and the following results are obtained:

	Trial 1	Trial 2	Trial 3
FVC (L)	4.4	4.9	5.0
FEV_1 (L)	2.3	3.3	2.6

The pulmonary function technologist should conclude which of the following:
a. Only the FVC is acceptable
b. Only the FEV_1 is acceptable
c. Both the FVC and FEV_1 are acceptable
d. The FEV_1/FVC is 52%

13. A patient whose FVC is 4 L performs two $D_{LCO}SB$ maneuvers with the following results:

	Trial 1	Trial 2
D_{LCO} (mL CO/mm Hg/min)	20.3	22.0
V_I (L)	3.7	3.8
Breathhold time (sec)	10.7	9.7

The pulmonary function technologist should:
a. Reject trial 1 because of the V_I
b. Reject trial 2 because of the breathhold time
c. Report the $D_{LCO}SB$ as 22.0 mL CO/mm Hg/min
d. Report the $D_{LCO}SB$ as 21.2 mL CO/mm Hg/min

14. Which of the following pulmonary function equipment must be disinfected between patient uses:

    I. Water-seal spirometers
    II. Dry rolling-seal spirometers
    III. Spirometry tubing
    IV. Small-volume nebulizers for inhalation challenge tests
    a. I, III, IV
    b. I, II, III
    c. I, II only
    d. III, IV only

15. Universal precautions, as published by the Centers for Disease Control (CDC) recommend that:
    I. Gloves be worn only for HIV or hepatitis B–infected blood
    II. Used needles should not be resheathed
    III. Lab coats or gowns be worn when handling blood
    IV. Hands should be washed after removing gloves
    a. I, II, III, IV
    b. I, II, III
    c. II, III, IV
    d. I, IV only

SELECTED BIBLIOGRAPHY

GENERAL REFERENCES

American Thoracic Society: Standardization of spirometry. *Am Rev Respir Dis* 119:831, 1979.

American Thoracic Society: Standardization of spirometry—1987 update. *Am Rev Respir Dis* 136:1285, 1987.

American Thoracic Society: Single breath carbon monoxide diffusing capacity (transfer factor)—recommendations for a standard technique. *Am Rev Respir Dis* 136:1299, 1987.

Clausen JL, editor: *Pulmonary function testing guidelines and controversies.* New York, 1982, Academic Press.

Morris AH, Kanner RE, Crapo RO, et al: *Clinical pulmonary function testing,* ed 2. Salt Lake City, 1984, Intermountain Thoracic Society.

CALIBRATION AND QUALITY CONTROL

Clausen JL, Hansen JE, Misuraca L, et al: Interlaboratory comparisons of blood gas measurements. *Am Rev Respir Dis* 123(suppl):104, 1981.

Gardner RM, Crapo RO, Billings RG, et al: Spirometry: what paper speed? *Chest* 84:161, 1983.

Gardner RM, Hankinson JL, West BJ: Evaluating commercially available spirometers. *Am Rev Respir Dis* 121:73, 1980.

Glindmeyer HW, Anderson ST, Kern RG, et al: A portable adjustable forced vital capacity simulator for routine spirometer calibration. *Am Rev Respir Dis* 121:599, 1980.

Hankinson JL, Gardner RM: Standard waveforms for spirometer testing. *Am Rev Respir Dis* 126:362, 1982.

Hankinson JL: Pulmonary function testing in the screening of workers: guidelines for instrumentation, performance, and interpretation. *J Occup Med* 28:1081, 1986.

Leary ET, Graham G, Kenny MA: Commercially available blood-gas quality controls compared with tonometered blood. *Clin Chem* 26:1309, 1980.

Leith DE, Mead J: *Principles of body plethysmography.* National Heart, Lung, and Blood Institute, Division of Lung Diseases, 1974.

Shigeoka JW: Calibration and quality control of spirometer systems. *Respir Care* 28:747, 1983.

Shigeoka JW, Gardner RM, Barkham HW: A portable volume/flow calibrating syringe. *Chest* 82:598, 1982.

Westgard JO, Groth T, Aronsson T, et al: Performance characteristics of rules for internal quality control: probabilities for false rejection and error detection. *Clin Chem* 23:1857, 1977.

CRITERIA FOR ACCEPTABILITY OF PULMONARY FUNCTION STUDIES

_____Office spirometry in clinical practice. ACCP Committee on clinic and office pulmonary function testing. *Chest* 74:298, 1978.

Ferris BG, editor: Epidemiology standardization project: recommended standardized procedures for pulmonary function testing. *Am Rev Respir Dis* 118(suppl 2):55, 1978.

Nathan SP, Lebowitz MD, Knudson RJ: Spirometric testing: number of tests required and selection of data. *Chest* 76:384, 1979.

Quanjer PhH, editor: Standardization of lung function testing. *Bull Eur Physiopathol Respir* 19(suppl 5), 1983.

Snow M: Determination of functional residual capacity. *Respir Care* 34:586, 1989.

Sorensen JB, Morris AH, Crapo RO, et al: Selection of the best spirometric values for interpretation. *Am Rev Respir Dis* 122:802, 1980.

Townsend MC, Duchene AG, Fallat RJ: The effects of underrecorded forced expirations on spirometric lung function indexes. *Am Rev Respir Dis* 126:734, 1982.

INFECTION CONTROL

Centers for Disease Control: Recommendations for prevention of HIV transmission in health-care settings. *MMWR* 36:3S, 1987.

Centers for Disease Control: Update: universal precautions for prevention of transmission of human immunodeficiency virus, Hepatitis B virus, and other bloodborne pathogens in healthcare settings. *MMWR* 37:377, 1988.

Chatburn RL: Decontamination of respiratory care equipment: what can be done, what should be done? *Respir Care* 34:98, 1989.

Garner JS, Favero MS: CDC guidelines for the prevention and control of nosocomial infections: guidelines for handwashing and hospital environmental control. *Am J Infect Control* 14:110, 1986.

National Committee for Clinical Laboratory Standards (NCCLS): *Protection of laboratory workers from infectious disease transmitted by blood, body fluids, and tissue,* ed 2. *Tentative guideline.* Publication M29-T2, 1992.

Simmons BP, Wong ES: Guidelines for prevention of nosocomial pneumonia. *Am J Infect Control* 11:230, 1983.

Tablan OC, Williams WW, Martone WJ: Infection control in pulmonary function laboratories. *Infect Control* 6:442, 1985.

Zibrak JD, O'Donnell CR, Wissler J, et al.: Infection control in the respiratory management of patients with HIV-related disorders. *Respir Care* 34:734, 1989.

12

Case Studies

The following cases are presented to illustrate the use of pulmonary function, exercise, and metabolic testing, and blood gas analysis to aid in the diagnosis and treatment of cardiopulmonary disorders. Each case includes a history, test data, interpretation, and discussion.

The subject's history accompanying each case provides clinical information pertinent to the numeric results. Readers are encouraged to evaluate the *History* and *Test* results sections, then to write down an interpretation, using the guidelines described in this section. Compare your assessment with that given in the *Interpretation* section. The *Discussion* section explains the comments given in the interpretation.

The first five cases deal with pulmonary function tests performed in most hospital laboratories. Case 6 is an inhalation challenge test. Cases 7, 8, and 9 are exercise tests that include exhaled gas analysis. Case 10 is an example of blood gas quality control interpretation. Case 11 describes the use of serial pulmonary function testing to follow a specific disease process. Case 12 concerns the use of pulse oximetry for simple exercise evaluation. Case 13 is a metabolic study.

GENERAL GUIDELINES FOR INTERPRETATION

These guidelines provide a framework for a systematic approach to interpreting pulmonary function and blood gas data.

1. *Acceptability of data.* Careful review of tracings and raw data should precede any interpretive steps. Two key elements that should be evaluated include proper equipment function and adequacy of subject effort. Malfunction of spirometers, gas analyzers, or other components can often be discerned from recorded tracings or raw data (i.e., analyzer readings or spirograms). Subject cooperation and effort also can be evaluated from tracings and raw data. Internal

consistency of the data also may be checked in order to detect problems. For example, the vital capacity (VC) may be measured as part of spirometry, as part of lung volume determination, during the $D_{L_{CO}}SB$ maneuver, and in conjunction with plethysmography. Each of these measures should be internally consistent. The VC measurements need not be identical, but differences, such as those between the FVC and slow VC (SVC), should be explained. A report by the technologist performing the study is invaluable if the interpreter is not present for the test. This report can be as simple as a set of notes describing the subject's cooperation and ability to perform the test maneuvers. The report also should include any problems that might affect the reported values. Criteria for acceptability of each test should be determined in advance by the laboratory. Guidelines for standardization such as those published by the ATS (see Chapter 11) should be the basis for these laboratory criteria. Nonacceptability of pulmonary function data should be documented in the interpretation, particularly if the reproducibility of the data is in question.

2. *Reference values.* The appropriateness of the reference values used in the interpretation should be verified. The interpreter should be familiar with the variability of the predicted values for each test. The population from which the predicted values were derived should ideally mirror the clients of the laboratory (see Using Predicted Values, Appendix). Laboratories should indicate the source of reference values on their reports. Prediction equations that provide lower limits of normal should be used whenever possible. "Abnormal" values for each test category may be enumerated, after ascertaining that the predicted values are appropriate for the subject tested. Incorrectly recording age, height, or sex commonly results in the wrong predicted values being used. Values falling outside expected limits should be examined in each test category:

- Spirometry before/after bronchodilator
- Lung volumes by gas dilution and/or plethysmography
- $D_{L_{CO}}$ (single breath or steady state)
- Blood gases
- Maximal inspiratory/expiratory pressures
- Airways resistance/conductance and compliance

Many computerized systems flag abnormal values. The method by which this is done should be determined by the laboratory based on evaluation of normal subjects and subjects with known disease. Other computerized functions that may be helpful include calculation of confidence intervals or percentiles.

3. *Type and severity of dysfunction.* Interpretation of pulmonary function tests of an individual patient should consider the clinical question to be answered by the test. The referring physician should indicate as precisely as possible the reason why the test is requested. Interpreters of pulmonary function studies should be conservative in suggesting a specific diagnosis based solely on

pulmonary function data. With "borderline" values, all available clinical information should be used to help decide what is normal or abnormal. If truly abnormal values are found, some general statement of the pattern of abnormality may be made. The simplest categorization is to describe the pattern as obstructive, restrictive, or as a combination of both. Obstructive diseases are characterized by reduction of maximal expiratory and/or inspiratory flows. Obstruction may be accompanied by increases in lung volumes, notably RV, FRC, and TLC. Reduced diffusing capacity and blood gas abnormalities also commonly accompany obstruction. Restrictive diseases are characterized by reduction in VC and TLC. Restriction also may be accompanied by abnormalities in diffusing capacity and blood gases. The severity of dysfunction is commonly classified by modifiers attached to the specific physiologic parameter measured. Examples are "severe reduction in flows," "moderately reduced TLC," and "mildly elevated Pco_2." The use of such modifiers is limited by the variability associated with the test performed. These terms may not adequately describe the severity of the disease, functional limitations to the subject, or the risk of morbidity/mortality. If such modifiers are used, the limits of normal for the test involved should be described. This is particularly important when the measured value falls close to the lower limit of normal. Extent of disease sometimes is also described by comparison with changes from previous tests. The variability of a specific physiologic parameter, and the variability of the testing technique, combine to determine how large a change can be considered significant. Subjects with disease often show increased variability in certain tests. Published studies are useful in determining the variation occurring in normal and diseased subjects. Each laboratory should determine the variability that results from their test methods.

4. *Clinical summary.* A summary statement that relates the acceptability of the data, the abnormal findings, and the type of dysfunction to the subject's clinical history is often useful. The summary statement should answer the clinical question asked of the test. This summary may be limited more by the history (or lack of it) than by the test data. In some cases, the interpretation may include questions. For example, an inquiry such as, "Does the subject have any history of exposure to . . . ," may assist in relating the observed values to the subject's symptoms. The summary also may include recommendations for further testing. Therapeutic recommendations, such as suggestions for oxygen, bronchodilators, or smoking cessation, may be included.

CASE 1

History

M.B. is a 27-year-old male high school teacher, whose chief complaint is dyspnea on exertion. The subject states that his breathlessness has worsened over the past several months. He has smoked one pack of cigarettes a day for approximately 10 years (10 pack/years). He denies a cough or sputum production. No one in his family ever had emphysema, asthma, chronic bronchitis, carcinoma, or tuberculosis. There is no history of exposure to extraordinary environmental pollutants.

Pulmonary Function Testing

1. Personal data

Sex:	Male
Age:	27 yrs
Height:	65 in
Weight:	297 lb
BSA:	2.28 M^2

2. Spirometry and airway resistance

	Before drug	Predicted	%
FVC (L)	2.90	4.70	62
FEV$_1$ (L)	2.47	3.86	64
FEV$_{1\%}$ (%)	85	82	—
FEF$_{25\%-75\%}$ (L/sec)	4.62	4.35	106
$\dot{V}_{max50}$ (L/sec)	4.94	5.82	85
$\dot{V}_{max25}$ (L/sec)	2.49	3.22	77
MVV (L/min)	178	137	130
Raw (cm H$_2$O/L/sec)	2.33	0.6–2.4	—
SGaw (L/sec/cm H$_2$O/L)	0.23	0.12–0.50	—

3. Lung volumes (by plethysmograph)

	Before drug	Predicted	%
VC (L)	2.90	4.70	62
IC (L)	1.96	2.91	67
ERV (L)	0.94	1.80	59
FRC (L)	1.87	3.29	57
RV (L)	0.93	1.49	57
TLC (L)	3.83	6.20	62
RV/TLC (%)	25	24	—

4. Diffusing capacity (single breath)

	Before drug	Predicted	%
D$_{LCO}$ (mL CO/min/mm Hg)	18.8	31.4	60
V$_A$ (L)	3.68	—	—
D$_L$/V$_A$	5.11	—	—

5. Blood gases (Fio_2 0.21)

pH	7.44
$Paco_2$	35
Pao_2	67
Sao_2	91%
HCO_3^-	23.6

Interpretation

All data from spirometry, lung volumes, diffusion, and blood gases are acceptable.

Spirometry shows a decreased FVC and FEV_1. Flows are within normal limits, as is the MVV. The Raw is near the upper limit of normal, but SGaw is normal.

Lung volumes are decreased, with the RV/TLC ratio preserved.

DL_{CO} SB is reduced. pH and $Paco_2$ are within normal limits, but the Pao_2 is decreased, representing a widened A-a difference.

Impression. Moderate restrictive lung disease without evidence of obstruction, with mild hypoxemia. Restrictive pattern may be related to subject's weight.

Discussion

This case offers a good example of what might be considered a "pure" restrictive defect. Characteristic of a restrictive process is a proportional decrease in all lung volumes, including FVC and FEV_1. There is little or no decrease in any of the flow measurements, such as $FEF_{25\%-75\%}$ or $\dot{V}_{max50}$. Also typical of simple restriction is the well-preserved ratio between FEV_1 and FVC. The volume expired in the first second was in correct proportion to the total volume exhaled, despite the decreases in the absolute volumes of each. The MVV demonstrates the subject's ability to move a normal maximal volume. This may be accomplished in spite of moderately severe restriction by an increase in the rate rather than the V_T.

The DL_{CO} SB confirms the effect of the decreased lung volume's impairment of gas transfer. The reduction in DL_{CO} is approximately proportional to the decrease in TLC. Another way of expressing this relationship is to divide the DL_{CO} by the lung volume at which the diffusion measurement was made. This ratio is called the DL/VA. The ratio in this case is 5.11 mL CO transferred per liter of lung volume. If the predicted $DL_{CO}SB$ is divided by the predicted TLC, a ratio of 5.06 mL CO transferred per liter of lung volume is obtained. The DL/VA may be helpful in defining the contribution of obstructive or restrictive components to reducing the DL_{CO}. In restrictive patterns, the DL/VA ratio is preserved, whereas in obstructive patterns it is decreased.

The widened A-a gradient of approximately 40 mm Hg is consistent with reduced lung volumes. The gradient is significant, particularly in view of the subject's complaint of exertional dyspnea and his age.

The explanation for the restrictive pattern lies in the subject's weight of 297 pounds. For his height, his actual weight is approximately 200% of his ideal weight. Obesity is a common cause of restrictive patterns. Further evaluation of this subject might include testing his response to hypoxia and hypercapnia, as chronically obese individuals often display patterns of decreased ventilatory drive resulting in CO_2 retention. The subject does not appear to be retaining CO_2 at this point, and treatment of the obesity might avoid future complications.

CASE 2

History

P.R. is a 21-year-old man in good health. He plays college football and has a chief complaint of shortness of breath following "wind sprints" and similar vigorous exercises. He denies any other symptoms, including cough or sputum production. He has never smoked. His grandfather had "lung problems," but there is no other history of pulmonary disease involving the family. He does state that his brothers and sisters have "hay fever." There is no history of exposure to extraordinary environmental pollutants.

Pulmonary Function Testing

1. Personal data
Sex: Male
Age: 21 yrs
Height: 73 in
Weight: 180 lb

2. Spirometry and airway resistance

	Before drug	Predicted	%	After drug	%
FVC (L)	6.85	6.04	111	6.73	111
FEV_1 (L)	4.65	4.78	97	5.45	114
FEV_1 (%)	70	79	—	81	—
$FEF_{25\%-75\%}$ (L/sec)	3.90	5.00	78	4.88	97
$\dot{V}_{max50}$ (L/sec)	5.01	6.52	77	6.10	94
$\dot{V}_{max25}$ (L/sec)	2.79	3.75	74	3.25	87
MVV (L/min)	218	166	131	215	130
Raw (cm H_2O/L/sec)	2.10	0.6–2.4	—	1.60	—
SGaw (L/sec/cm H_2O/L)	0.14	0.10–0.39	—	0.18	—

3. Lung volumes (open-circuit method)

	Before drug	**Predicted**	**%**
VC (L)	6.58	6.04	109
IC (L)	4.63	3.65	127
ERV (L)	1.95	2.39	82
FRC (L)	3.60	4.33	83
RV (L)	1.65	1.94	85
TLC (L)	8.23	7.98	103
RV/TLC (%)	20	24	—

4. Diffusing capacity (single breath)

	Before drug	**Predicted**	**%**
$D_{L_{CO}}$ (ml CO/min/mm Hg)	28.2	34.5	82
V_A (L)	7.90	—	—
D_L/V_A	3.57	4.32	—

5. Blood gases (Fio_2 0.21)

pH	7.41
$Paco_2$ (mm Hg)	39
Pao_2 (mm Hg)	94
Sao_2 (%)	97
HCO_3^- (mEq/L)	24.4

Interpretation

All data for spirometry, lung volumes, diffusing capacity, and blood gases are acceptable.

Spirometry is within normal limits except for a decrease in the FEV_1. There is a significant increase in the FEV_1, $\dot{V}_{max50}$, $\dot{V}_{max25}$, $FEV_{1\%}$, and $FEF_{25\%-75\%}$ following administration of the bronchodilator. The MVV is normal, as are the Raw and SGaw. The Raw and SGaw showed a significant improvement following bronchodilator. All lung volumes are within normal limits, as are the blood gases and $D_{L_{CO}}$ SB.

Impression. Mild obstructive defect with significant response to bronchodilator; otherwise normal lung function. Evaluation for exercise-induced bronchospasm is recommended.

Discussion

This subject is an example of an individual with normal, or slightly above normal, values for almost every lung function parameter. The exception is the $FEV_{1\%}$, which is consistent with a mild obstructive pattern. Simple evaluation of the FVC and $FEV_{1\%}$ in relation to their predicted values might give the impression that this subject is normal; but the FEV_1 indicates that the subject, whose lung volumes are slightly larger than normal, expired a disproportionately small volume in the first second. This pattern of supranormal volumes with lower than normal $FEV_{1\%}$ is sometimes seen in healthy young adults, especially athletes. The slightly decreased values for $FEF_{25\%-75\%}$, $\dot{V}_{max50}$, and $\dot{V}_{max25}$, however, suggest an obstructive process. In addition, there is a 17% increase in FEV_1 following administration of a beta-adrenergic bronchodilator. This response is significant in view of the subject's chief complaint of shortness of breath following exercise. The subject appears to exhibit reversible airway obstruction triggered by exercise.

Further evaluation of P.R. included an exercise test to try to demonstrate exercise-induced asthma (EIA). After 6 minutes of treadmill jogging at 88% of his predicted maximal heart rate, the subject's FEV_1 began to fall. The FEV_1 fell to 4.10, with an $FEV_{1\%}$ of 62%, 5 minutes after termination of the test. Scattered wheezes were heard on auscultation. The obstruction was readily reversed by inhaled bronchodilator.

Measurement of the closing volume (CV) by the SBN_2 method revealed a CV/VC ratio of 16%, compared with an expected value of 8.1%. The CV further suggests the presence of small airway abnormality. Methacholine challenge testing was deferred because the obstructive defect was adequately demonstrated by the exercise test.

CASE 3

History

F.H. is a 47-year-old loading dock foreman, whose chief complaint is shortness of breath on moderate exertion. He claims that his dyspnea has become worse recently, but has been present for over 5 years. F.H. has smoked 1½ packs of cigarettes a day since age 15 years (48 pack/years). He admits of a cough on waking. He states that he produces a "small amount of grayish sputum" usually in the morning. F.H.'s father had tuberculosis. One brother had multiple cases of pneumonia as a child and now has bronchiectasis. He denies any extraordinary exposure to environmental dusts or fumes.

Pulmonary Function Testing

1. Personal data
   Sex: Male
   Age: 47 yrs
   Height: 70 in
   Weight: 185 lb

2. Spirometry and airway resistance

	Before drug	Predicted	%	After drug	%
FVC (L)	4.01	4.97	81	4.49	90
FEV_1 (L)	2.05	3.67	56	2.20	60
$FEV_{1\%}$ (%)	51	74	—	49	—
$FEF_{25\%-75\%}$ (L/sec)	1.20	3.69	33	1.30	35
$\dot{V}_{max50}$ (L/sec)	1.35	5.54	24	1.67	30
$\dot{V}_{max25}$ (L/sec)	0.55	2.58	21	1.02	40
MVV (L/min)	71	136	52	85	63
Raw (cm H_2O/L/sec)	3.10	0.6–2.4	—	2.90	—
SGaw (L/sec/cm H_2O/L)	0.07	0.11–0.42	—	0.08	—

3. Lung volumes (by plethysmograph)

	Before drug	Predicted	%
VC (L)	4.01	4.97	81
IC (L)	2.71	3.18	85
ERV (L)	1.30	1.76	74
FRC (L)	4.60	3.94	117
RV (L)	3.30	2.18	151
TLC (L)	7.31	7.12	103
RV/TLC (%)	45	31	—

4. Diffusing capacity (single breath)

	Before drug	Predicted	%
$D_{L_{CO}}$ (mL CO/min/ mm Hg)	6.7	29.1	23
V_A	7.16	—	—
D_L/V_A	0.94	—	—

5. Blood gases (Fio_2 0.21)

pH	7.37
$Paco_2$ (mm Hg)	51
Pao_2 (mm Hg)	54
Sao_2 (%)	86
HCO_3^- (mEq/L)	32
Hb (g%)	18.3 vol%

Interpretation

All data were acceptable. The breathhold time on the $D_{L_{CO}}$ was longer than acceptable (11.2 seconds) because of prolonged expiratory time.

The subject has a decreased FEV_1 with only a slightly decreased FVC. The $FEF_{25\%-75\%}$ is decreased, as are the $\dot{V}_{max50}$ and $\dot{V}_{max25}$. The MVV is reduced, and the Raw is slightly above the expected. The SGaw is below the lower limit of normal. There is little or no response to the bronchodilator.

Lung volumes show an increased RV, with concomitant increases in the FRC and TLC. The RV/TLC is elevated.

The $D_{L_{CO}}$ is reduced and the D_L/V_A is less than 1.0. Arterial blood gases reveal a compensated respiratory acidosis with moderate hypoxemia and an elevated Hb.

Impression. Moderate airway obstruction with minimal response to inhaled bronchodilator. A trial of bronchodilators may be clinically indicated. Moderate air trapping is present and diffusing capacity is markedly reduced. There is hypoxemia and hypercapnia with polycythemia.

Discussion

F.H. typifies a smoker who has developed a moderate degree of airway obstruction. His spirometry reveals the extent of the obstruction: FEV_1, 56% of predicted; $FEF_{25\%-75\%}$, 33% of predicted; and MVV, 52% of predicted. The FVC is relatively well preserved. It even increased following inhalation of the bronchodilator. The $FEF_{25\%-75\%}$, despite being 33% of predicted, must be interpreted cautiously because of its variability in normal subjects. The 95% confidence limits for this subject would include values between 1.45 L/sec and 5.93 L/sec — a large range. (See the Appendix for predicted values and the SEE.) Flows do not increase significantly following the bronchodilator. The $FEV_{1\%}$ actually decreases as a result of a larger increase in the FVC than the FEV_1. This pattern occurs commonly in irreversible obstructive disease.

The MVV is reduced as might be expected. To ascertain that a valid MVV maneuver was obtained, the FEV_1 may be multiplied by a factor of 40. If the MVV approximates the resulting value as it does here, a good effort was made by the subject.

The Raw is slightly increased, consistent with moderate airway obstruction and a productive cough. Specific conductance is less than the lower limit of normal, consistent with increased resistance and increased lung volumes.

The lung volumes reveal air trapping, as indicated by the increased RV and RV/TLC ratio. The RV has increased at the expense of the VC. The remaining lung volumes (i.e., TLC and FRC) are close to their expected values.

The $D_{L_{CO}}$ is markedly reduced. This is a typical result when there is mismatching of ventilation and perfusion caused by airway obstruction. The loss of diffusing capacity per liter of lung volume (0.94) is typical of moderate or severe obstructive disease. This D_L/V_A may be contrasted to the value presented in Case 1. In that case, the $D_{L_{CO}}$ was reduced, but the ratio was close to the expected, consistent with a restrictive defect. In the present case the ratio is low. This suggests that the decreased $D_{L_{CO}}$ is not a result of loss of lung volume. In addition, a $D_{L_{CO}}$ that is 23% of predicted warns that oxygenation may be further impaired during exercise. It is not possible, however, to predict the extent of exercise desaturation that might occur. Although the $D_{L_{CO}}$ is sometimes used to distinguish emphysema (i.e., decreased $D_{L_{CO}}$) from bronchitis (i.e., normal $D_{L_{CO}}$), the diseases often overlap in such a way as to limit the usefulness of this distinction.

Blood gas results reveal resting hypoxemia consistent with $\dot{V}/\dot{Q}$ mismatching. There is a slightly elevated Hb, which may be secondary to the hypoxemia. In addition, there is a mild degree of CO_2 retention with renal compensation.

The lung function of this subject exemplifies the pattern seen in chronic obstructive airway disease with both emphysema and chronic bronchitis. Although air trapping is consistent with emphysematous changes, it may be present in bronchitis and asthma, particularly during acute exacerbations.

Further evaluation of F.H. included a chest x-ray film and a ventilation-perfusion scan. The chest film showed increased hilar markings and right ventricular enlargement. The $\dot{V}/\dot{Q}$ scan showed areas of low $\dot{V}/\dot{Q}$ in both lower lobes, perhaps explaining the hypoxemia. He was recommended for exercise evaluation to determine whether further desaturation occurred with an increased work load and to determine his potential for pulmonary rehabilitation.

CASE 4

History

R.B. is a 37-year-old pipe fitter whose chief complaint is shortness of breath at rest and on exertion. His dyspnea has worsened in the past 6 months, so much so that he is no longer able to work. Additional symptoms include a dry cough. He admits some sputum production when he has a "chest cold." He has smoked one pack of cigarettes a day since age 18 (19 pack/years). He quit smoking about 3 weeks prior to the tests. His father died of emphysema and his mother of lung cancer. An only brother is in good health. His occupational exposure includes working for the past 13 years in the assembly room of a boiler plant, where boilers are put together. He admits to seldom using the respirators provided despite the "dusty" environment.

Pulmonary Function Tests

1. Personal data

Sex: Male
Age: 37 yrs
Height: 69 in
Weight: 143 lb

2. Spirometry

	Before drug	Predicted	%	After drug	%
FVC (L)	3.04	5.05	60	3.10	61
FEV$_1$ (L)	2.03	3.90	52	2.26	58
FEV$_{1\%}$ (%)	67	77	—	73	—
FEF$_{25\%-75\%}$ (L/sec)	1.30	4.09	32	1.60	39
$\dot{V}_{max50}$ (L/sec)	2.12	5.78	37	2.42	42
$\dot{V}_{max25}$ (L/sec)	0.78	2.95	26	1.20	41
MVV (L/min)	83	141	59	91	65
Raw (cm H$_2$O/L/sec)	2.51	0.6–2.4	—	2.47	—
SGaw (L/sec/cm H$_2$O/L)	0.14	0.11–0.44	—	0.15	—

3. Lung volumes (by plethysmograph)

	Before drug	Predicted	%
VC (L)	3.04	5.05	60
IC (L)	1.62	3.18	51
ERV (L)	1.42	1.87	76
FRC (L)	2.75	3.81	72
RV (L)	0.33	1.94	69
TLC (L)	4.37	6.99	63
RV/TLC (%)	30	28	—

4. Diffusing capacity (single breath)

	Before drug	Predicted	%
D$_{LCO}$ (mL CO/min/ mm Hg)	8.1	30.6	25
V$_A$ (L)	4.22	—	—
D$_L$/V$_A$	1.91	4.38	—

5. Blood gases (Fio$_2$ 0.21)

pH	7.43
Paco$_2$ (mm Hg)	36
Pao$_2$ (mm Hg)	52
Sao$_2$ (%)	87
HCO$_3^-$ (mEq/L)	23.0

Interpretation

All data from spirometry, lung volumes, diffusing capacity and blood gases are acceptable.

Spirometry shows a reduced FVC and FEV$_1$. The FEF$_{25\%-75\%}$, $\dot{V}_{max50}$, and $\dot{V}_{max25}$ are all reduced. The MVV is low. The Raw and SGaw are at their respective limits of normal. Response to bronchodilators is borderline, with an increase in the FEV$_1$ of only 11%. The $\dot{V}_{max25}$ improved somewhat more than the other flows.

The lung volumes are all decreased. The RV/TLC ratio is normal.

The $D_{L_{CO}}SB$ is reduced as is the D_L/V_A. The blood gases indicate resting hypoxemia with a normal acid-base status.

Impression. Combined moderate obstructive and restrictive pattern without borderline bronchodilator response. Hypoxemia is present and oxygen supplementation is indicated. Further desaturation may occur with exertion.

Discussion

R.B. typifies the subject with combined obstructive and restrictive disease. His spirometry indicates that a rather serious obstructive component is present, as revealed by the $FEF_{25\%-75\%}$ and $\dot{V}_{max50}$. The $FEV_{1\%}$, however, is close to normal, because the FVC is also reduced. Airway narrowing as a result of restriction is sometimes responsible for decreased flows. This is particularly the case when the restriction is severe. R.B.'s symptoms of cough and sputum suggest a genuine obstructive process. He has a smoking and family history that place him at risk. Because the FVC can be reduced in either obstructive and restrictive processes, spirometry alone does not adequately define the exact nature of this subject's disease.

The lung volume measurements confirm the presence of a restrictive component. All lung volumes are reduced in similar proportions. The reduction in VC matches decreases in FRC, RV, and TLC. The reduced $D_{L_{CO}}$ and hypoxemia are presumably results of the combined disease patterns. The subject's history and symptoms suggest the possibility of restrictive or obstructive disease, or both. The obstructive component may be related to the subject's smoking history, but the etiology of the restrictive component is less clear. On further investigation, it was learned that the subject's occupation involved exposure to asbestos, which can cause fibrosis and/or carcinoma. Chest roentgenograms revealed linear calcifications of the diaphragmatic pleura and pleural thickening, as well as fibrotic changes. These findings are all consistent with asbestos exposure.

Asbestos bodies were identified from the subject's sputum. Open lung biopsy was deferred because it was felt that the causes of both the obstructive and restrictive components were adequately identified. Measurement of compliance (C_L) could have been used to document the severity of the fibrosis.

CASE 5

History

P.W. is a 27-year-old auto mechanic whose chief complaint is "breathing problems." He describes "attacks" of breathlessness that occur suddenly and then subside. He has no other symptoms and no personal history of lung disease. No other immediate family has had any lung disease. He has smoked a pack of cigarettes a day for the last 10 years. He has no unusual environmental exposure, but claims that gasoline fumes sometimes bring on the episodes of shortness of breath.

Pulmonary Function Tests

1. Personal data

Sex: Male
Age: 27 yrs
Height: 68 in
Weight: 150 lb

2. Spirometry

	Before drug	Predicted	%
FVC (L)	3.80	5.15	74
FEV_1 (L)	3.70	4.13	90
$FEV_{1\%}$ (%)	97	80	—
$FEF_{25\%-75\%}$ (L/sec)	4.62	4.49	103
$\dot{V}_{max50}$ (L/sec)	4.81	6.01	80
$\dot{V}_{max25}$ (L/sec)	3.12	3.33	94
MVV (L/min)	162	146	111

3. Lung volumes (closed-circuit technique)

	Before drug	Predicted	%
VC (L)	4.97	5.15	97
IC (L)	3.30	3.17	104
ERV (L)	1.67	1.98	84
FRC (L)	3.72	3.68	101
RV (L)	2.05	1.70	121
TLC (L)	7.02	6.85	102
RV/TLC (%)	29	25	—

4. Diffusing capacity (single breath; corrected for COHb of 8.3%)

	Before drug	Predicted	%
$D_{L_{CO}}$ (mL CO/min/mm Hg)	18.8	32.2	58
V_A (L)	4.62	—	—
D_L/V_A	4.10	4.70	—

5. Blood gases (Fio_2 0.21)

pH	7.44
$Paco_2$ (mm Hg)	36
Pao_2 (mm Hg)	92
Sao_2 (%)	87.1
COHb (%)	8.3

Interpretation

Spirometry, lung volumes, and $D_{L_{CO}}$ are unacceptable because of poor patient effort or technical errors.

Spirometry shows a reduced FVC, with all other flows and the MVV being normal. Lung volumes are normal, with a slight increase in the RV. The $D_{L_{CO}}$ is reduced. Blood gases are within normal limits except for a markedly elevated carboxyhemoglobin and concomitant reduction in Sa_{O_2}.

Impression. Spirometry is inconsistent. The FVC and SVC differ markedly, and the $D_{L_{CO}}$ is inconsistent. Inadequate subject effort or technical errors are present.

Discussion

These test data are good examples of poor reproducibility, particularly on maneuvers that may be influenced by subject effort.

The spirometric data seem to be consistent with a mild restrictive process. However, the FVC is much smaller than the VC. Because the subject cannot "overshoot" on the VC maneuver, the FVC can be presumed to be inaccurate. The FVC is sometimes less than the VC in severe obstruction when there is dynamic compression of the airways. The FVC also may be smaller than the VC if repeated forced expiratory maneuvers induce bronchospasm. All of this subject's flows and his MVV appear normal. Flows whose measurement depend on the FVC, such as the $FEF_{25\%-75\%}$ or $\dot{V}_{max50}$, also might be erroneous if the FVC is incorrect. The FEV_1 and MVV do not depend on the FVC, and they appear to be normal.

The lung volumes appear normal. Because the closed-circuit technique for determination of FRC requires only tidal breathing, it is not usually influenced by poor effort unless the subject introduces a leak. If the VC is used to calculate $FEV_{1\%}$ (i.e., FEV_1/VC rather than FEV_1/FVC), the ratio becomes 74% in comparison to the 97% estimated from the FVC maneuver itself.

The $D_{L_{CO}}$ is much lower than one might expect, particularly in relation to the "normal" blood gases. An acceptable $D_{L_{CO}}SB$ maneuver depends on the subject rapidly inspiring a VC breath from RV. A poor inspiratory effort could result in an underestimate of the true diffusing capacity. The effect of the elevated COHb would be to reduce the driving pressure of CO across the lung and to further reduce the measured $D_{L_{CO}}$. In this case, the $D_{L_{CO}}$ has been corrected for the carboxyhemoglobin.

Because of the inconsistencies in the reported data, further evaluation of the available raw test data was performed. Closer examination of the volume-time spirograms revealed that during the spirometry the subject terminated each FVC maneuver after approximately 2 seconds. The suboptimal maneuver explains the discrepancy between FVC and VC. Each of the three recorded spirograms had widely varying FVC values. The two best FVC values were not within 5%, confirming poor subject cooperation. Lack of reproducibility of the FVC maneuvers is not sufficient reason for discarding the test results, provided that at least three acceptable tests are obtained. This subject's FVC maneuvers lasted only 2 seconds. The efforts did not meet the criteria of continuing for at least 6 seconds or showing an obvious plateau (i.e., no volume change for at least 2 seconds). The $D_{L_{CO}}$ maneuver also showed inconsistent inspiratory volumes, with the largest V_I equalling only 66% of the VC.

Careful attention to these inaccuracies at the time of the test might have prevented the inconsistencies from appearing on the final report. The subject was requested to return for a second test. (Criteria for determining acceptability of various tests may be found in Chapter 11.)

CASE 6

History

M.M. is a 39-year-old secretary who has recently begun experiencing episodes of "choking and coughing." She was referred by an industrial health specialist who suspected reactive airways involvement. She relates that cigarette smoke and strong odors seem to bring on the episodes. She has never smoked, and has no history of lung disease. She had some childhood allergies that disappeared at puberty. There is no history of lung involvement in any of her immediate family. She is not currently on any medications.

Pulmonary Function Tests

1. Personal data

Sex: Female
Age: 39 yrs
Height: 66 in
Weight: 130 lb

2. Spirometry

	Before drug	Predicted	%
FVC (L)	3.71	3.80	98
FEV_1 (L)	2.80	2.97	94
$FEV_{1\%}$ (%)	75	78	—
$FEF_{25\%-75\%}$ (L/sec)	2.99	3.34	90
$\dot{V}_{max50}$ (L/sec)	3.93	4.62	85
$\dot{V}_{max25}$ (L/sec)	1.01	2.36	43
MVV (L/min)	106.4	109.7	97
Raw (cm H_2O/L/sec)	2.51	0.6–2.4	—
SGaw (L/sec/cm H_2O/L)	0.12	0.14–0.56	—

3. Lung volumes (by plethysmograph)

	Before drug	**Predicted**	**%**
VC (L)	3.70	3.80	97
IC (L)	2.03	2.60	78
ERV (L)	1.67	1.20	139
FRC (L)	3.11	3.00	104
RV (L)	1.44	1.80	80
TLC (L)	5.14	5.60	92
RV/TLC (%)	28	32	—

4. Diffusing capacity (single breath)

	Before drug	**Predicted**	**%**
$D_{L_{CO}}$ (mL CO/min/mm Hg)	18.9	21.9	86
V_A (L)	4.99	—	—
D_L/V_A	3.79	3.91	—

5. Blood gases (Fio_2 0.21)

pH	7.43
$Paco_2$ (mm Hg)	37
Pao_2 (mm Hg)	98
Sao_2 (%)	97.3%
HCO_3^- (mEq/L)	23.3

Methacholine Challenge

Methacholine (mg/mL)	**FEV_1**	**%Control**	**Cumulative breaths**	**Cumulative units/5 breaths**
Baseline	2.97	—	—	—
Control	2.92	100	—	—
0.075	2.93	100	5	0.375
0.150	2.90	99	10	1.125
0.310	2.75	94	15	2.68
0.62	2.41	83	20	5.78
1.25	1.99	68	25	12.00

One methacholine unit is arbitrarily defined as 1 mg/mL of methacholine in diluent.

Interpretation

Spirometry, lung volumes, diffusing capacity, and blood gas data are all acceptable, as are the data collected during the inhalation challenge.

Spirometry is within normal limits, except for the $\dot{V}_{max25}$, which is reduced. The Raw and SGaw are at their respective limits of normal, consistent with some airflow obstruction. Lung volumes are within normal limits, although the ERV is larger than expected. The $D_{L_{CO}}$ and blood gases are normal.

The methacholine challenge test is *positive* with a PD_{20} of 1.25 mg/mL, representing a total dose of 12 methacholine units. The test was terminated because the subject's FEV_1 fell below 80% of the control value. Wheezing was present on auscultation for the last two methacholine dosages, and the subject experienced symptoms similar to her chief complaint when the test became positive.

Impression.   Normal lung function with a positive methacholine challenge, consistent with hyperreactive airway disease.

Discussion

This subject is an ideal candidate for an inhalation challenge test. Her baseline pulmonary function studies are normal, with possible small airway involvement. Her complaint of episodic coughing and choking suggests some form of hyperreactive airways abnormality. Many subjects who develop an asthmatic response to inhaled irritants complain of cough as the primary symptom, while wheezing may or may not be present.

If obvious airway obstruction were present on the baseline spirometry, the challenge test would have been contraindicated. A simple before and after bronchodilator trial might have sufficed to demonstrate reversible obstruction. Methacholine challenge testing may be used in subjects with known obstruction to quantify the degree of airway hyperreactivity. In this case, the objective of the test was to determine if the subject had hyperreactivity.

The FEV_1 is commonly used as the index of obstruction for inhalation challenge tests because it is simple to perform and highly reproducible. Other parameters also may be evaluated, as the forced expiratory maneuver is repeated at each dosage. The $FEF_{25\%-75\%}$, $\dot{V}_{max50}$, $\dot{V}_{max25}$, Raw, and SGaw are sometimes used to define the extent of airway reactivity. The SGaw is sensitive and reproducible, and is often used to quantify changes occurring during challenge testing. A fall of 35% to 40% in the SGaw is usually considered indicative of a positive response. The variability of the $FEF_{25\%-75\%}$, $\dot{V}_{max50}$, and $\dot{V}_{max25}$ make interpretation of changes during challenge testing somewhat difficult. In some instances, the peak flow (PEF) may fall as the challenge is performed, particularly if the large airways are involved.

Results of a methacholine challenge test should be interpreted cautiously. The subject should be largely symptom free at the time of the test. Beta-adrenergic, anti-cholinergic, or methylxanthine bronchodilators that might influence the results must be withheld before testing (see Chapter 8). These conditions were met in this subject. Because the FEV_1 fell precipitously at a moderate methacholine dosage, the test can be interpreted as positive with some certainty. In order to better manage this patient, a portable peak flow meter was dispensed. The subject was instructed in its use, and her PEF using it correlated well with that measured during spirometry. She was requested to use the device every morning and evening, or when symptoms appeared. Any significant change in PEF was treated using a metered-dose inhaler. Subsequent reports indicated that her peak flow fell in excess of the level demonstrated on the challenge, but the symptoms were promptly relieved with use of the inhaler.

CASE 7

History

T.S. is a 65-year-old man with a history of COPD who was referred for exercise evaluation for pulmonary rehabilitation. He admits experiencing shortness of breath and dyspnea on exertion, and claims that these have grown worse over the last year. He has a smoking history of 72 pack/years and has recently quit smoking. A chest x-ray film shows emphysematous changes and some flattening of the diaphragms. Family history and occupational exposure were not significant.

Pulmonary Function Tests

1. Personal data

Sex:	Male
Age:	65 yrs
Height:	69 in
Weight:	125 lb

2. Spirometry

	Before drug	Predicted	%	After drug	% Change
FVC (L)	2.42	4.35	56	2.51	4
FEV_1 (L)	1.20	3.01	40	1.30	8
$FEV_{1\%}$ (%)	50	69	—	52	—
$FEF_{25\%-75\%}$ (L/sec)	0.77	2.83	27	0.85	10
$\dot{V}_{max50}$ (L/sec)	1.37	4.94	28	1.51	10
$\dot{V}_{max25}$ (L/sec)	0.59	1.80	33	0.57	−3
MVV (L/min)	45	118	38	48	7
Raw (cm H_2O/L/sec)	2.80	0.6–2.4	—	2.71	−3
SGaw (L/sec/cm H_2O/L)	0.07	0.11–0.44	—	0.07	0

3. Lung volumes (by plethysmograph)

	Before drug	Predicted	%
VC (L)	2.42	4.35	56
IC (L)	1.74	2.96	59
ERV (L)	0.68	1.39	49
FRC (L)	5.11	3.81	134
RV (L)	4.43	2.42	183
TLC (L)	6.85	6.77	101
RV/TLC (%)	65	36	—

4. Diffusing capacity (single breath)

	Before drug	Predicted	%
$D_{L_{CO}}$ (mL CO/min/ mm Hg)	11.8	25.7	46
V_A (L)	6.70	—	—
D_L/V_A	1.76	3.79	—

Interpretation (Pulmonary Function Study)

Seven acceptable FVC maneuvers were obtained but the two best FVC values were not within 5%. Lung volumes and diffusing capacity tests were acceptable.

Spirometry is consistent with severe obstructive lung disease without significant response to bronchodilators. Lung volumes show marked air trapping with RV replacement of the VC. The diffusing capacity is severely reduced.

Interpretation (Exercise Evaluation)

The exercise test (Table 12–1) was terminated because the subject exceeded 85% of his age-related predicted maximum heart rate (HR). He was also very short of breath. His maximum $\dot{V}_E$ exceeded his MVV. The V_T increased with exercise, as did V_D, and the V_D/V_T fell slightly. His gas exchange shows a $\dot{V}_{O_2}$ of 1.2 L/min, which is approximately 57% of expected. The $\dot{V}_{CO_2}$ rose so that an R slightly greater than 1 occurred at the highest work load. The ventilatory equivalent for oxygen ($\dot{V}_E/\dot{V}_{O_2}$) is elevated, and the O_2 pulse is slightly reduced.

Blood gases during exercise reveal a mild hypoxemia that worsened slightly with exercise. Saturation remained adequate. No hypercapnia or acidosis occurred.

No arrhythmias or ischemic changes were observed. The highest HR achieved was 88% of his predicted maximum. There was mild systolic hypertension.

TABLE 12–1

Exercise Test: Case 7

Exercise level	1	2	3	4	5	6
Work load						
mph	0	1.5	2	2	2.5	3
%Grade	0	0	4	8	8	8
Duration (min)	10	3	3	3	3	3
METS	1	3.144	3.365	4.030	4.459	5.082
Ventilation						
f (b/min)	30	24	26	30	36	39
$\dot{V}_E$ (L BTPS)	13.52	24.83	27.57	33.30	48.08	51.98
$\dot{V}_A$ (L BTPS)	5.99	14.37	17.34	21.57	31.64	34.31
V_T (L BTPS)	0.451	1.035	1.055	1.110	1.335	1.340
V_D (L BTPS)	0.251	0.436	0.391	0.392	0.457	0.456
V_D/V_T	0.556	0.421	0.371	0.352	0.342	0.340
Gas exchange						
$\dot{V}_{O_2}$ (L STPD)	0.237	0.745	0.797	0.954	1.056	1.204
$\dot{V}_{CO_2}$ (L STPD)	0.244	0.655	0.733	0.896	1.044	1.298
R	1.030	0.880	0.920	0.940	0.989	1.078
$\dot{V}_E/\dot{V}_{O_2}$ (L/L)	57	33.35	34.60	34.90	45.53	43.18
$\dot{V}_{O_2}$/HR (mL/beat)	2.786	7.838	8.390	9.090	8.516	8.916
Blood gases						
pH	7.47	7.43	7.42	7.39	7.39	7.38
Pa_{CO_2} (mm Hg)	33	35	34	36	33	35
Pa_{O_2} (mm Hg)	74	72	72	70	73	68
Sa_{O_2} (%)	95.5	95	95	94	94	93
$P (A - a)O_2$ (mm Hg)	36	31	38	38	41	46
Hemodynamics						
HR (beats/min)	85	95	95	105	124	135
Systolic BP (mm Hg)	124	162	178	194	200	210
Diastolic BP (mm Hg)	90	86	90	100	104	108

Impression.   1. Marked aerobic impairment; 2. ventilatory limitation with hypoxemia; and 3. inappropriate cardiovascular response for the work load achieved.

Discussion

T.S. walked a total of 15 minutes on the treadmill, reaching a rate of 3 mph at 8% grade. This equaled an energy production of 5.08 METS.

His ventilatory pattern is characteristic of a subject with moderate airway obstruction. His respiratory rate is elevated at the beginning of the procedure, falls slightly and then increases, particularly at the last two levels of work. The minute ventilation increases dramatically from rest to the beginning of exercise. It then increases slowly until the last two levels. The $\dot{V}_A$ increases in approximately the same pattern. His V_T increases to about 1 L and stays near that level throughout the test. This is a normal response. Healthy subjects generally accomplish increases in ventilation by increasing their V_T until they are using about 60% of their VC. Further increases are obtained by increasing the rate of breathing. In this case, the subject immediately increased his V_T to 50% to 60% of his VC. He then increased $\dot{V}_E$ by raising his rate, particularly at the end of the test. His MVV was measured as 45 L/min and the $FEV_1 \times 35$ was 42 L/min. Compared with these values, the subject exceeded the maximal level of total ventilation that might have been expected. The V_D rose during the exercise and fluctuated somewhat. The V_D/V_T ratio decreased slightly, as might be expected, even with moderate obstruction. The ratio fell because the V_T increased more rapidly than the V_D.

At the resting exercise level (level 1), the subject has an R slightly greater than 1.0. The $\dot{V}_{CO_2}$ is elevated in relation to $\dot{V}_{O_2}$. The subject also has a respiratory alkalosis, indicating hyperventilation. This pattern is not uncommon in resting subjects before beginning exercise. Once he begins walking on the treadmill, his gas exchange parameters return to a normal pattern. There is a steady increase in both $\dot{V}_{O_2}$ and $\dot{V}_{CO_2}$, with an R exceeding 1.0 at the final level. The subject may have reached his anaerobic threshold at this point, although the arterial pH is well within normal limits. The marked increase in $\dot{V}_E$ during the last two levels may have resulted from the increased $\dot{V}_{CO_2}$ of anaerobic metabolism.

The ventilatory equivalent for oxygen is inappropriately high at rest (level 1). This finding might be expected for someone with moderate airway obstruction. The $\dot{V}_E/\dot{V}_{O_2}$ falls during the first few stages of exercise, but rises again at the higher work loads. At all levels, the subject is performing an abnormally high level of ventilation compared with the work being performed. This finding is also consistent with airway obstruction.

The O_2 pulse ($\dot{V}_{O_2}/HR$) rose with exercise, but not to 10 to 15 mL/beat, as might be expected. This suggests an inappropriate cardiovascular response. The O_2 pulse is a function of the stroke volume (SV) and the $C(a-\bar{v})_{O_2}$. It is uncertain which factor was responsible for the low ratio of $\dot{V}_{O_2}$ to HR in this case. Cardiac pathology usually results in decreased SV. Deconditioning can be accompanied by a reduced SV. Deconditioning also results in a low $C(a-\bar{v})_{O_2}$ caused by poor extraction of O_2 at the muscle level. Because the subject's HR and blood pressure (BP) rose to near maximal levels without arrhythmias or S-T segment changes on the ECG, there may be some element of deconditioning involved.

Despite a ventilatory limitation to exercise, the arterial blood gas levels did not change dramatically. The pH was slightly alkalotic at rest, consistent with hyperventilation. The pH fell with exercise, but remained within a normal range. The $Paco_2$ remained constant. The Pao_2, slightly low at rest, fell minimally. The subject used his remaining cardiopulmonary reserves to maintain normal blood gas levels.

The subject demonstrated a marked reduction in his exercise capacity based on his $\dot{V}_{O_{2max}}$ of 57% of expected. This reduction was caused primarily by a ventilatory limitation, but with possible evidence of deconditioning. His rehabilitation program was subsequently directed toward conditioning exercises within the limits of his pulmonary system.

CASE 8

History

J.Y. is a 69-year-old woman with a history of chronic bronchitis who was referred for exercise evaluation. She complained of shortness of breath on exertion. Her smoking history is 56 pack/years, but she quit over 1 year prior to this test. Her chest x-ray film is consistent with chronic bronchitis, showing increased vascular markings and an enlarged heart. She had no significant family history or occupational exposure. She admitted to a morning cough that produced thick white sputum.

Pulmonary Function Tests

1. Personal data

Sex:	Female
Age:	69 yrs
Height:	64 in
Weight:	128 lb

2. Spirometry

	Before drug	Predicted	%
FVC (L)	1.30	2.85	46
FEV_1 (L)	0.73	2.04	36
$FEV_{1\%}$ (%)	56	72	—
$FEF_{25\%-75\%}$ (L/sec)	0.43	2.32	18
$\dot{V}_{max50}$ (L/sec)	0.55	3.80	14
$\dot{V}_{max25}$ (L/sec)	0.25	1.27	20
MVV (L/min)	31	85	36
Raw (cm H_2O/L/sec)	2.77	0.6–2.4	—
SGaw (L/sec/cm H_2O/L)	0.09	0.15–0.60	—

3. Lung volumes (by plethysmograph)

	Before drug	Predicted	%
VC (L)	1.30	2.85	46
IC (L)	1.08	1.99	54
ERV (L)	0.23	0.86	26
FRC (L)	3.78	2.77	137
RV (L)	3.55	1.91	186
TLC (L)	4.85	4.76	102
RV/TLC (%)	73	40	—

4. Diffusing capacity (single breath)

	Before drug	**Predicted**	**%**
$D_{L_{CO}}$ (mL CO/min/mm Hg)	8.3	17.4	48
V_A (L)	4.70	—	—
D_L/V_A	1.77	3.77	—

A multistage exercise test was performed with a treadmill and an arterial catheter in place. Level 1 was a 10-minute baseline at rest (Table 12–2).

Interpretation (Pulmonary Function Studies)

All spirometry data were acceptable, as were the data for the diffusing capacity. Several plethysmographic lung volume maneuvers had to be discarded before three acceptable measurements were obtained.

TABLE 12–2

Exercise Test: Case 8

Exercise level	1	2	3
Work load			
mph	0	1.5	3
%Grade	0	0	0
Duration (min)	10	3	3
METS	1	3.3	3.4
Ventilation			
f (breaths/min)	12	27	33
$\dot{V}_E$ (L BTPS)	8.020	21.220	22.630
$\dot{V}_A$ (L BTPS)	4.17	11.671	12.447
V_T (L BTPS)	0.668	0.768	0.686
V_D (L BTPS)	0.321	0.350	0.309
V_D/V_T	0.48	0.45	0.45
Gas exchange			
$\dot{V}_{O_2}$ (L STPD)	0.160	0.530	0.548
$\dot{V}_{CO_2}$ (L STPD)	0.149	0.489	0.498
R	0.930	0.923	0.908
$\dot{V}_E/\dot{V}_{O_2}$ (L/L)	50.14	40.04	41.28
$\dot{V}_{O_2}/HR$ (mL/beat)	2.459	5.047	5.221
Blood gases			
pH	7.48	7.42	7.41
Pa_{CO_2} (mm Hg)	34	39	37
Pa_{O_2} (mm Hg)	74	60	63
Sa_{O_2} (%)	94.9	89.9	91.0
P (A–a)O_2 (mm Hg)	39	48	45
Hemodynamics			
HR (beats/min)	65	105	105
Systolic BP (mm Hg)	160	212	250
Diastolic BP (mm Hg)	80	100	102

Spirometry is consistent with obstructive airway disease. Lung volumes indicate air trapping with a normal TLC. The diffusing capacity is reduced. Blood gas analysis was deferred because this study immediately preceded the exercise test. Bronchodilator studies were not performed because the patient had used her usual regimen immediately prior to the pulmonary function study.

Interpretation (Exercise Test)

The reason for termination of the test was a systolic BP of 250 mm Hg. The subject's respiratory rate increased from 12 to 33 breaths/min, with an increase in ventilation from 8 to 22 L/min. The V_T was relatively fixed at about 700 mL. The $\dot{V}_A$ increased in proportion to $\dot{V}_E$.

Her $\dot{V}_{O_2}$ rose to only 0.548 L/min, or 34% of her predicted maximum (1.634). Her ventilatory equivalent for O_2 ($\dot{V}_E/\dot{V}_{O_2}$) remained elevated throughout the test. Her O_2 pulse was low, but elevated normally with exercise, though not to maximal levels.

Blood gas studies indicate a mild hypoxemia during exercise with an increased A-a gradient ($P(A-a)_{O_2}$). Her Pa_{CO_2} rose slightly, and the pH changed accordingly, but without evidence of anaerobic metabolism.

Her HR rose to 105 beats/min, which is only 72% of her age-related predicted maximum. The systolic BP rose dramatically from 160/80 to 250/102, at which point the test was terminated. There were no arrhythmias, S-T segment changes, or other evidence of ischemia noted.

Impression. 1. Exercise limited by marked hypertension; 2. ventilatory reserve is present despite moderately severe airway obstruction; and 3. mild impairment of oxygenation during exercise, but not significantly limiting.

Discussion

J.Y. presents an example of an individual with well-documented airway obstruction in whom exercise limitation is caused primarily by an inappropriate cardiovascular response.

Comparison of her maximal ventilation of 22.63 L/min with her MVV of 31 L/min indicates very little ventilatory reserve. Because her MVV is so markedly reduced, there must be some ventilatory limitation to work. Her V_T, both at rest and during the mild exercise, remained relatively fixed near 700 mL. Because this volume was already 50% to 60% of her VC, she could only increase her ventilation by increasing her rate. Her V_D/V_T ratio decreased only slightly, probably as a direct result of the fixed V_T. In instances in which both the V_T and V_D increase proportionately, the V_D/V_T ratio does not decrease. This pattern may be consistent with pulmonary vascular disorders, but is probably not evidenced here, as neither the V_T nor the V_D increased significantly.

J.Y. has marked aerobic impairment as indicated by the low $\dot{V}_{O_2}$ of 0.548 L/min, at 3.0 mph and 0% grade on the treadmill. Her R appears to fall, perhaps because she was hyperventilating at the resting level. Her ventilation is inappropriately elevated for the work loads evaluated, as shown by the $\dot{V}_E/\dot{V}_{O_2}$. This pattern is consistent with the increased V_D/V_T ratio. High ventilation is required to maintain an adequate $\dot{V}_A$.

Her O_2 pulse (i.e., $\dot{V}_{O_2}/HR$) was low at rest, and increased only slightly during the mild exercise. The maximal O_2 pulse that might have been attained can be estimated by dividing her predicted $\dot{V}_{O_{2max}}$ by her predicted maximum HR × 1000. In this case, the calculation would be 1.634/148 × 1000, or 11.

J.Y. failed to increase her O_2 pulse because she was limited by other factors at an HR significantly lower than her predicted maximum. An inappropriate rise in systolic BP to 250 mm Hg led to termination of the test. Peripheral vasodilatation normally redirects the cardiac output to exercising muscles. The hypertensive response observed here indicates a failure of this mechanism. Local lesions, such as claudication, and diffuse disease, such as essential hypertension, can result in anaerobic metabolism in the exercising muscles. As a result, metabolic acidosis develops, with stimulation of respiration, and dyspnea. J.Y. did not develop acidosis (i.e., pH of 7.41) or dyspnea during the test. Her presenting complaint of increasing shortness of breath may well have been related to both the hypertensive response and her pulmonary limitations.

Because of the results of the exercise evaluation and her slight hypertension at rest, the subject was referred for further evaluation of her hypertension.

CASE 9

History

C.J. is a 53-year-old office worker who was referred for evaluation of shortness of breath. She has a 44 pack/year history of smoking and continued to smoke up to the time of her test. She admits a morning cough that produces 50 to 100 mL of thick white sputum per day. Her chest x-ray film shows increased vascular markings and mild hyperinflation. She was taking no medications at the time of this test. No familial history of lung disease or cancer was found, and she had no unusual environmental exposure.

Pulmonary Function Tests

1. Personal data
   Sex: Female
   Age: 53 yrs
   Height: 65 in
   Weight: 131 lb

2. Spirometry

	Before drug	Predicted	%	After drug	%
FVC (L)	3.24	3.35	97	3.34	100
FEV_1 (L)	1.49	2.53	59	1.56	62
$FEV_{1\%}$ (%)	46	75	–	47	–
$FEF_{25\%-75\%}$ (L/sec)	0.79	2.86	27	1.19	42
$\dot{V}_{max50}$ (L/sec)	1.99	4.24	47	2.25	53
$\dot{V}_{max25}$ (L/sec)	0.68	1.86	37	0.99	53
MVV (L/min)	52	97.9	53	55	56
Raw (cm H_2O/L/sec)	2.22	0.6–2.4	–	2.10	–
SGaw (L/sec/cm H_2O/L)	0.12	0.14–0.58	–	0.13	–

3. Lung volumes (by plethysmograph)

	Before drug	Predicted	%
VC (L)	3.27	3.35	98
IC (L)	1.80	2.31	78
ERV (L)	0.99	1.04	95
FRC (L)	3.54	2.88	123
RV (L)	2.55	1.84	136
TLC (L)	5.82	5.20	112
RV/TLC (%)	44	35	–

4. Diffusing capacity (single breath)

	Before drug	Predicted	%
$D_{L_{CO}}$ (mL CO/min/ mm Hg)	8.8	20.0	44
V_A (L)	5.67	–	–
D_L/V_A	1.55	3.85	–

5. Blood gases (Fio_2 0.21)

pH	7.38
$Paco_2$ (mm Hg)	43
Pao_2 (mm Hg)	59
Sao_2 (%)	85.1
COHb (%)	5.7

Interpretation (Pulmonary Function Study)

All spirometry, lung volume, diffusing capacity, and blood gas measurement were acceptable.

Spirometry shows an obstructive process, with a well-preserved FVC. There is only a 5% improvement in the FEV_1 following bronchodilator.

Lung volumes by plethysmography show an increased FRC and RV consistent with air trapping. The TLC is close to normal, so there is little hyperinflation.

The $D_{L_{CO}}$SB is reduced. Arterial blood gases on air show hypoxemia complicated by an elevated COHb.

Impression. Moderately severe obstructive disease with no significant response to bronchodilators. Air trapping is present, and the $D_{L_{CO}}$ is severely reduced. Exercise evaluation for oxygen desaturation is recommended.

Three days later, a treadmill exercise test was performed with an arterial catheter in place. The test was repeated with O_2 supplementation. Gas with an Fi_{O_2} of 0.28 was prepared in a meteorologic balloon for the portion of the exercise test on O_2 (Table 12–3).

Interpretation (Exercise Evaluation)

The exercise test was performed in two parts. The first part of the test was terminated because the subject's Pa_{O_2} fell to 46 mm Hg with an Sa_{O_2} of 77.3%. The second phase, on O_2, was terminated because of shortness of breath on the part of the subject. The subject tolerated very low work loads even with supplementary oxygen.

Ventilation was slightly elevated at rest but increased in a normal fashion. On O_2, ventilation was slightly lower both at rest and at similar work loads. The V_D/V_T ratio was mildly elevated but decreased with exercise, on both air and O_2. The subject's minute ventilation was only 51% of her observed MVV after bronchodilator administration, indicating some ventilatory reserve.

The subject achieved a maximal $\dot{V}_{O_2}$ of only 0.986 L/min on O_2, which is 53% of her age-related predicted of 1.858 L/min. This is consistent with moderately severe exercise impairment. The ventilatory equivalent for O_2 is within normal limits, and the O_2 pulse increased normally, though not to maximal values.

Blood gas analysis during exercise shows borderline hypoxemia at rest because of a Pa_{O_2} of 61 mm Hg in combination with an elevated COHb. The Pa_{O_2} fell to 47 mm Hg with only slight exertion. On 28% O_2, the Pa_{O_2} improved to 84 mm Hg at rest, but decreased as the work load increased. Her Pa_{CO_2} increased slightly during O_2 breathing, possibly as a result of respiratory depression. The COHb was elevated, likely because of the subject's continued smoking. Pulse oximetry (Sp_{O_2}) during exercise shows readings higher than the actual saturation, presumably as a result of the subject's COHb.

The HR and BP responses were appropriate for the work loads achieved breathing both air and O_2. The low maximal HR suggests an exercise limitation

TABLE 12–3.

Exercise Test: Case 9

Exercise level	1	2	3	4	5
		Air		Oxygen	
Work load					
mph	0	1.5	0	1.5	2
%Grade	0	0	0	0	4
Duration (min)	10	3	10	3	3
METS	1.48	4.00	1.34	3.11	4.73
Ventilation					
f (breaths/min)	16	28	13	20	31
$\dot{V}_E$ (L BTPS)	10.20	23.40	6.23	16.59	27.81
$\dot{V}_A$ (L BTPS)	6.02	14.74	3.74	10.45	17.80
V_t (L BTPS)	0.638	0.836	0.479	0.830	0.897
V_D (L BTPS)	0.262	0.309	0.190	0.307	0.323
V_D/V_T	0.41	0.37	0.40	0.37	0.36
Gas exchange					
$\dot{V}_{O_2}$ (L STPD)	0.310	0.835	0.279	0.649	0.986
$\dot{V}_{CO_2}$ (L STPD)	0.303	0.743	0.251	0.617	0.976
R	0.98	0.89	0.90	0.95	0.99
$\dot{V}_E/\dot{V}_{O_2}$ (L/L)	32.90	28.00	22.33	25.50	28.20
$\dot{V}_{O_2}$/HR (mL/beat)	3.44	7.59	3.29	6.18	8.57
Pulse oximeter					
Sp_{O_2} (%)	92	87	97	93	93
Blood gases					
pH	7.45	7.39	7.38	7.36	
Pa_{CO_2} (mm Hg)	34	39	44	45	46
Pa_{O_2} (mm Hg)	61	47	84	71	66
Sa_{O_2} (%)	87.4	77.3	91.4	88.9	87.0
COHb (%)	5.1	4.7	4.8	4.7	4.6
$P(A-a)_{O_2}$ (mm Hg)	51	56	64	78	84
Hemodynamics					
HR (beats/min)	90	110	92	105	115
Systolic BP (mm Hg)	130	145	134	145	150
Diastolic BP (mm Hg)	85	88	90	90	90

other than cardiovascular pathology or deconditioning. The ECG was unremarkable.

Impression and Recommendations. Moderately severe exercise impairment resulting primarily from desaturation during exercise. Some ventilatory limitation is probably present as well. The desaturation is aggravated by an elevated COHb. The subject should begin a formal effort for smoking cessation. She should use O_2 at 1 to 2 L/min for exertion. A follow-up evaluation is recommended 1 to 3 months following smoking cessation.

Discussion

This patient characterizes the subject with obstructive lung disease in whom derangement of blood gases limits exercise more than impaired ventilation does. C.J.'s ventilation and gas exchange are fairly normal at rest and at 1.5 mph, 0% grade. The Po_2 is low, however, and falls abruptly with just a small increase in work load. The decrease is severe enough to cause concern that desaturation might occur with simple daily activities or during sleep. The elevated COHb further impairs O_2 delivery. Although a pulse oximeter was used during the exercise test, it read falsely high because of the elevated COHb. Even if the pulse oximeter readings are corrected for the COHb, there is still a discrepancy between Spo_2 and Sao_2 during exercise. This "error" in the pulse oximeter reading may be the result of changes in blood flow at the sensor site or motion artifact during exercise (see Case 12 also, this chapter). The desaturation might be expected because of her low Dl_{CO}. There is some evidence that Dl_{CO} values less than 50% of expected may predict exercise desaturation.

In order to evaluate the effect of O_2 therapy, a controlled trial of walking while breathing supplementary O_2 was performed. The subject breathed from a balloon containing a gas blended to have an Fio_2 of 0.28. The most notable change was the increase in resting Pao_2 from 61 to 84 mm Hg. The pattern of desaturation persisted, however. Her O_2 tension fell dramatically, just as when she breathed room air. Because her Pao_2 was elevated by the supplementary O_2, it remained above 55 mm Hg. This is the level at which serious symptoms of hypoxemia begin to occur. Breathing supplementary O_2 also may be responsible for the decrease in total ventilation at rest and during exercise exhibited by the patient. The mild increase in $Paco_2$ is evidence of an increased sensitivity of the subject to hypoxemia. When she breathes O_2, her respiratory drive decreases slightly, allowing CO_2 to rise. Abnormal $\dot{V}/\dot{Q}$ is the most likely explanation of the pattern of desaturation observed in the subject. The bronchitic component of her obstructive disease results in shunting and venous admixture.

While she was breathing O_2, she did not desaturate to a level where hypoxemia might be considered as a cause of the exercise limitation. She did not increase her ventilation to her maximal level. This might suggest that deconditioning was responsible for the low maximal work load achieved. However, her HR and BP did not increase as typical in significant deconditioning. Other possible causes for the low work load achieved while breathing O_2 might be inadequate subject effort, the development of bronchospasm, or a greatly increased work of breathing.

The subject was referred for pulmonary rehabilitation, which included smoking cessation, bronchial hygiene, and exercise with supplementary O_2.

CASE 10

This case concerns the use of blood gas quality control to detect analytical errors.

Background

F.F. is a 30-year-old fireman referred for pulmonary function tests and arterial blood gases as part of a 5-year physical examination required by his fire district. He has no extraordinary symptoms or history suggestive of pulmonary disease. He has never smoked. He performed all portions of the spirometry, lung volumes, and $D_{L_{CO}}$ maneuvers acceptably. All results were within normal limits for his age and height.

Blood Gases (Fio_2 0.21)

pH	7.41
Pco_2 (mm Hg)	39
Pao_2 (mm Hg)	54
Sao_2 (%)	96.0
COHb (%)	1.2
HCO_3^- (mEq/L)	24.1

Because of the low arterial Po_2 in an otherwise normal subject, and because the Sao_2, measured discretely by co-oximetry, showed a normal saturation, the Po_2 electrode of the automated blood gas analyzer was questioned.

A review of the two most recent automatic calibrations revealed the following:

	Calibration	**Expected**	**Drift**
09:00			
pH	7.387	7.384	0.003
Pco_2 (mm Hg)	39.1	38.6	0.5
Po_2 (mm Hg)	132.0	140.1	-8.1
10:00			
pH	7.383	7.384	-0.001
Pco_2 (mm Hg)	38.4	38.6	-0.2
Po_2 (mm Hg)	151.2	140.1	11.1

For each automatic calibration, the instrument analyzes a calibration gas or buffer and compares the measured value to an expected value. The drift is the amount of adjustment that must be applied to a particular electrode to bring it within calibration limits. The excessive drift exhibited by the Po_2 electrode prompted a review of the most recent quality control runs performed on the analyzer.

Blood gas quality control (five most recent runs)

Control	Mean (mm Hg)	SD	RUNS* 1	2	3	4	5
Level A	45	±2	46	47	49	42	50
Level B	100	±2	101	99	97	96	105
Level C	150	±3	147	151	151	149	143

*Control runs performed every 8 hours

Discussion

The findings in this case regarding the function of the O_2 electrode are not unusual. An abnormally low Pao_2 in an otherwise healthy person with normal lung function suggested that an analytic error had occurred. If the subject had presented with evidence of lung disease or abnormalities in his pulmonary function test, the inaccuracy of the Pao_2 might have gone unnoticed, or led to inappropriate therapy.

Excessive drift of the O_2 electrode should have prompted the immediate attention of the technologist performing the blood gas analyses. A common problem with automated analyzers is their apparent simplicity. Because calibrations are performed automatically, there is a tendency to overlook the corrections that the analyzer makes. Automated analyzers adjust the zero and gain of each electrode to correct for small changes that occur in electrode performance. These small changes may result from a buildup of protein at the tip, electrolyte exhaustion, or slight temperature alterations. If there is a large change in electrode performance, such as electrode failure, the instrument attempts to correct the electrode's output just as it would for small changes that occur normally. Some automated analyzers flag a large "drift" in electrode performance as an error, while others simply report the "drift." In this case, the reported drifts signaled that the Po_2 electrode was fluctuating. One calibration reading was high, while the next one was lower than the expected value.

The change in electrode performance should have been detected by the routine quality control run before the excessive drift was observed during the automatic calibrations. Blood gas quality control used in this laboratory consisted of multiple levels of control materials. Means and standard deviations had been determined for each level.

Examination of control runs 1 through 4 reveal acceptable electrode performance. All values are within ±2 SDs of the established mean. Run 5 (the most recent run) shows values that are all 2 or more SDs away from the mean. In comparison to the mean of Levels A, B, or C, each Po_2 control value from run 5 is between 2 and 3 SDs from its respective mean. These control results might be expected to occur 5% of the time simply because of the random error associated with sampling. If run 5 is considered in conjunction with the previous four runs, and multiple rules (see Chapter 11) are applied, then the electrode is clearly "out-of-control." When multiple levels of controls are evaluated, more than one control value outside of the 2 SD limit suggests an out-of-control situation. For both Level A and Level B, there is a change of 4 SDs from run 4 to run 5. Changes of this magnitude are not consistent with random error, and are detected only when a control history is kept. Similarly, there are inconsistencies within run 5 across the three levels of controls. Levels A and B both show control values that are more than 2 SDs *above* their respective means, while Level C shows a value that is more than 2 SDs *below* its mean. This pattern suggests fluctuating electrode performance, as displayed during the automatic calibrations that followed.

The Po_2 electrode was removed from the instrument. A new membrane was installed after the tip was polished with an abrasive to expose the platinum cathode. The electrode was refilled with fresh electrolyte. The instrument was recalibrated and multiple levels of controls were run. All Po_2 values fell within 2 SDs of the established means. The subject's blood, which had been kept in an ice water bath, was re-analyzed, and a Pao_2 of 89 mm Hg was obtained.

CASE 11

History

D.M. is a 44-year-old account executive. He has idiopathic pulmonary fibrosis, which has been followed for several years. Treatment has included steroid therapy. He has had increasing shortness of breath over the past 3 months. He denies cough or sputum production. He has never smoked and his family history is unremarkable.

Pulmonary Function Testing

1. Personal data
   Sex: Male
   Age: 44 yrs
   Height: 65 in
   Weight: 146 lb

2. Spirometry

	Before drug	Predicted	%
FVC (L)	1.89	4.85	39
FEV_1 (L)	1.80	3.75	48
$FEV_{1\%}$ (%)	95	77	—
$FEF_{25\%-75\%}$ (L/sec)	5.10	3.95	129
MVV (L/min)	95	137	69
Raw (cm H_2O/L/sec)	1.03	0.6–2.4	—

3. Lung volumes (N_2 washout)

	Before drug	Predicted	%
RV (L)	1.65	1.86	89
TLC (L)	3.54	6.44	55
RV/TLC (%)	47	29	—

4. Diffusing capacity (single breath)

	Before drug	Predicted	%
$D_{L_{CO}}$ (mL CO/min/mm Hg)	*unable to perform		
V_A (L)	—		
D_L/V_A	—		

5. Blood gases (Fio_2 0.21)

pH	7.45
$Paco_2$ (mm Hg)	37
Pao_2 (mm Hg)	75
Sao_2	96

Interpretation

All data from spirometry and lung volumes are acceptable. The patient was unable to perform a $D_{L_{CO}}$ maneuver because of shortness of breath.

Spirometry shows a severely reduced FVC and FEV_1. The $FEV_{1\%}$ is increased. Airway resistance is within normal limits.

Lung volumes are markedly reduced with the RV close to normal.

Blood gases show mild hypoxemia at rest.

Impression.   Severe restrictive lung disease with mild hypoxemia. Exercise evaluation is recommended to assess possible desaturation on exertion.

Discussion

This patient had rapidly progressing pulmonary fibrosis. An exercise test with an arterial catheter was performed, as recommended. Exercise caused a rapid fall in the Pao$_2$ to 46 mm Hg at a very low work load. The patient was subsequently evaluated for possible lung transplantation. Pulmonary function studies 2 months later indicated further reduction in all lung volumes. Three months after the pulmonary function study listed above, D.M. received a single lung transplant of the left lung.

D.M. was followed with routine pulmonary function studies after his lung transplant. Table 12–4 lists spirometry values for the patient for 25 months. Figure 12–1 presents the flow-volume curves obtained at the time of each test listed in Table 12–4.

D.M. followed a pattern that is not unusual in patients who have received transplanted lungs. The first flow-volume curve, 3 months before transplantation, is typical of severe restriction. One month after transplantation, there was improvement in the patient's FVC, FEV$_1$, and TLC. A moderately severe restrictive process was still present. This is not unusual following thoracic surgery and lung transplantation. The FEV$_1$/FVC ratio decreased to a normal range (86%). The FEF$_{25\%-75\%}$ was somewhat reduced, but consistent with the reduction in lung volumes.

By 6 months posttransplantation, the patient showed significant improvement in FVC, FEV$_1$, and FEF$_{25\%-75\%}$. The flow-volume curve has assumed a relatively normal appearance, with some slight decrease in flows at low lung volumes.

At 12 months posttransplantation, the FVC had increased to 81% of the expected value. The FEV$_1$ had increased to 82% of the patient's predicted value. The FEV$_1$ was completely normal. The FEF$_{25\%-75\%}$, however, had fallen slightly over the 6-month interval. The MEFV curve also showed a definite pattern of small airway obstruction. The patient had few complaints, but did experience

TABLE 12–4.

Serial Pulmonary Function Studies: Case 11*

Months posttransplant	– 3	1	6	12	21	22
FVC (L BTPS)	1.89	2.31	3.40	3.78	2.91	2.24
	(39)	(49)	(77)	(81)	(63)	(48)
FEV$_1$ (L BTPS)	1.80	2.00	2.86	2.98	1.51	1.30
	(48)	(55)	(79)	(82)	(42)	(36)
FEV$_1$/FVC (%)	95	86	84	79	52	58
FEF$_{25\%-75\%}$ (L/sec)	5.10	2.29	2.54	2.38	0.49	0.54
	(129)	(59)	(66)	(62)	(13)	(14)
RV (L BTPS)	1.65	1.63	–	1.66	2.38	2.15
	(89)	(88)		(90)	(129)	(116)
TLC (L BTPS)	3.54	3.94	–	5.44	5.29	4.39
	(55)	(63)		(91)	(89)	(73)

*Numbers in parentheses are percents of predicted.

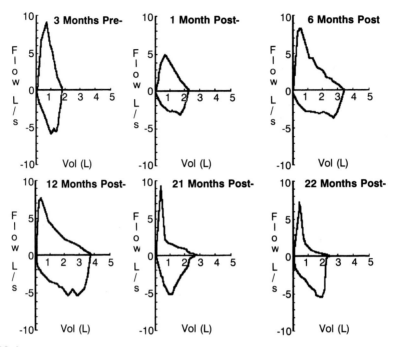

FIG 12-1
Serial flow-volume curves for a patient receiving a single lung transplant. See **Table 12-4** for pulmonary function values, and text for explanation.

some shortness of breath on exertion. An exercise test revealed adequate oxygenation although the subject did not reach his predicted maximal work load.

By 20 months after transplantation, the patient's complaint of breathlessness had worsened. A biopsy of the transplanted left lung revealed a pattern consistent with progressive obliteration and obstruction of the small airways (bronchiolitis obliterans). Pulmonary function studies were performed at 21 months after the patient had been treated with corticosteroids. The FVC and FEV$_1$ had each decreased significantly compared with the values at 12 months posttransplantation. The FEF$_{25\%-75\%}$ dropped from 2.38 L/sec to 0.49 L/sec within 9 months. All flows at low lung volumes were similarly decreased, as demonstrated by the MEFV curve at 21 months (see Fig 12–1). The RV had increased to 129% of expected, even though the TLC decreased slightly. The increased RV was consistent with the rapidly progressive development of small airway obstruction.

Within 1 month (i.e., 22 months posttransplantation), the FVC, FEV$_1$, and TLC had all decreased further (see Table 12–4). The patient was extremely short of breath with mild exertion. An exercise test revealed values similar to those observed before the single lung transplant. Twenty-four months after the single lung transplant, the patient received a double lung transplant.

This case is representative of many lung transplant recipients. The development of bronchiolitis obliterans has been noted to occur in approximately 40% to 50% of patients receiving lung transplants. The exact cause of bronchiolitis obliterans in lung transplant recipients is not clear. All transplant recipients are treated with drugs to suppress rejection of the transplanted organ. The suppression of their immune systems makes them candidates for opportunistic lung infections, such as cytomegalovirus (CMV). If immunosuppression is withheld, the transplanted lung tissue is rejected by the body. Repeated episodes of acute rejection seem to correlate with the development of bronchiolitis obliterans. There is some evidence that the small airway changes observed may be caused by a chronic, subacute type of rejection. Some combination of opportunistic infections and tissue rejection may be responsible for the rapid obliteration of the small airways. The results are not unlike those seen in advanced emphysema.

Serial pulmonary function studies demonstrate the rapid improvement that occurs with lung transplantation. They also provide one means of tracking the changes known to occur in bronchiolitis obliterans. Flow measurements that represent small airway function may be the most useful. In this patient, the $FEF_{25\%-75\%}$ and MEFV curves indicated changes in the small airways as early as 12 months following transplantation. The FVC, FEV_1, and TLC were still improving in D.M. even though small airway function was decreasing. $D_{L_{CO}}$ measurements were not particularly revealing in this patient. The diffusing capacity remained in the range of 40% to 50% of predicted following transplantation. Lack of improvement in $D_{L_{CO}}$ may have resulted because of the fact that only one lung was transplanted. Before his bronchiolitis obliterans had developed, the patient had a $\dot{V}/\dot{Q}$ scan indicating 80% of gas exchange occurring in the transplanted lung. A poorly functioning native lung and a transplanted lung developing bronchiolitis obliterans may have been responsible for gas exchange abnormalities. Exercise testing with arterial blood gases confirmed what might have been expected as the patient developed severe obstruction. Desaturation occurred with even moderate work loads. The cause of hypoxemia in this patient was most likely the shift of ventilation from the transplanted lung to the native lung as bronchiolar obliterans developed. Perfusion to the transplanted lung continued, creating $\dot{V}/\dot{Q}$ mismatching and shunting.

Rapidly progressive disease, such as bronchiolitis obliterans, can be detected clinically using appropriate pulmonary function tests. Care must be taken to interpret serial measurements in light of the multiple processes that may occur simultaneously. In lung transplantation, these processes include recovery from thoracic surgery, type of transplant (i.e., single or double lung), level of immunosuppression, occurrence of opportunistic infections, and episodes of acute rejection. If spirometry indicates that bronchiolitis obliterans may be developing, histologic documentation by biopsy is required. Appropriate treatment depends on the presence or absence of opportunistic infections.

CASE 12

History

E.E. is a 65-year-old man who was referred to the pulmonary function laboratory. He had spirometry in the referring physician's office that indicated obstruction. Because of his chief complaint of dyspnea on exertion, his physician recommended that he get full pulmonary function studies. The referring physician also requested a simple exercise test with pulse oximetry to determine if E.E. might require supplementary O_2. The patient was not currently taking any medications for heart or lung disease. He confirmed that he had been a smoker until about 6 months ago. He had smoked approximately one pack of cigarettes a day for 30 years.

Pulmonary Function Tests

1. Personal data

Sex:	Male
Age:	65 yrs
Height:	69 in
Weight:	185 lb

2. Spirometry

	Before drug	Predicted	%	After drug	% Change
FVC (L)	4.03	4.35	92	4.11	2
FEV_1 (L)	2.62	3.01	87	2.65	1
$FEV_{1\%}$ (%)	65	69	—	64	—
$FEF_{25\%-75\%}$ (L/sec)	1.75	2.83	62	1.85	6
$\dot{V}_{max50}$ (L/sec)	3.01	4.94	61	3.11	3
$\dot{V}_{max25}$ (L/sec)	1.56	1.80	87	1.47	−6
MVV (L/min)	92	118	77	89	−2
Raw (cm H_2O/L/sec)	2.01	0.6–2.4	—	1.71	−15
SGaw (L/sec/cm H_2O/L)	0.17	0.11–0.44	—	0.27	59

3. Lung volumes (by He dilution)

	Before drug	Predicted	%
VC (L)	4.03	4.35	93
IC (L)	3.01	2.96	102
ERV (L)	1.02	1.39	73
FRC (L)	4.11	3.81	108
RV (L)	3.09	2.42	128
TLC (L)	7.12	6.77	105
RV/TLC (%)	43	36	—

4. Diffusing capacity (single breath)

	Before drug	Predicted	%
D_{LCO} (mL CO/ min/mm Hg)	19.3	25.7	75
V_A (L)	6.80	—	—
D_L/V_A	2.84	3.80	—

Interpretation (Pulmonary Function Study)

All spirometry, lung volume, and diffusing capacity maneuvers were performed acceptably. All data were reproducible.

Spirometry indicates a slightly reduced FEV_1, consistent with mild obstruction. The $FEF_{25\%-75\%}$ and all other flows are also slightly reduced. There is no significant improvement following administration of inhaled bronchodilators. Airway resistance and conductance are within normal limits. Lung volumes show a slight elevation of the FRC and RV, indicating that there may be some air trapping. The D_{LCO} also is mildly reduced.

Impression. There is mild obstruction and air trapping without significant response to bronchodilators.

A cycle ergometer exercise test was then performed. The subject was monitored using a modified 12-lead ECG system and a pulse oximeter attached to his finger (Table 12–5).

Interpretation (Exercise Test)

The patient exercised on a cycle ergometer for a total of 8 minutes. After 3 minutes at 50 WATTS, the patient's pulse oximeter reading was 83%. E.E. gave no sign of distress as might have been expected with a low O_2 saturation. The ergometer resistance was advanced to 75 WATTS and the patient pedaled for 2 more minutes. When the patient signaled that he was becoming very short of breath, an arterial blood gas was obtained by radial puncture. The patient

TABLE 12–5

Exercise Test: Case 12

Exercise Level	1	2	3	4
Activity (cycle)	Sit	Pedal	Pedal	Pedal
WATTS	0	25	50	75
Duration (min)	5	3	3	2
Respiratory rate (b/min)	18	22	30	32
Spo_2 (%)	92	88	83	84
HR (beats/min)	98	122	147	151
Systolic BP (mm Hg)	128	154	190	200
Diastolic BP (mm Hg)	80	88	100	100
pH	—	—	—	7.31
Pco_2 (mm Hg)	—	—	—	31
Po_2 (mm Hg)	—	—	—	77
SaO_2	—	—	—	90

achieved an HR of 151 beats per minute, or 89% of his predicted maximum. There were no arrhythmias or ST-T wave changes. His blood pressure increased to 200/100 at peak exercise. His respiratory rate was 30 breaths per minute. Arterial blood gases revealed a metabolic acidosis, consistent with anaerobic metabolism. The Pao_2 was 77 mm Hg, with an Sao_2 of 90% measured by co-oximeter. The co-oximeter saturation value did not support the value of 84% obtained by pulse oximeter.

Impression.   1. Exercise was limited by cardiovascular system. Absence of arrhythmias and slight hypertensive response suggests deconditioning. 2. There was no O_2 desaturation at this time. A program of aerobic conditioning, including adequate warm-up and cool-down, is recommended. A target HR of 120 to 130 beats per minute would be appropriate.

Discussion

This patient is typical of those referred to a full-function laboratory after screening spirometry and symptoms indicate pulmonary disease. In this case, the subject had mild obstructive airways disease with little response to bronchodilators. The complaint of shortness of breath prompted the referring physician to suggest a simple exercise evaluation to assess possible O_2 desaturation. The exercise test revealed cardiovascular limitations rather than hypoxemia as the cause of the shortness of breath.

The discrepancy between the pulse oximeter and the measured blood saturation by co-oximeter is noteworthy. Pulse oximeters offer a simple, inexpensive means of assessing O_2 saturation of hemoglobin. The limitations of the pulse oximeter should be considered, especially when used in conjunction with exercise tests. Motion artifact, incident light, local perfusion, and skin pigmentation have all been demonstrated to affect the accuracy of the pulse oximeter. Carboxyhemoglobin is also known to cause erroneously elevated readings (see Chapter 6). The reason that the pulse oximeter read lower than the co-oximeter in this case was not readily apparent. Motion and changes in local perfusion are most the likely factors during exercise. Because the patient was exercised with an ergometer, his hand was relatively stable on the handle bar. Squeezing the handle bar may have caused the problem, even though the subject was coached to relax his hand.

In order to reduce the possibility of false-positive (as in this case) or false-negative results of pulse oximetry, several steps can be taken. The sight of sensor placement should be chosen to minimize motion. The connecting cable between the sensor and oximeter should be stabilized to prevent pulling or twisting during exercise. A pulse oximeter capable of displaying pulse waveforms and HR is preferable. Visualization of the pulse waveform can help the technologist or physician judge the validity of the saturation reading. If there is not a good pulse waveform, or if the HR differs significantly from the ECG, the saturation values should be suspect.

As was done in this case, a single arterial blood gas measurement at peak exercise may be necessary to completely answer the clinical question. A blood gas drawn at rest may correlate with pulse oximetry readings. The same may not be true during exercise. A radial puncture may be performed at peak exercise, or within 15 seconds of termination of exercise. A modified Allen's test (see Chapter 6) should be performed to assess the sample site before exercise begins. A cycle ergometer provides a good platform for performing a radial puncture because there is minimal body movement. A blood gas at peak exercise can be obtained from a subject on a treadmill, but may require the use of a side-rail to stabilize the wrist. The specimen should be obtained within 15 seconds after the end of exercise, before recirculation occurs. If the co-oximeter saturation verifies the pulse oximeter reading, additional arterial specimens should not be necessary. If there is a significant discrepancy between blood and pulse oximeter values, further sampling may be required. If blood cannot be obtained within 15 seconds, the exercise session may need to be repeated. For patients in whom there is difficulty obtaining blood by radial puncture, an arterial catheter may be indicated. Radial artery cannulation may be less traumatic if multiple blood gases need to be obtained, as in titration of O_2 therapy for exercise.

CASE 13

History

J.P. is a 53-year-old woman who suffered multiple abdominal injuries in a motor vehicle accident. Following surgical repair of a perforated bowel, she developed acute renal failure, then respiratory failure. She was placed on mechanically supported ventilation. She became increasingly dependent on the ventilator. After 13 days, a metabolic study was requested to assess the adequacy of parenteral nutrition.

Metabolic Assessment

1. Personal data

Sex: Female
Age: 53 yrs
Height: 157 cm
Weight: 50 kg

2. Nutritional information

	Total cal	Nonprotein cal	Grams protein
Parenteral	1717	1393	75
Enteral	(none)	—	—
24-hour urinary N_2	9 g		
Basal metabolic rate	1176 kcal/24 hours (estimated)		

3. Ventilator settings

Fio_2 0.35
V_T 750 mL
Rate   10
Mode   SIMV*
Status   Awake, resting

*(*Synchronized Intermittent Mandatory Ventilation)*

4. Metabolic measurements

$\dot{V}co_2$ (mL/min)   205
$\dot{V}o_2$ (mL/min)   200
RER   1.03
$\dot{V}e$ (L/min)   10.2
REE   1442 kcal/day
RQnp*   1.07

*(*Non Protein RQ. See Chapter 8.)*

Energy substrate utilization
Carbohydrate (kcal/day)   1495
Fat (kcal/day)   − 296
Protein (kcal/day)   243

5. Blood Gases

pH	7.37
Pa_{CO_2}	51
Pa_{O_2}	71
HCO_3^-	29

Interpretation

The data for this study were collected over 26 minutes and appear to represent a steady state. A urinary N_2 was collected for 24 hours prior to the test. The patient was receiving 1717 kcal/day of parenteral nutrition. Estimated energy expenditure as determined by metabolic assessment indicates a requirement of 1442 kcal/24 hours. Substrate utilization showed carbohydrate oxidation (104%). The negative value for fat utilization is consistent with lipogenesis. Replacement of glucose with lipids and reduction of total calories to approximately 1450 kcal/day are recommended. The patient should be reassessed within 24 hours.

Discussion

This study involves factors commonly encountered in the nutritional support of critically ill patients. These factors include the patient's clinical status, the estimated and actual caloric requirements, and the role of nutritional status in ventilatory support.

This patient was critically ill and required ventilatory support. Parenteral nutrition was being supplied approximately 45% above the estimated resting caloric requirements. Estimation of caloric requirements is often performed by calculating the basal rate using the Harris-Benedict equations (see Chapter 8). The basal rate is then adjusted using factors that consider the clinical status of the patient (i.e., disease state, trauma).

The metabolic assessment indicated that the patient required fewer calories per day than were currently being administered. In addition, carbohydrates were supplying the entire caloric need. The negative value calculated for fat utilization indicates that some of the carbohydrates were probably being stored as fat (i.e., lipogenesis). When carbohydrates are oxidized, CO_2 is produced. The RER of 1.03 supports the presence of an excess CO_2 production in relation to metabolic demands.

The metabolic assessment was performed with the patient on a ventilator. The patient's minute ventilation during the assessment was 10.2 L, slightly higher than the ventilator settings. Difficulty weaning this patient from mechanically supported ventilation may have been a result of the CO_2 load induced by parenteral nutrition in excess of metabolic demand. The arterial blood gases support increased CO_2 production. The Pa_{CO_2} is increased despite mechanically supported ventilation. The patient was unable to ventilate enough to return the

Pa_{CO_2} to a value near 40 mm Hg. The excess CO_2 produced contributed directly to the inability to wean the patient from mechanical ventilation.

The interpretation notes that the data was representative of a steady state. Steady-state measurements are essential in order to estimate caloric requirements for the entire 24-hour period. Each metabolic assessment should include adequate data so that steady-state conditions can be verified. The length of the study should be appropriate to establish that a steady state existed. Analysis of the variability of the $\dot{V}_{O_2}$ and $\dot{V}_{CO_2}$ may be helpful. The O_2 consumption and CO_2 production should ideally vary less than 10% during the measurement. Values for the RER that are outside of the normal range of 0.70 to 1.00 should be carefully evaluated to assure that measurement errors did not occur. Difficulty measuring $\dot{V}_{O_2}$ on subjects receiving supplementary O_2 is well documented. Calorimetry using open-circuit methods (see Chapter 8) is usually limited to measurements when the Fi_{O_2} is 0.50 or less.

J.P. was switched to a 50/50 mixture of lipid and carbohydrate. The total caloric intake was also reduced to 1450 kcal/day. Her ventilation decreased, and ventilatory support was gradually reduced. An additional metabolic study indicated good agreement between the prescribed nutritional support and her metabolic demands. Her RER on the subsequent study was 0.79 with an REE of 1395 kcal/day. This RER value compares favorably with 0.82, which is a target value for metabolism of appropriate amounts of carbohydrate, fat, and protein. She was successfully weaned from the ventilator 4 days after the initial assessment.

SELECTED BIBLIOGRAPHY

PULMONARY FUNCTION INTERPRETATION

American Thoracic Society: Lung function testing: selection of reference values and interpretive strategies. *Am Rev Respir Dis* 144:1202, 1991.

Bates DV, Macklem PT, Christie RV: *Respiratory function in disease,* ed 2. Philadelphia, 1971, WB Saunders.

Becklake MR, Permutt S: Evaluation of tests of lung function for "screening" of early detection of chronic obstructive lung disease. In Macklem PT, Permutt S, editors: *The lung in transition between health and disease.* New York, 1979, Marcel Dekker.

Clausen JL: Clinical interpretation of pulmonary function tests. *Respir Care* 34:638, 1989.

Morris AH, Kanner RE, Crapo RO, et al: *Clinical pulmonary function testing,* ed 2. Salt Lake City, 1984, Intermountain Thoracic Society.

West JB: *Pulmonary pathophysiology—the essentials,* ed 4. Baltimore, 1992, Williams and Wilkins.

EXERCISE TEST INTERPRETATION

American College of Sports Medicine: *Guidelines for exercise testing and prescription,* ed 4. Philadelphia, 1991, Lea and Febiger.

Astrand PO, Rodahl K: *Textbook of work physiology,* ed 2. New York, 1977, McGraw-Hill.

Bell CW: Pulmonary rehabilitation and exercise testing. In Wilson PK, Bell CW, Norton AC, editors: *Rehabilitation of the heart and lungs.* Fullerton, Calif, 1980, Beckman Instruments.

Jones NL: *Clinical exercise testing,* ed 3. Philadelphia, 1988, WB Saunders.

Jones NL: Exercise testing in pulmonary evaluation: rationale, methods, and the normal respiratory response to exercise. *N Engl J Med* 293:541, 647, 1975.

Kattus AA: *Exercise testing and training of apparently healthy individuals.* New York, 1972, American Heart Association.

Spiro SG: Exercise testing in clinical medicine. *Br J Dis Chest* 71:145, 1977.

Wasserman K, Whipp BJ: Exercise physiology in health and disease. *Am Rev Respir Dis* 112:219, 1975.

BLOOD GAS INTERPRETATION

Shapiro BA: *Clinical applications of blood gases.* Chicago, 1989, Mosby–Year Book, Inc.

Appendix

SYMBOLS AND ABBREVIATIONS USED IN PULMONARY FUNCTION TESTING

(Where two symbols are given, both are commonly used)

General Symbols

P	Pressure, blood or gas
V	Gas volume
$\dot{V}$	Gas volume per unit time, or flow
F	Fractional concentration of gas
I	Inspired
E	Expired
A	Alveolar
T	Tidal
D	Dead space
Q	Blood volume
$\dot{Q}$	Blood flow
C	Content in blood
S	Saturation
a	Arterial
c	Capillary

v	Venous
$\bar{v}$	Mixed venous
BTPS	Body temperature and pressure saturated with water vapor
ATPS	Ambient temperature, pressure, saturated with water vapor
STPD	0°C, 760 mm Hg, dry

Lung Volumes

VC	Vital capacity, slow vital capacity
IC	Inspiratory capacity
IRV	Inspiratory reserve volume
ERV	Expiratory reserve volume
FRC	Functional residual capacity
RV	Residual volume
TLC	Total lung capacity
RV/TLC (%)	Residual volume to total lung capacity ratio expressed as a percentage
V_{TG}	Thoracic gas volume
V_T	Tidal volume
V_A	Alveolar volume
V_D	Dead space volume
V_L	Actual lung volume

Ventilation and Ventilatory Control

$\dot{V}_E$	Expired volume per minute, minute volume (BTPS)
$\dot{V}_A$	Alveolar ventilation per minute (BTPS)
$\dot{V}_D$	Dead space ventilation per minute (BTPS)
f_b, f	Respiratory rate per minute, breathing frequency
V_D/V_T	Dead space to tidal volume ratio

P_{100}, $P_{0.1}$ — Pressure in the first 100 msec of an occluded breath, occlusion pressure

Spirometry

FVC — Forced vital capacity with maximally forced expiratory effort

FIVC — Forced inspiratory vital capacity with maximally forced inspiratory effort

FEV_T — Forced expiratory volume for a specific interval T

$FEV_T/FVC\%$, $FEV_{T\%}$ — Forced expiratory volume to forced vital capacity ratio expressed as a percentage

FEF_X — Forced expiratory flow related to some specific portion of the FVC, denoted as subscript X, referring to the volume of FVC already exhaled at the time of measurement

$FEF_{25\%-75\%}$ — Forced expiratory flow during the middle half of the FVC (formerly the MMF)

PEF — Peak expiratory flow

MEFV — Maximum expiratory flow-volume curve

MIFV — Maximum inspiratory flow-volume curve

PEFV — Partial expiratory flow-volume curve

$\dot{V}_{max_x}$ — Forced expiratory flow related to the actual volume of the lungs denoted by subscript X, referring to the lung volume remaining when measurement is made

MVV_X — Maximal voluntary ventilation as the volume of air expired in a specified interval, denoted by subscript X (formerly MBC)

Viso$\dot{V}$ — Volume of isoflow

Pulmonary Mechanics

C — Compliance, volume change per unit of pressure change

Cdyn — Dynamic compliance, measured during breathing

Cst	Static compliance, measured during periods of no airflow
Crs	Compliance of the respiratory system
C/V_L	Specific compliance
Raw	Airway resistance, pressure per unit flow
Gaw	Airway conductance, flow per unit of pressure (1/Raw)
Raw/V_L, SRaw	Specific resistance
Gaw/V_L, SGaw	Specific conductance
MEP	Maximum expiratory pressure
MIP	Maximum inspiratory pressure

Gas Distribution

$\Delta N_{2_{750-1250}}$	Change in percent N_2 over the 750 to 1250 mL portion of the SBN_2 test
SBN_2, SBO_2	Single-breath nitrogen elimination
Slope of Phase III	Slope of best-fit line through alveolar portion of the SBN_2 from 30% of VC to onset of Phase IV
CV	Closing volume
CV/VC (%)	Closing volume to vital capacity ratio expressed as a percentage
CC	Closing capacity
CC/TLC (%)	Closing capacity to total lung capacity ratio expressed as a percentage

Diffusion

$D_{L_{CO}}$	Diffusing capacity for carbon monoxide
1/Dm	Diffusion resistance of the alveolocapillary membrane
$1/\Theta Vc$	Diffusion resistance of the red cell and Hb reaction rate
D_L/V_A, D_L/V_L	Specific diffusion per unit of alveolar lung volume

Exercise and Metabolic Studies

$\dot{V}_{O_2}$	Oxygen consumption or uptake per minute (STPD)
METS	Multiples of the resting oxygen uptake (usually 3.5 mL/Kg)
$\dot{V}_{CO_2}$	Carbon dioxide production per minute (STPD)
$\dot{V}_E/\dot{V}_{O_2}$	Ventilatory equivalent for oxygen
$\dot{V}_E/\dot{V}_{CO_2}$	Ventilatory equivalent for CO_2
$\dot{V}_{O_2}/HR$	Oxygen pulse
kpm	Kilopond-meters, a unit of power output
R, RER	Respiratory exchange ratio
RQ	Respiratory quotient
REE	Resting energy expenditure
Kcal	Kilocalorie

Blood Gases and Monitoring

P_{AO_2}	Alveolar oxygen tension
Pa_{O_2}	Arterial oxygen tension
$P\bar{v}_{O_2}$	Mixed venous oxygen tension
tcP_{O_2}	Transcutaneous oxygen tension
Sa_{O_2}	Arterial oxygen saturation
$S\bar{v}_{O_2}$	Mixed venous oxygen saturation
Sp_{O_2}	Pulse oximeter saturation
Ca_{O_2}	Arterial oxygen content
$C\bar{v}_{O_2}$	Mixed venous oxygen content
$P(A\text{-}a)_{O_2}$	Alveolar-arteral O_2 tension difference
$C(a\text{-}\bar{v})_{O_2}$	Arterial-venous O_2 content difference
P_{ACO_2}	Alveolar carbon dioxide tension
Pa_{CO_2}	Arterial carbon dioxide tension

$P_{ET_{CO_2}}$	End-tidal carbon dioxide tension
tcP_{CO_2}	Transcutaneous carbon dioxide tension
pH	Negative logarithm of the H^+ concentration used as a positive number
HCO_3^-	Plasma bicarbonate concentration
BE	Base excess, base deficit
COHb	Carboxyhemoglobin
MetHb	Methemoglobin
P_{50}	Partial pressure of oxygen at which hemoglobin is 50% saturated

---

GLOSSARY

accuracy	(1) Freedom from mistake or error; (2) conformity to truth or to a standard or model; degree of conformity of a measure to a standard or a true value.
acidosis	Pathologic condition resulting from accumulation of acid in, or loss of base from, the body.
A/D converter	Analog-to-digital converter; a device for translating an analog signal into a digital value.
airway resistance	Opposition of the air passages to conduction of gas.
alkalosis	Pathologic condition resulting from accumulation of base in, or loss of acid from, the body.
alveolar	Pertaining to an alveolus (a small sac-like dilatation).
back-extrapolation	Process of determining the true beginning of a forced expiratory maneuver by extrapolating the steepest portion of the volume-time curve backwards.
bit	Binary digit, a 0 or 1.
breath-by-breath	Describing analysis of expired gas as air taken in and expelled by expansion and contraction of the thorax.

bronchodilator	(1) Dilating or expanding the lumina of air passages of the lungs; (2) agent that causes expansion of the lumina of the air passages of the lungs.
byte	Series of eight bits
calibration	Act of determining, rectifying or marking the graduations of an instrument or device.
capnograph	Instrument for recording the concentration of carbon dioxide, especially in exhaled gas.
closing volume	Absolute lung volume at which small airways begin to close.
compliance	Quality of yielding to pressure or force without disruption, or an expression of the measure of the ability to do so, as an expression of the distensibility of an air- or fluid-filled organ (e.g., lung).
control	Mechanism used to regulate or guide the operation of a machine, apparatus, or system.
co-oximeter	Instrument that measures various forms of hemoglobin using spectrophotometric methods.
CRT	Cathode ray tube, as used for computer displays.
data base	Organized array of records or files.
dead space	Volume of gas in the lungs that does not participate in gas exchange.
diffusion	Tendency of molecules of a substance (gaseous, liquid, or solid) to move from a region of high concentration to one of lower concentration.
disability	Lack of ability to function normally, physically or mentally; incapacity; anything that causes disability.
distribution	Pattern of branching and termination of a ramifying structure, e.g., the airways.
DOS	Disk operating system, used to describe the software which allows data to be stored and retrieved on hard or floppy disks.
EIA	Exercise-induced asthma; bronchospasm thought to accompany heat and/or water loss from the upper airways during increased ventilation, as with exercise.

electrocardiogram	Graphic tracing of the electrical potentials caused by the excitation of the heart muscle, as detected at the body surface.
electrode	Device used to measure current or voltage due to chemical changes with the interconversion of chemical and electrical energy.
end-tidal	Describing gas collected that represents the last gas to leave the lungs during tidal breathing.
ergometer	Apparatus for measuring the muscular, metabolic, and respiratory effects of exercise.
floppy disk	A thin, flexible medium used for computer data storage.
frequency response	Characteristic of an instrument as to how accurately it can record or reproduce the number of times that a periodic function repeats a sequence.
gas chromatograph	Device for separating gases by allowing absorption or passage of different gases at varying rates.
hard disk	Metal platter or series of platters, used for magnetic data storage.
HR$_{MAX}$	Maximal heart rate achieved during high levels of exercise.
hypercapnia	Excess of carbon dioxide in the blood.
hyperventilation	State in which there is an increased amount of air entering the pulmonary alveoli (increased alveolar ventilation), resulting in reduction of carbon dioxide tension and eventually leading to alkalosis.
hypocapnia	Deficiency of carbon dioxide in the blood, resulting from hyperventilation and eventually leading to alkalosis.
hypoventilation	State in which there is a reduced amount of air entering the pulmonary alveoli, eventually leading to acidosis.
hypoxemia	Deficient oxygenation of the blood; low oxygen content or tension.

indirect calorimetry	Measurement of the amount of heat produced by a subject by determining the amount of oxygen consumed and the quantity of nitrogen and carbon dioxide eliminated.
infrared	Lying outside the visible spectrum at its red end- used of thermal radiation of wavelengths longer than those of visible light; relating to, producing, or employing infrared radiation.
I/O	Input and/or output; any device that communicates with a computer.
isocapnia	State in which the carbon dioxide tension of arterial blood remains constant.
kilobyte	1024 bytes Kb.
kymograph	Recording device on which a graphic record of motion or pressure may be traced.
linearity	Property of having a response or output that is directly proportional to the input.
lung scan	Diagnostic procedure for imaging the lung or its components, usually involving radioisotopes.
mass spectrometer	Apparatus that separates a stream of charged particles into a spectrum according to the masses of the particles by means of electric and magnetic fields.
megabyte	1024 kilobytes Mb.
methacholine	Cholinergic agonist, acetyl-b-methylcholine, having a longer duration of action than acetylcholine and predominantly muscarinic effects; used to test for hyperreactive airway disease.
microprocesor	An electronic device capable of executing commands to perform digital operations; the central processing unit (CPU) of a computerized device.
obstruction	Act of blocking or clogging; state or condition of being clogged.

OS

Operating system; the software that controls input/output operations of a computer.

pathogen

Specific cause of a disease, such as a bacterium or virus.

peak flow

Upper limit of flow from the lungs, either inspiratory or expiratory.

plethysmograph

Instrument for determining and registering variations in volume of an organ, part, or limb and in amount of blood passing through it; device for measuring change in body volume, used especially in pulmonary function measurements.

pneumonectomy

Excision of lung tissue, especially an entire lung.

pneumotachometer

Device for measuring the speed of the flow of gas into or out of the lungs.

polarographic

Method of qualitative or quantitative analysis based on current/voltage curves obtained during electrolysis of a solution with a steadily increasing electromotive force.

potentiometer

Instrument for measuring electromotive forces; a voltage divider.

precision

Quality or state of being precise; the degree of refinement with which an operation is performed or a measurement stated; reproducibility of a measurement.

preoperative

Preceding a surgical procedure.

pulse oximeter

Photoelectric device for determining the oxygen saturation of blood, usually attached to a site where pulsatile capillary blood flow can be obtained (i.e., finger or ear).

RAM

Random access memory; memory that may have digital data stored and read back.

range

Sequence, series or scale between limits; the difference between the least and the greatest values of the attribute or variable in a distribution.

rebreathing

Describing a situation in which the same gas is breathed repeatedly.

reproducibility	Characteristic of causing or seem to be causing to be repeated.
restriction	Constraint or limitation; pulmonary disease characterized by reduction of lung volumes.
ROM	Read-only memory; memory that has data permanently coded into it.
shunt	In the cardiovascular system, an abnormality of blood flow between the sides of the heart or between the systemic and pulmonary circulations.
software	The programs that a computer uses to function.
spectroscopy	Method using any of various instruments for forming and examining optical spectra.
spirogram	Tracing or graph of respiratory movements.
spirometer	Instrument for measuring the air taken into and exhaled from the lungs.
spreadsheet	Array of rows and columns used for data manipulation; a computer program that allows numbers or labels to be manipulated by their position.
steady-state	Not fluctuating or varying widely; constant, when used in regard to gas exchange.
thermistor	Electrical resistor made of a material whose resistance varies sharply in a known manner with the temperature.
tidal volume	Volume of air exchanged on each breath during normal breathing.
tonometry	Using a device that measures the pressure of gas in a liquid.
transcutaneous	Transdermal; taken through the dermis or skin.
transducer	Device that is actuated by power from one system and supplies power in any other form to a second system.
treadmill	Device that allows walking or running in place for the purpose of exercise or stress testing.

turbine	Device that rotates when actuated by the reaction or impulse of a current of fluid or gas under pressure; usually made with a series of curved vanes on a central rotating spindle.
Universal Precautions	Set of guidelines related to the handling of blood and blood-contaminated instruments or equipment.
ventilation	In respiratory physiology, the process of exchange of air between the lungs and the ambient air.
ventilatory equivalent	(1) Ratio of the total volume of ventilation to the volume of expired CO_2 per minute; (2) ratio of the total volume of ventilation to the volume of oxygen consumed per minute.
VPC	Ventricular premature contraction; an ectopic heart beat arising from an irritable focus in the ventricle, characterized by a wide, high voltage QRS complex.
water-sealed	Spirometer bell that rests in or floats on water.

TYPICAL VALUES FOR PULMONARY FUNCTION TESTS (VALUES FOR A HEALTHY YOUNG MAN, 1.7 M² BODY SURFACE AREA)

Test	Value
Lung volumes (BTPS)	
IC	3.60 L
ERV	1.20 L
VC	4.80 L
RV	1.20 L
FRC	2.40 L
V_{TG}	2.40 L
TLC	6.00 L
(RV/TLC) × 100	20%
Ventilation (BTPS)	
V_T	0.50 L
f	12 breaths/min
$\dot{V}_E$	6.00 L/min
V_D	0.15 L
$\dot{V}_A$	4.20 L/min
V_D/V_T	0.30

Pulmonary mechanics

FVC	4.80 L
FEV_1	4.00 L
$FEV_{1.0\%}$	83%
$FEF_{25\%-75\%}$	4.7 L/sec
$\dot{V}_{max50}$	5.0 L/sec
PEF	10.0 L/sec
MVV	170 L/min
C_L	0.2 L/cm H_2O
C_{LT}	0.1 L/cm H_2O
Raw	1.5 cm H_2O/L/sec
SGaw	0.25 L/sec/cm H_2O
MIP	130 cm H_2O
MEP	250 cm H_2O

Gas distribution

$\Delta N_{2_{750-1250}}$	Less than 1.5% N_2
7-minute N_2	Less than 2.5% N_2

Diffusion

$D_{L_{CO}}SB$	25 mL CO/min/mm Hg
D_L/V_A	4.2 mL CO/min/mm Hg/L

Blood gases and related tests

$\dot{V}_A/\dot{Q}_C$	0.8
$\dot{Q}_S/\dot{Q}_T$	Less than 7%
pH	7.40
Pa_{CO_2}	40 mm Hg
HCO_3^-	24.0 mEq/L
Pa_{O_2}	95 mm Hg
Sa_{O_2}	97%
COHb	Less than 1.5%
MetHb	Less than 1.5%

SELECTING AND USING REFERENCE VALUES

Reference values for each test of pulmonary function are derived from a statistical analysis of a population of "normal" subjects. These subjects are classified as normal (healthy) because there is no history of lung disease in themselves or their families. Minimal exposure to risk factors, such as smoking or environmental pollution, is usually considered in selecting "normals." In some studies, smokers were included as normals, and this may have affected the resulting reference values.

All pulmonary function parameters vary in the normal population. Some parameters vary much more than others. The arterial pH and Pa_{CO_2} have a very narrow range in normal subjects. The $FEF_{25\%-75\%}$, however, may vary by almost ±2 L/sec. This variability must be considered when comparing a measured value to a reference value. Most parameters "regress," or vary, in a predictable fashion in relation to one or more physical factors. The physical characteristics that most influence pulmonary function are:

- Age
- Sex
- Height (standing/sitting)
- Race or Ethnic Origin
- Weight or Body Surface Area

The altitude at which subjects reside also influences their lung function development. By analyzing each parameter in regard to the subject's physical characteristics, regression equations can be generated in order to predict the expected value. Most regression analyses presume that lung function changes are *linearly* related to the physical characteristics of age, height, and sex. This may not be accurate, particularly in subjects who are very old or young, or very tall or short.

Race or ethnic origin influences stature and body proportions. Lung function parameters, particularly lung volumes and $D_{L_{CO}}$, differ significantly among races. Some computerized pulmonary function systems allow proportional changes to be applied to reference values derived from normal Caucasians in order to "correct" the reference value. Although the lung function differences between races is well documented, there is no single "correction factor" that is applicable to all measurements. Some laboratories correct the reference values for volumes such as FVC and TLC by factors of 10% to 15% for Blacks. Race-specific regression equations may be used if they produce reference values representative of normal subjects in the population which the laboratory tests.

Several methods of utilizing reference values are in common use:

1. Tables of normal values
2. Nomograms
3. Graphs
4. Regression equations

In instances where a calculator or computer is unavailable or not practical, tables, nomograms, or graphs may be used. Figures A–1, A–2, and A–3 are examples of nomograms used for obtaining a reference value. Figures A–4, A–5, and A–6 are examples of graphs that may be used to obtain reference values. The use of calculators and computers allows the employment of complex regression equations.

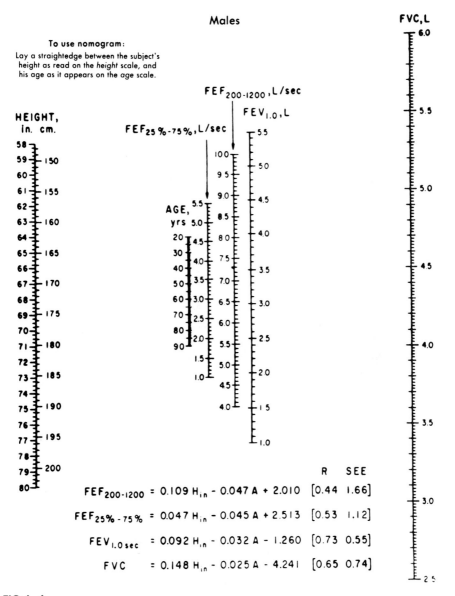

FIG A–1.

Prediction nomograms (BTPS), spirometric values in normal males. (From Morris JF, Koski WA, Johnson LD: *Am Rev Respir Dis* 103(1):57, 1971.)

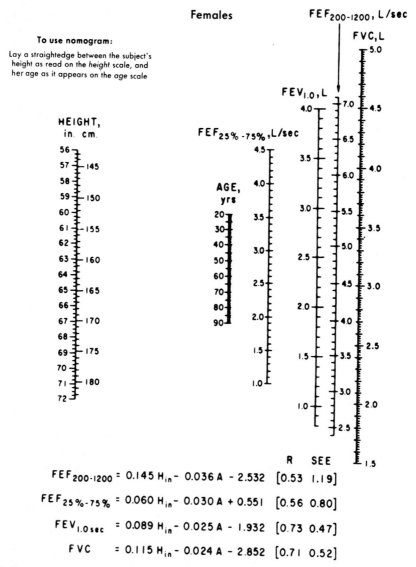

To use nomogram:

Lay a straightedge between the subject's height as read on the *height* scale, and her age as it appears on the age scale

Females

FEF$_{200-1200}$, L/sec

FVC,L

FEV$_{1.0}$,L

HEIGHT, in. cm.

FEF$_{25\%-75\%}$,L/sec

AGE, yrs

R   SEE

FEF$_{200-1200} = 0.145\ H_{in} - 0.036\ A - 2.532$ [0.53 1.19]

FEF$_{25\%-75\%} = 0.060\ H_{in} - 0.030\ A + 0.551$ [0.56 0.80]

FEV$_{1.0 sec} = 0.089\ H_{in} - 0.025\ A - 1.932$ [0.73 0.47]

FVC $= 0.115\ H_{in} - 0.024\ A - 2.852$ [0.71 0.52]

FIG A–2.

Prediction nomograms (BTPS), spirometric values in normal females. (From Morris, JF, Koski WA, Johnson LD: *Am Rev Respir Dis* 103(1):57, 1971.)

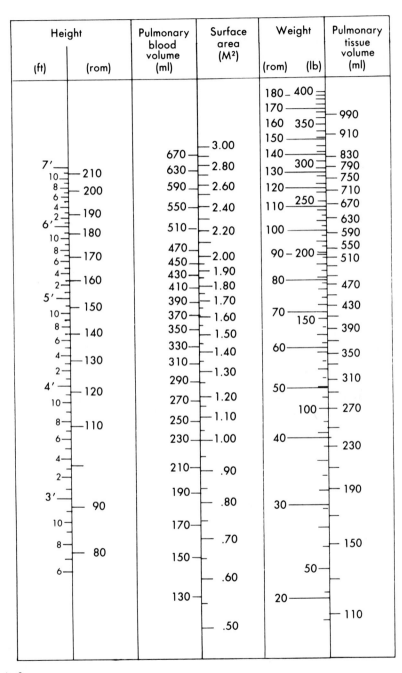

FIG A–3.
Pulmonary tissue/blood volume nomogram (for use with the radiologic method of estimating TLC [see Chapter 1]). (From Ferris BG: *Am Rev Respir Dis* Suppl 118:109, 1978.)

SUMMARY CURVES FOR PREDICTING
NORMAL VALUES IN CHILDREN

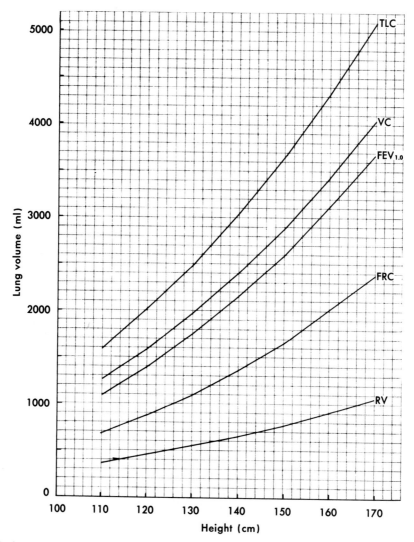

FIG A–4.

Summary curves for lung volumes and FEV$_1$, in milliliters, for boys, as a function of height in centimeters. Summary curves are derived from regression equations from several different studies. (From Polgar G, Promadhat V: *Pulmonary function testing in children*. Philadelphia, 1971, WB Saunders, p. 209.)

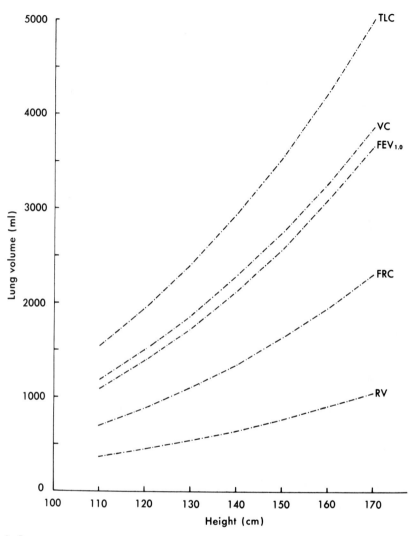

FIG A–5.
Summary curves for lung volumes and FEV$_1$, in milliliters, for girls, as a function of height in centimeters. Summary curves are derived from regression equations from several different studies. (From Polgar G, Promadhat V: *Pulmonary function testing in children.* Philadelphia, 1971, WB Saunders, p. 210.)

Establishing a lower limit of normal is done in one of several ways. Many clinicians use a *fixed percentage of the reference value* (measured/reference × 100) to determine the degree of abnormality, often with ± 20% as the limit of normal. This method is simple and produces approximate lower limits of normal for adults of average age and height for FVC and FEV$_1$. Eighty

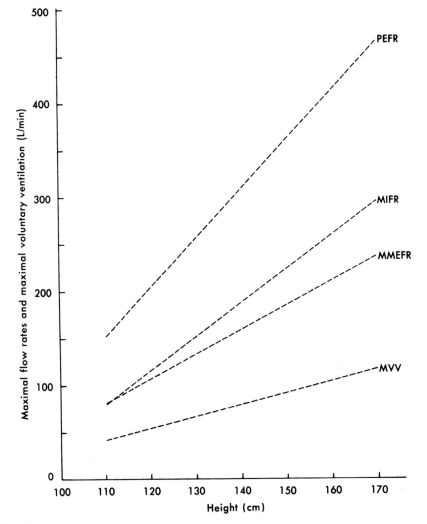

FIG A–6.
Summary curves for maximal midexpiratory flow rate (FEF$_{25\%-75\%}$), peak expiratory flow (PEF), maximal voluntary ventilation (MVV), and maximal inspiratory flow rate (MIFR) in liters per minute, as a function of height for boys and girls. Summary curves are derived from regression equations from several different studies. (From Polgar G, Promadhat V: *Pulmonary function testing in children.* Philadelphia, 1971, WB Saunders, p. 211.)

percent of predicted is close to the fifth percentile in these subjects. Using a fixed percentage will result in shorter, older subjects being classified as abnormal. Tall, younger subjects may be erroneously classified as normal. The fixed percentage of reference produces erroneous lower limits however for the FEF$_{25\%-75\%}$ and for instantaneous flows ($\dot{V}_{max}$). The lower limit of normal for these flow measurements is approximately 50% of the predicted value. Fixed percentages may be acceptable in children, if the variability is proportional to the predicted mean value.

A more precise approach is to define a lower limit based on the *reference value and the variability.* Assuming that the lung function parameter varies in normal fashion (a Gaussian or bell-shaped distribution curve), the mean ± 1.96 standard deviations (SDs) defines the 95% confidence limits. Statistically, 95% of the normal population falls within 1.96 SDs of the mean. If a subject's measured value is outside of the range defined by his expected value ± 1.96 SDs, there is less than a 5% chance that the parameter is normal. Certain pulmonary function parameters require consideration of only the *lower* limit of normal, that is, below the mean. In these cases, 1.65 SDs may be used to define the lower limit of normal. Those parameters that can be abnormal by being either too high or too low (i.e., RV, TLC, $Paco_2$) must use the 1.96-SD method.

A more sophisticated means of representing the abnormality is to express the difference between the reference value and the subject's measured value in terms of confidence intervals (CI). In this method, the difference between the reference value and measured value is divided by the value representing one CI (either 1.96 or 1.65 SD) and expressing the result as a ratio:

$$\frac{\text{Reference} - \text{Measured}}{\text{CI}}$$

Using this method, a normal value is always less than or equal to 1.00, while abnormal values are greater. The degree of abnormality also can be quantified by relating the confidence interval ratio to the degree of obstruction or restriction. For example, the $FEV_{1\%}$ may be evaluated:

$FEV_{1\%}$	(CI)
Normal	< 1 CI
Mild obstruction	> 1 < 2 CI
Moderate obstruction	> 2 < 4 CI
Severe obstruction	> 4 CI

Degrees of abnormality are not always expressed in terms of whole units of confidence intervals. Parameters that display a wide variability, such as $FEF_{25\%-75\%}$, may have confidence intervals that in some instances are larger than the expected value. As a result, the lower limit of normal may be zero or even a negative value. Though statistically valid, the use of the CI may not be applicable in every situation.

A third method of determining lower limits of normal uses the *fifth percentile.* The fifth percentile for any pulmonary function parameter may be calculated as the percent of reference above which 95% of the healthy population falls. Although the fifth percentile method requires a large sample population, it does not require that the pulmonary function parameter be normally distributed throughout the population. Lower limits of normal by the fifth percentile method are usually expressed in relation to specific age groupings. Both the CI and fifth percentile methods yield similar results for lower limits of normal, if the parameter is normally distributed in the population.

In selecting reference values, individual laboratories should attempt to choose reference studies that closely approximate the population to be tested. The following factors may be considerations in selecting reference values:

1. *Type of equipment* used for the reference study—does it comply with the most recent recommendations (1987) of the American Thoracic Society? (See Chapter 11.)

2. *Methodologies*—were the instrumentation and procedures used in the reference study similar to those to be employed, particularly for flows, lung volumes, and $D_{L_{CO}}$?

3. *Sample population*—what age ranges were included? Did the study generate different regressions for different ethnic origins? Did the study include smokers or other "at-risk" individuals as normals?

4. *Statistical data*—are lower limits of normal defined? Are adequate data available, so that lower limits of normal can be calculated?

5. *Conditions of the study*—was the study performed at a different altitude or under different environmental conditions?

6. *Published reference equations*—do reference values generated using the study's regressions differ markedly from other published reports?

Each laboratory should perform measurements on 20 to 40 subjects who represent a healthy cross section of the population the laboratory usually tests. Measured values from these subjects may be compared with values from various reference equations. The equations with the smallest average differences and the smallest range of differences should be selected. An evaluation based on a small number of subjects may not show marked differences between equations for parameters such as the FVC and FEV_1, but may show noticeable discrepancies for $D_{L_{CO}}$ and for maximal flow measurements. Equations for similar tests (i.e., spirometry, lung volumes) should all be taken from a single reference, if possible. If healthy subjects fall outside the limits of normal, the laboratory should question its testing methodology, the selection of the normal subjects, or the prediction equations selected.

Although there are no universally accepted reference values, several excellent studies are available to provide a diverse combination of regressions, so that many of the considerations discussed can be addressed. The reference equations included here are widely used regressions and compare favorably with other published studies. Other acceptable studies are included in the references. Laboratories are encouraged to evaluate these and other equations in selecting references.

PREDICTION REGRESSIONS FOR PULMONARY FUNCTION TESTS (ALL VALUES BTPS UNLESS OTHERWISE STATED)*

Test	Formula	SD	Source
VC (L)			
Males	$0.148H - 0.025A - 4.24$	0.74	1
Females	$0.115H - 0.024A - 2.85$	0.52	1
FRC (L)			
Males	$0.130H - 5.16$	—	2
Females	$0.119H - 4.85$	—	2
RV (L)			
Males	$0.069H + 0.017A - 3.45$	—	3
Females	$0.081H + 0.009A - 3.90$	—	3
Derived Lung Volumes			
	TLC (L) = VC + RV		
	IC(L) = TLC − FRC		
	ERV(L) = VC − IC		
FVC (L)			
Males	(same as VC)	—	1
Females	(same as VC)	—	1
$FEV_{0.5}$ (L)			
Males	$0.24 + 0.02H - 0.024A$	0.51	4
FEV_1 (L)			
Males	$0.092H - 0.032A - 1.260$	0.55	1
Females	$0.089H - 0.025A - 1.93$	0.47	1
$FEF_{25\%-75\%}$ (L/sec)			
Males	$0.047H - 0.045A + 2.513$	1.12	1
Females	$0.060H - 0.030A + 0.551$	0.80	1
PEF (L/sec)			
Males	$0.144H - 0.024A + 0.225$	—	5
Females	$0.090H - 0.018A + 1.130$	—	5
$\dot{V}_{max75}$ (L/sec)			
Males	$0.090H - 0.020A + 2.726$	—	5
Females	$0.069H - 0.019A + 2.147$	—	5
$\dot{V}_{max50}$ (L/sec)			
Males	$0.065H - 0.030A + 2.403$	—	5
Females	$0.062H - 0.035A + 1.426$	—	5
$\dot{V}_{max25}$ (L/sec)			
Males	$0.036H - 0.041A + 1.984$	—	5
Females	$0.023H - 0.035A + 2.216$	—	5
MVV (L/min)			
Males	$3.03H - 0.816A - 37.9$	—	5
Females	$2.14H - 0.685A - 4.87$	—	5

CV/VC (%)

Males	$0.357A + 0.562$	4.15	6
Females	$0.293A + 2.812$	4.90	6

CC/TLC (%)

Males	$0.496A + 14.878$	4.09	6
Females	$0.536A + 14.420$	4.43	6

Viso$\dot{V}$/FVC (%)

All ages	$0.450A + 4.69$	5.27	7
> 50 years	$0.303A + 13.43$	4.31	7

$D_{L_{CO}}SB$ (mL CO/min/mm Hg STPD)

Males	$0.250H - 0.177A + 19.93$	—	8
Females	$0.284H - 0.177A + 7.72$	—	8

Maximal Expiratory Pressure (cm H_2O)

Males	$268 - 1.03A$	—	9
Females	$170 - 0.53A$	—	9

Maximal Inspiratory Pressure (cm H_2O)

Males	$143 - 0.55A$	—	9
Females	$104 - 0.51A$	—	9

$\dot{V}_{O_{2max}}$ (L/min STPD)

Males	$4.2 - 0.032A$	0.4	10
Females	$2.6 - 0.014A$	0.4	10

HR_{max} (beats/min)

Males and Females	$210 - 0.65A$	10–15	10

Pa_{O_2} (mm Hg)

Males and Females	$-0.279A + 0.113P_B + 14.632$	—	11

H is height in inches; A is age in years; P_B is barometric pressure.

SOURCES FOR PREDICTION REGRESSIONS

1. Morris JF, Koski A, Johnson LC: Spirometric standards for healthy non-smoking adults. *Am Rev Respir Dis* 103:57, 1971.
2. Bates DV, Macklem PT, Christie RV: *Respiratory function in disease*, ed 2. Philadelphia, 1971, WB Saunders.
3. Goldman HI, Becklake MR: Respiratory function tests: normal values at median altitudes and the prediction of normal results. *Am Rev Tuberculosis* 79:457, 1959.
4. Kory RC, Callahan R, Synder JC: The veterans administration–army cooperative study of pulmonary function: I. Clinical spirometry in normal men. *Am J Med* 30:243, 1961.
5. Cherniack RM, Raber MD: Normal standards for ventilatory function using an automated wedge spirometer. *Am Rev Respir Dis* 106:38, 1972.
6. Buist SA, Ross BB: Predicted values for closing volumes using a modified single breath nitrogen test. *Am Rev Respir Dis* 111:405, 1975.

7. Gelb AF, Maloney PA, Klein E, et al: Sensitivity of volume of isoflow in the detection of mild airway obstruction. *Am Rev Respir Dis* 112:401, 1975.
8. Gaensler EA, Wright GW: Evaluation of respiratory impairment. *Arch Environ Health* 12:146, 1966.
9. Black LF, Hyatt RE: Maximal respiratory pressures: normal values and relationship to age and sex. *Am Rev Respir Dis* 99:696, 1969.
10. Jones NL, Campbell EJM, Edwards RHT, et al: *Clinical exercise testing,* ed 2. Philadelphia, 1983, WB Saunders.
11. Morris AH, Kanner RE, Crapo RO, et al: *Clinical pulmonary function testing,* ed 2. Salt Lake City, 1984, Intermountain Thoracic Society.

ADDITIONAL RECOMMENDED SOURCES FOR PULMONARY FUNCTION PREDICTED VALUES

GENERAL

American Thoracic Society: Lung function testing: selection of reference values and interpretive strategies. *Am Rev Respir Dis* 144:1202, 1991.

SPIROMETRY

Crapo RO, Morris AH, Gardner RM: Reference spirometric values using techniques and equipment that meets ATS recommendations. *Am Rev Respir Dis* 123:659, 1981.

Knudson RJ, Slatin RC, Lebowitz MD: The maximal expiratory flow-volume curve: normal standards, variability, and effects of age. *Am Rev Respir Dis* 113:587, 1976.

Quanjer PH, editor: Report of working party—European community for coal and steel. Standardized lung function testing. *Bull Eur Physiopathol Respir* 19(suppl 5):7, 1983.

Schoenberg JB, Beck GJ, Bouhuys A: Growth and decay of pulmonary function in healthy blacks and whites. *Respir Physiol* 33:367, 1978.

LUNG VOLUMES

Crapo RO, Morris AH, Clayton PD, et al: Lung volumes in healthy non-smoking adults. *Bull Eur Physiopathol Respir* 18:419, 1982.

Grimby G, Soderholm B: Spirometric studies in normal subjects: III. Static lung volumes and maximum voluntary ventilation in adults with a note on physical fitness. *Acta Med Scand* 173:199, 1963.

DIFFUSING CAPACITY

Bates DV, Macklem PT, Christie RV: *Respiratory function in disease.* Philadelphia, 1971, WB Saunders.

Crapo RO, Morris AH: Standardized single breath normal values for carbon monoxide diffusing capacity. *Am Rev Respir Dis* 123:185, 1981.

PEDIATRIC PULMONARY FUNCTION

Hsu KHK, Bartholomew PH, Thompson V, et al: Ventilatory functions of normal children and young adults—Mexican-American, white, and black: I. Spirometry. *J Pediatr* 95:14, 1979.

Polgar G, Promadhat V: *Pulmonary function testing in children: techniques and standards.* Philadelphia, 1971, WB Saunders.

NORMAL VALUES FOR PULMONARY FUNCTION STUDIES IN CHILDREN (ALL VALUES BTPS UNLESS OTHERWISE NOTED)*

Test	Formula	SD	Source
(Children 42–59 inches, 5–17 years old)			
FVC (L)			
Males	$0.094H - 3.04$	0.176	1
Females	$0.077H - 2.37$	0.171	1
FEV_1 (L)			
Males	$0.085H - 2.86$	0.159	1
Females	$0.074H - 2.48$	0.166	1
$FEF_{25\%-75\%}$ (L)			
Males	$0.094H - 2.61$	0.388	1
Females	$0.087H - 2.39$	0.347	1
PEF (L/Sec)			
Males	$0.161H - 5.88$	0.451	1
Females	$0.130H - 4.51$	0.487	1
MVV (L/Min)			
Males and Females	$3.81H - 134$	—	1
Children 60–78 inches, 5–17 years old)			
FVC (L)			
Males	$0.174A + 0.164H - 9.43$	0.354	1
Females	$0.102A + 0.117H - 5.87$	0.287	1
FEV_1 (L/Sec)			
Males	$0.126A + 0.143H - 7.86$	0.303	1
Females	$0.085A + 0.100H - 4.94$	0.290	1
$FEF_{25\%-75\%}$ (L/Sec)			
Males	$0.126A + 0.135H - 6.50$	0.612	1
Females	$0.083A + 0.093H - 3.50$	0.621	1
PEF (L/Sec)			
Males	$0.205A + 0.181H - 9.54$	0.780	1
Females	$0.139A + 0.100H - 4.12$	0.798	1
MVV (L/Min)			
Males and Females	$3.81H - 134$	—	1

Most of the factors of this equation can be combined to give an approximate value for a conversion factor. Local P_B causes slight differences.

Conversion factor	Gas temperature (°C)	P_{H_2O}
1.112	18	15.6
1.107	19	16.5
1.102	20	17.5
1.096	21	18.7
1.091	22	19.8
1.085	23	21.1
1.080	24	22.4
1.075	25	23.8
1.068	26	23.8
1.063	27	26.7
1.057	28	28.3
1.051	29	30.0
1.045	30	31.8
1.039	31	31.8
1.032	32	35.7
1.026	33	35.7
1.020	34	35.7
1.014	35	42.2
1.007	36	44.6
1.000	37	47.0

Converting Gas Volumes from ATPS to STPD

$$\text{Volume (STPD)} = \text{Volume (ATPS)} \times \frac{P_B - P_{H_2O}}{760} \times \frac{273}{273 + T}$$

where:

P_B = barometric pressure

P_{H_2O} = water vapor pressure at spirometer temperature

T = temperature of the spirometer

760 = standard barometric pressure at sea level

273 = absolute temperature equal to 0°C

Calculating Water Vapor Pressure

$$P_{H_2O} = 47.07 \times 10^{\left[\frac{6.36(T-37)}{232+T}\right]}$$

VC (L)
    Males   (same as FVC)   1
    Females   (same as FVC)   1

FRC (L)
    Males and Females $0.067 \times e^{0.05334H}$ —   2

RV (L)
    Males and Females $0.033 \times e^{0.05334H}$ —   2

Derived Lung Volumes (L)

$$TLC = VC + RV$$
$$IC = TLC - FRC$$
$$ERV = VC - IC$$

$D_{L_{CO}}SB$ (mL CO/min/mm Hg STPD)
    Males and Females $0.693H - 20.13$ —   3

SOURCES FOR NORMAL VALUES FOR CHILDREN

1. Dickman M, Schmidt CD, Gardner RM: Spirometric standards for normal children and adolescent (ages 5 years through 18 years). *Am Rev Respir Dis* 104:680, 1971.
2. Weng TR, Levison H: Standards of pulmonary function in children. *Am Rev Respir Dis* 99:879, 1969.
3. Gaensler EA, Wright GW: Evaluation of respiratory impairment. *Arch Environ Health* 12:146, 1966.

(See also Additional Recommended Sources for Pulmonary Function Predicteds.)

CONVERSION AND CORRECTIONS FACTORS

Converting Gas Volumes from ATPS to BTPS

$$\text{Volume (BTPS)} = \text{Volume (ATPS)} \times \frac{P_B - P_{H_2O}}{P_B - 47} \times \frac{310}{273 + T}$$

where:

P_B = barometric pressure, mm Hg

P_{H_2O} = vapor pressure of water at spirometer temperature

T = Temperature in degrees Celsius

47   = vapor pressure of water at 37°C

310 = absolute body temperature

where:

P_{H_2O} = water vapor pressure in mm Hg
T = temperature, from 0 to 40°C

Calculating Barometric Pressure at Altitude

$$P_B = 760 \times [1 - (6.873 \times 10^{-6} \times \text{Altitude})]^{5.256}$$

where:

P_B = barometric pressure in mm Hg

Altitude = altitude in feet above sea level

SI (SYSTÈME INTERNATIONAL) UNITS

Conversion factors for units of measurement commonly used in pulmonary function testing. (Except for temperature, to convert a value expressed in conventional units to its equivalent in SI units, *multiply* the conventional units by the conversion factor. To convert from SI to conventional units, *divide* by the factor.)

Measurement	Conventional Unit	SI Unit	Conversion Factor
Temperature	°C	°K	°C + 273.15
Length	inch (in)	meter (m)	0.0254
	foot (ft)	m	0.3048
Area	in^2	cm^2	6.452
	ft^2	m^2	0.0929
Volume	ft^3	L	28.32
Pressure	cm H_2O	kilopascal (kPa)	0.09806
	mm Hg (torr)	kPa	0.1333
	pounds/in^2 (psi)	kPa	6.895
Work	kilogram meter (kg m)	joule (J)	9.807
Power	kg m/min	(J)	0.1634
Energy	kilocalorie (Kcal)	(J)	4185.0
Compliance	L/cm H_2O	L/kPa	10.20
Resistance	cm H_2O/L/sec	kPa/L/sec	0.09806

REGULATIONS AND REGULATORY AGENCIES

Several agencies regulate operations in pulmonary function and/or blood gas laboratories. These regulations concern laboratory procedures, infection control, safety, and reimbursement.

Occupational Safety and Health Administration (OSHA)

OSHA is an agency of the U.S. Government charged with developing and implementing policies to address hazards in the workplace. OSHA regulations apply to two main areas in pulmonary function and blood gas laboratories:

1. *Hazard communication* relates to all chemicals or substances used in the laboratory. Laboratories are required to maintain lists of hazardous substances. In addition, Material Safety Data Sheets must be kept. Employees must be trained regarding, and kept informed of, hazardous chemicals in their workplace.

2. Training regarding *blood-borne pathogens* is mandated. Employees who may be exposed to blood or blood products must receive training regarding the transmission of blood-borne pathogens. Methods of preventing exposure, identification of tasks involving risk of exposure, and actions to be taken must be documented. Plans for removal of blood and blood products are necessary, as are explanations of personal protective equipment, such as gloves and gowns.

Regulations mandated by OSHA are published in the Federal Register and are continually updated.

National Institute for Occupational Safety and Health (NIOSH)

NIOSH is an agency of the U.S. Government that enforces standards set by OSHA. NIOSH regulations concerning pulmonary function measurements are related to the "Cotton Dust Standard." The federal regulations (29 CFR: 1910.1043) describe how spirometry is to be performed in the examination of individuals exposed to cotton dust. The appendix to this statute lists the standards for the spirometer and recorder used, the measurement technique, the interpretation of the spirogram, and the qualifications for personnel performing spirometry. Guidelines for a minimal spirometry training are included. These NIOSH regulations regarding spirometry are often applied in areas of occupational exposure other than cotton dust, making them de facto standards. Updates to NIOSH regulations are published in the Federal Register.

Health and Human Services (HHS)

Health and Human Services is a department of the U.S. Government. Programs impacting pulmonary function and blood gas laboratories are administered by the Health Care Financing Administration (HCFA).
Clinical Laboratory Improvement Amendments of 1988 (CLIA 88)
CLIA 88 (42 CFR: 405, et al) consists of a series of rules regarding laboratory practices. These rules apply to blood gas laboratories, and may have ramifications for pulmonary function testing as well. Under CLIA 88 rules:

1. Laboratories must register and apply for certification. Level of certification depends on the complexity of tests performed.

2. Three categories of testing based on complexity of the testing method have been established:

Waived tests   These include simple nonautomated tests such as pH measurement by dipstick method.

Tests of moderate complexity   These include automated tests or manual procedures with limited steps. Automated blood gas analyses that do not require operator intervention during the analytic process are included in the moderate complexity group.

Tests of high complexity   These include semiautomated or manual procedures that require multiple steps, preparation of complex reagents, and operator intervention in the analytic process.

3. Personnel requirements are linked to the complexity model for testing. For moderately complex tests, standards for laboratory directors, technical consultants, clinical consultants, and testing personnel are defined. For high-complexity tests, standards for technical and general supervisors are added to the list. The regulations list specific functions and qualifications for each position. Qualified individuals can fill more than one position in either moderate- or high-complexity testing.

4. Proficiency testing is required to externally evaluate each laboratory's performance. Each laboratory performing moderate- or high-complexity tests must participate in proficiency testing. Proficiency tests must be performed for each regulated analyte for which the laboratory reports results. Proficiency testing samples must include five samples for each analyte or test. The laboratory must participate in the program at least three times per year. A separate grading formula is established for each analyte. For most analytes or tests, a score of 80% (i.e., acceptable measurement on four of five samples) is required. Laboratories who are unsuccessful, that is score less than 80%, on two of three testing events will be subject to sanctions for the involved test.

5. Each laboratory must establish a quality control program. The rules require that for tests of moderate complexity, such as blood gases, the manufacturer's instructions be followed, a procedure manual be available, and calibrations be performed. Quality control runs with at least two levels must be performed daily. Instruments and test systems will be evaluated by the Food and Drug Administration (FDA) to determine the applicable levels of quality control required.

In addition to the laboratory regulations defined by CLIA 88, HHS sets standards for reimbursement under the DRG (Diagnosis Related Groups) system for Medicare patients. Reimbursement requires that charges for procedures performed be correctly classified using Current Procedural Terminology (CPT) codes. HHS also lists requirements for disability according to the Social Security Administration (SSA). These regulations specify levels of pulmonary function impairment that qualify candidates for disability reimbursement (see Chapter 8).

Updates to CLIA 88 regulations are published in the Federal Register. Regulations related to reimbursement under HCFA or SSA are published by those agencies respectively.

Joint Committee on Accreditation of Healthcare Organizations (JCAHO)

The JCAHO is a voluntary accrediting agency that develops standards of quality for health care organizations. The JCAHO has published standards for all areas of the hospital environment. The standards that affect pulmonary function laboratories are listed primarily under Respiratory Care Services. JCAHO standards require:

1. Pulmonary function studies and blood gas analysis capability should be appropriate for the level of respiratory care services provided and are readily available to meet the needs of patients. Blood gases should be available 24 hours per day.

2. The scope of diagnostic services is defined in writing, and is related to other hospital departments by an organizational plan.

3. Services provided from outside of the hospital meet all necessary requirements.

4. Medical direction should be provided by a physician qualified by special training or interest in respiratory problems, and should be readily available for consultation.

5. Trained personnel should be available to meet the needs of the patients served. Hazardous procedures, such as arterial puncture, must be authorized in writing according to medical staff policy.

6. There must be written policies and procedures for pulmonary function testing, and obtaining and analyzing blood samples. Policies and procedures should address equipment maintenance, safety, infection control, and administration of medications.

7. There must be sufficient facilities (equipment, space) for performing pulmonary function studies and blood gas analyses. Requirements regarding performance of pulmonary function or blood gas studies must be met regardless of which hospital department performs them. Equipment must be calibrated and maintained according to the manufacturer's specifications.

Standards developed by the JCAHO are published annually in their document entitled *Accreditation Manual for Hospitals.*

Certifying and Standards Organizations

The following are organizations that offer certification or publish standards related to pulmonary function testing and/or blood gas analysis:

Organization	Certification/Standards
American College of Sports Medicine (ACSM)	Provides training courses and certification for exercise technologists; publishes guidelines for exercise testing and training
American Thoracic Society (ATS)	Publishes standards for spirometry, single-breath $D_{L_{CO}}$, pulmonary function personnel qualifications, use of computers in pulmonary function testing, guidelines for quality assurance, and interpretive strategies. Standards are published in the *American Review of Respiratory Disease*
Center for Disease Control and Prevention (CDCP)	Promulgates standards related to infection control and disease prevention; regulations are published in *Morbidity and Mortality Weekly Report*
College of American Pathologists (CAP)	Accredits clinical and research laboratories, including blood gas laboratories; provides quality control programs and proficiency testing survey materials
National Board for Respiratory Care (NBRC)	Provides national certification for respiratory care practitioners, including pulmonary function technologists; offers Certified Pulmonary Function Technologist (CPFT) and Registered Pulmonary Function Technologist (RPFT) credentials
National Committee for Clinical Laboratory Standards (NC-CLS)	Publishes standards for all areas of laboratory medicine, including blood gas laboratories

SOME USEFUL EQUATIONS

Alveolar air equation

It is often necessary to determine the composition of alveolar gas. Estimations of the partial pressure of CO_2, N_2, and H_2O can be done rather easily, but the $P_{A_{O_2}}$ is somewhat more difficult to obtain. One practical application of the alveolar air equation is determination of $P_{A_{O_2}}$ for calculation of the percent of shunt. The formula for the alveolar equation is as follows:

$$P_{A_{O_2}} = (F_{I_{O_2}} \times (P_B - 47)) - Pa_{CO_2}\left(F_{I_{O_2}} + \frac{1 - F_{I_{O_2}}}{R}\right)$$

where:

$F_{I_{O_2}}$ = fractional concentration of inspired O_2

P_B = barometric pressure

47 = partial pressure of water vapor at 37°C

Pa_{CO_2} = arterial CO_2 tension, presumed equal to alveolar CO_2 tension

R = respiratory exchange ratio ($\dot{V}_{CO_2}/\dot{V}_{O_2}$)

If the fraction of inspired O_2 is 1.0, the entire factor in the right-hand parentheses becomes 1 and can be deleted. R varies between 0.70 and 1.00 and is often assumed to be about 0.80.

Poiseuille's Law

Poiseuille's law describes the flow of gas through a tube. The law has many applications in pulmonary physiology. It applies to laminar flow of gas through the conducting airways. It is also utilized in pneumotachography to relate flow and pressure changes within a tube. The law is stated thus:

$$\Delta P = \frac{\dot{V}8\eta l}{\pi r^4}$$

where:

ΔP = change in pressure from one end of the tube to the other

$\dot{V}$ = flow through the tube

η = coefficient of viscosity of the gas

l = length of the tube

r = radius of the tube

The equation can be rearranged thus:

$$\frac{\Delta P}{\dot{V}} = \frac{8\eta l}{\pi r^4}$$

The ratio of the pressure differences at the ends of the tube (ΔP) and the flow through the tube ($\dot{V}$), which defines *resistance,* is equated to the length and radius of the tube. Resistance varies directly with the length of the conducting tube. It varies inversely with the fourth power of the radius. A twofold increase in the length of the tube doubles the resistance. A reduction of the radius by half increases the pressure difference 16 times. In the airways, narrowing caused by secretions or other lesions can significantly increase airway resistance. Poiseuille's law holds true for any round tube in which laminar flow is possible, and pneumotachography is based directly on this law (see "Pressure Differential Flow Sensors," Chapter 9). The length and radius of a pressure differential flow sensor remain constant. The viscosity of respiratory gases varies only slightly. Therefore, the variables in Poiseuille's equation can be reduced to a single constant, except for ΔP and $\dot{V}$, by rearranging:

$$\dot{V} = \frac{\Delta P}{K_R}$$

where:

K_R = a resistance constant determined by the length and radius of the flow tube

Using this equation, to measure $\dot{V}$, all that is required is to determine the pressure differential. This is easily accomplished by means of pressure transducers.

Thoracic Gas Volume Equation

Measurement of the V_{TG} with the body plethysmograph is based on Boyle's law:

$$P_1 V_1 = P_2 V_2$$

or by expanding:

$$P_1 V_1 = (P_1 + \Delta P)(V_1 + \Delta V)$$

where:

P_1 = initial pressure in the lungs (713 mm Hg or 970 cm H_2O)

V_1 = V_{TG} or thoracic gas volume

ΔV = change in lung volume

ΔP = change in lung pressure

Then by rearranging:

$$P_1 \Delta V + V_1 \Delta P + \Delta V \Delta P = 0$$

solving for V_1:

$$V_1 = -\frac{\Delta V}{\Delta P}(P_1 + \Delta P)$$

Because ΔP is small compared with P_1, $P_1 + \Delta P \approx P_1$, therefore:

$$V_1 = -\frac{P_1(\Delta V)}{(\Delta P)}$$

In terms of the plethysmographic method (and disregarding the sign):

$$V_{TG} = 970\frac{(\Delta V)}{(\Delta P)}$$

A sloping line is recorded on an oscilloscope or computer screen. The line represents the change in mouth pressure per unit change in box volume ($\Delta P/\Delta V$) or λV_{TG}, as the subject breathes against an occluded airway. The equation them becomes:

$$V_{TG} = \frac{970}{\lambda V_{TG}}$$

This is the working form of the equation. Box pressure and mouth pressure calibration factors are also required to complete the calculation (see Sample Calculations). Simple measurements of the slope of the tracing allows rapid calculations of V_{TG}.

Fick's Law of Diffusion (Modified)

In reference to gas exchange across a membrane, Fick's law states that:

$$\dot{V}_{gas} = \frac{A}{T} \times D \times (P_1 - P_2)$$

where:

$$A = \text{area of the membrane}$$

$$T = \text{thickness of the membrane}$$

$$P_1 - P_2 = \text{pressure gradient across the membrane}$$

$$D = \text{diffusion constant}$$

D is related to the molecular weight and solubility of the gas to which it refers by:

$$D \propto \frac{\text{Solubility}}{\sqrt{\text{Molecular weight}}}$$

Because A and T remain relatively constant in the lung system:

$$D_L \propto \frac{\dot{V}_{gas}}{P_A - P_C}$$

where:

D_L = diffusion constant for the lung

P_A = alveolar gas pressure

P_C = capillary gas pressure

When D_L is measured with carbon monoxide (CO), the capillary partial pressure is assumed to be zero, thus:

$$D_L = \frac{\dot{V}_{CO}}{P_{A_{CO}}}$$

All CO methods of measuring D_L use this basic equation. The single-breath and steady-state methods differ in that the former measures $\dot{V}_{CO}$ during breath holding, while the latter measures it during "normal" breathing. The steady-state methods vary by the way in which they measure $P_{A_{CO}}$.

Fick Principle (Cardiac Output Determination)

The Fick principle relates $\dot{V}_{O_2}$ to arterial mixed venous O_2 content difference $(C[a\text{-}\bar{v}]_{O_2})$ to determine cardiac output $(\dot{Q})$:

$$\dot{Q}_T = \frac{\dot{V}_{O_2}}{Ca_{O_2} - C\bar{v}_{O_2}}$$

This equation forms the basis for determining various fractions of the cardiac output, namely, the shunt fraction $(\dot{Q}_S)$ and the fraction participating in ideal gas exchange $(\dot{Q}_C)$. The relationship between $\dot{Q}_S$ and the total cardiac output $\dot{Q}_T$ can be expressed as a ratio using the concept of O_2 content differences:

$$\frac{\dot{Q}_S}{\dot{Q}_T} = \frac{Cc_{O_2} - Ca_{O_2}}{Cc_{O_2} - C\bar{v}_{O_2}}$$

where:

$Cc_{O_2} - Ca_{O_2}$ = content difference between pulmonary end capillary blood, Cc_{O_2}, and arterial blood, Ca_{O_2}, which increases when blood passes through the pulmonary system without coming into contact with alveolar gas (a shunt)

$Cc_{O_2} - C\bar{v}_{O_2}$ = content difference between blood returning to the lungs by way of the pulmonary artery and the pulmonary end-capillary blood; the total change reflects the arterialization of mixed venous blood

In a system in which all blood equilibrates with alveolar gas, Cc_{O_2} and Ca_{O_2} become identical, no matter what the value of the denominator, so that the ratio becomes zero and the shunt must be zero. If some blood does not equilibrate, the numerator becomes larger in relation to the denominator and an increased $\dot{Q}s/\dot{Q}\tau$ results.

Pulmonary end-capillary O_2 content, Cc_{O_2}, is impossible to sample, and represents a mathematical entity rather than an actual phenomenon. A modified form of the equation is used clinically (as described in Chapter 6):

$$\frac{\dot{Q}s}{\dot{Q}\tau} = \frac{(P_{A_{O_2}} - Pa_{O_2})(0.0031)}{(C[a - \bar{v}]_{O_2}) + (P_{A_{O_2}} - Pa_{O_2})(0.0031)}$$

where:

$P_{A_{O_2}} - Pa_{O_2}$ = difference on O_2 tension between the alveoli and arterial blood

0.0031 = solubility factor to convert O_2 tension to volume percent

The equation is implemented by having the subject breathe 100% O_2 long enough to completely saturate the Hb (Pa_{O_2} greater than 150 mm Hg). The only difference between pulmonary end-capillary blood (assumed to be in equilibrium with the $P_{A_{O_2}}$ and arterial blood exists in the difference in O_2 content in the dissolved form. This difference is related to the normal a-$\bar{v}$ content difference ($C[a-\bar{v}]_{O_2}$) plus the actual dissolved content difference, denoted by the same term in both numerator and denominator. A ratio is thus derived between the content difference of shunted blood and the total difference, in this case determined by using dissolved O_2 differences. $P_{A_{O_2}}$ is determined by the alveolar air equation outlined previously in the Appendix.

Calculated Bicarbonate (HCO_3^-)

The bicarbonate concentration in plasma can be calculated from the Henderson-Hasselbalch equation if the pH and Pco_2 are known:

$$pH = pK + \log\frac{(HCO_3^-)}{(H_2CO_3)}$$

The working form of the equation becomes:

$$(HCO_3^-) = 0.0306 \times Pco_2 \times 10^{((pH - 6.161)/(0.9524))}$$

where:

HCO_3^- = bicarbonate concentration, in mEq/L

0.0306 = solubility coefficient for CO_2

$$6.161 = \text{the pK of carbonic acid}$$

$$0.9524 = \text{an empirically determined constant}$$

The total CO_2 concentration can then be determined by summing the HCO_3^- and the dissolved CO_2:

$$T_{CO_2} = 0.0306 \times P_{CO_2} + (HCO_3^-)$$

Calculated Oxygen Saturation

Although it is preferable to actually measure oxygen saturation (see Chapter 6), the saturation of Hb with O_2 can be calculated if the pH and P_{O_2} are known. Assuming that the Hb is normal, (i.e., having a P_{50} of 26.6), the saturation may be calculated:

$$\text{Saturation} = \frac{Z^{2.60}}{(26.6)^{2.60} + Z^{2.60}} \times 100$$

where:

$$Z = P_{O_2} \times 10^{(-0.48\ (7.40\ -\ pH))}$$

where:

P_{O_2} = the partial pressure of O_2 in the sample

pH = the negative log of the hydrogen ion concentration in the sample

-0.48 = the Bohr factor (normal blood)

Because of the assumptions concerning normality of the hemoglobin as well as its P_{50}, calculated saturations may be in error if the true factors are different.

SAMPLE CALCULATIONS

Open-circuit FRC determination (N_2 washout) (see Chapter 1)

FRC	Unknown
% N_2 final:	6% (0.06 as a fraction)
% $N_{2_{alveolar1}}$:	76% (0.76 as a fraction)
% $N_{2_{alveolar2}}$:	1% (0.01 as a fraction)
Volume expired (V_E):	27.5 L
Test time (T):	7 minutes

Blood/tissue N_2 washout factor: 0.04 L/min (correction factor)
Spirometer temperature: 24°C
System deadspace: 1.0 L

1.

$$\text{FRC} = \frac{[\%N_{2_{final}} \times (V_E + V_D)] - (T \times N_2 \text{ correction})}{\%N_{2_{alveolar1}} - \%N_{2_{alveolar2}}}$$

2.

$$= \frac{[0.06 \times (27.5 + 1.0L) - (7.0\text{min} \times 0.04 \text{ L/min})}{0.76 - 0.01}$$

3.

$$= \frac{(0.06 \times 28.5 - (0.28 \text{ L})}{0.75}$$

4.

$$= \frac{1.71L - 0.28L}{0.75}$$

5.

$$= \frac{1.43}{0.75}$$

6.

$$\text{FRC} = 1.91L \text{ (ATPS)}$$

This value is ATPS and must be corrected to BTPS. The spirometer temperature was 24°C. Using the appropriate correction factor from page 685:

7.

$$\text{FRC(BTPS)} = 1.91 \times 1.08$$

8.

$$\text{FRC (BTPS)} = 2.06$$

Closed-Circuit FRC Determination (Helium Dilution) (see Chapter 1)

FRC   Unknown
He added: 0.5L

% He$_{initial}$:	9.5% (0.095 as a fraction)
% He$_{final}$:	5.5% (0.055 as a fraction)
He absorption correction:	0.1 L
Spirometer temperature:	24°C

1.

$$FRC = \left[\frac{(\%He_{initial} - \%He_{final})}{\%He_{final}} \times \text{Initial volume} \right] - \text{He correction}$$

2.

$$\text{Initial volume} = \frac{He_{added}}{\%He_{initial}} \text{(spirometer and circuitry)}$$

$$= \frac{0.05L}{0.095}$$

$$= 5.26L$$

3.

$$FRC = \left[\frac{(0.095 - 0.055)}{0.055} \times 5.26L \right] - 0.1L$$

4.

$$= (0.73 \times 5.26L) - 0.1L$$

5.

$$= 3.84L - 0.1L$$

6.

$$FRC = 3.74 \text{ L (ATPS)}$$

Correcting to BTPS with appropriate correction factor from page 685:

7.

$$FRC \text{ (BTPS)} = 3.74 \times 1.08$$

8.

$$FRC \text{ (BTPS)} = 4.04L$$

Single-Breath D$_{L_{CO}}$ (see Chapter 5)

Volume inspired (V$_I$):	4.0 L
F$_{I_{CO}}$:	0.3% (0.003 as a fraction)
F$_{A_{CO_{T2}}}$:	0.125% (0.00125 as a fraction)
F$_{I_{He}}$:	10.0% (0.10 as a fraction)
F$_{E_{He}}$:	7.5% (0.075 as a fraction)
P$_B$:	760 mm Hg
Breath-hold time (T$_2$ − T$_1$):	10.0 sec
Spirometer temperature:	25°C
Hb:	10.0 g/dL
COHb:	5.5%

1.

$$D_{L_{CO}}SB = \frac{V_A \times 60}{(P_B - 47)(T_2 - T_1)} \times Ln \frac{(F_{A_{CO_{T1}}})}{(F_{A_{CO_{T2}}})}$$

2.

$$V_A = \frac{V_I}{F_{E_{He}} / F_{I_{He}}}$$

$$= 5.33L \quad (5333 \text{ mL})$$

$$= \frac{4.0L}{0.075 / 0.10}$$

3.

$$F_{A_{CO_{T1}}} = F_{I_{CO}} \times F_{E_{He}}/F_{I_{He}}$$

$$= 0.003 \times \frac{0.075}{0.10}$$

$$= 0.0025$$

4.

$$D_{L_{CO}}SB = \frac{5333 \text{ mL} \times 60 \text{ sec}}{(713 \text{ mm Hg}) \times (10.0 \text{ sec})} \times Ln \frac{(0.0025)}{(0.00125)}$$

5.

$$= \frac{319980}{7130} \times Ln (1.8)$$

6.

$$= 44.9 \text{ mL/min/mm Hg} \times (0.5878)$$

7.

$$D_{L_{CO}}SB = 26.38 \text{ mL CO/min/mm Hg (ATPS)}$$

This value is ATPS and is normally converted to STPS (0°C, 760 mm Hg, dry). The correction factor can be calculated:

8.

$$\text{STPD correction factor} = \frac{273}{273 + T°C} \times \frac{P_B - P_{H_2O} \ T°C}{760}$$

where:

$T°C$ = spirometer temperature

$P_{H_2O} \ T°C$ = partial pressure of water vapor at the spirometer temperature (in this case: 24 mm Hg at 25°C)

9.

$$\text{STPD Correction factor} = \frac{273}{273 + 25} \times \frac{760 - 24}{760}$$

10.

$$= 0.916 \times 0.968 = 0.887$$

11.

$$D_{L_{co}}SB = (26.38 \text{ mL CO/min/mm Hg}) \times (0.887)$$
$$= 23.4 \text{ mL CO/min/mm Hg (STPD)}$$

This value also should be corrected for the Hb, in this case 10 g/dL:

12.

$$\text{Hb correction} = \frac{10.22 + Hb}{1.7 \times Hb}$$
$$= \frac{10.22 + 10.0}{1.7 \times 10.0}$$
$$= 1.19$$

13.

$$D_{L_{CO}}SB \text{ (corrected)} = (1.19) \times (23.4)$$

14.

$$= 27.9 \text{ mL CO/min/mm Hg (STPD)}$$

If the COHB level is known, the $D_{L_{CO}}SB$ can be corrected for the back pressure of CO:

15.

$$\text{COHb adjusted } D_{L_{CO}} = \text{Measured } D_{L_{CO}} \times \left(1.00 + \frac{\%COHb}{100} \right)$$

16.

$$= 27.9 \times \left(1.00 + \frac{5.5}{100} \right)$$

17.

$$\text{COHb adjusted } D_{L_{CO}} = 29.4 \text{ mL CO/min/mm Hg (STPD)}$$

Thoracic Gas Volume (V$_{TG}$) (see Chapter 1)

(Data for V$_{TG}$ and Raw are from the same subject)

V$_{TG}$:	Unknown
V$_{TG}$ tangents:	0.71 (angle 35.4)
	0.73 (angle 36.1)
	0.73 (angle 36.1)
P$_B$:	755 mm Hg
Subject weight:	71 kg
P$_{mouth}$ calibration:	10 cm H$_2$O/cm
P$_{box}$ calibration:	30 mL/cm
Deadspace correction:	100 mL
Plethysmograph volume:	530L

1.

$$\text{Average V}_{TG} \text{ tangent (TAN)} = \frac{(0.71 + 0.73 + 0.73)}{3}$$

$$= 0.72$$

The barometric pressure correction is calculated:

2.

$$P_{B_{corr}} = (P_B - 47) \times 1.36$$
$$= (755 \text{ mm Hg} - 47 \text{ mm Hg}) \times 1.36$$
$$= 963 \text{ cm H}_2O$$

The subject volume correction (K) is calculated:

3.

$$K = \frac{[\text{Pleth volume} - (\text{Subject weight}/1.07)]}{\text{Pleth volume}}$$
$$= \frac{[530 \text{ L} - (71 \text{ kg}/1.07)]}{530 \text{ L}}$$
$$= 0.874$$

4.

$$V_{TG} = \left(\frac{P_{B_{corr}}}{\text{TAN}} \times \frac{P_{box_{cal}}}{P_{mouth_{cal}}} \times K \right) - \text{Dead space}$$

5.

$$= \left(\frac{963 \text{ cm H}_2O}{0.72} \times \frac{30 \text{ mL/cm}}{10 \text{ cm H}_2O/\text{cm}} \times 0.874 \right) - 100 \text{ mL}$$

6.

$$= (1338 \times 3 \text{ mL} \times 0.874 - 100 \text{ mL}$$
$$V_{TG} = 3408 \text{ mL } (3.41 \text{ L})$$

Airway Resistance (Raw) (see Chapter 3)

Raw: Unknown
P_mP_{box} TAN: 0.61 (angle = 31)
$\dot{V}/P_{box}$ TAN: 3.0 (angle = 72)
P_{mouth} calibration: 10 cm H_2O/cm
P_{box} calibration: 30 mL/cm
$\dot{V}$ calibration: 1.0 L/sec/min
R_{sys}:   0.25 cm H_2O/L/sec

1.

$$\text{Raw} = \left(\frac{P_{mouth}/P_{box} \text{ TAN}}{\dot{V}/P_{box} \text{TAN}} \times \frac{P_{mouth_{cal}}}{\dot{V}_{cal}} \right) - R_{sys}$$

2.

$$= \left(\frac{0.61}{3.0} \times \frac{10 \text{ cm } H_2O/cm}{1.0 \text{ L/sec/cm}} \right) - 0.25$$

3.

$$= (0.203 \times 10) - 0.25$$

4.

$$\text{Raw} = 1.78 \text{ cm } H_2O/L/sec$$

Several repetitions of the panting maneuver are usually performed. Unlike the V_{TG} maneuver, however, the tangents are not averaged. Because the flow and volume tangents influence each other, the Raw is calculated and then averaged. In order to calculate the SGaw (specific airway conductance), the volume at which each Raw maneuver performed is calculcated as for the V_{TG}, using the P_{mouth}/P_{box} tangent from the specific maneuver. For the above example:

1.

$$\text{SGaw} = (1/\text{Raw})/V_{TG}$$

2.

$$V_{TG} = \left(\frac{963 \text{ cm } H_2O}{0.61} \times \frac{30 \text{ mL/cm}}{10 \text{ cm } H_2O/cm} \times 0.874 \right) - 100$$

3.

$$= (1579 \times 3 \text{ mL} \times 0.874) - 100$$

4.

$$= 4040 \text{ mL } (4.04 \text{ L})$$

Calculating the SGaw:

5.

$$\text{SGaw} = (1/1.78 \text{ cm } H_2O/L/sec)/4.04 \text{ L}$$

6.

$$= 0.14 \text{ cm } H_2O/L/sec/L$$

The average of 3 to 5 maneuvers is usually reported, after the SGaw for individual efforts has been calculated.

Exercise Study (see Chapter 7)*

Volume exhaled (V):	20.0 L (ATPS)
Collection time (sec):	60 seconds
Temperature (T):	24°C
F_{EO_2}:	17.0% (0.17 as a fraction)
F_{ECO_2}:	3.0% (0.03 as a fraction)
f:	25/min
HR:	100/min
P_{aO_2}:	95 mm Hg
P_{aCO_2}:	35 mm Hg
P_B:	750 mm Hg
Mechanical V_D:	18 mL (0.018 L)
Subject's weight:	55 kg

*Values as might be obtained at a submaximal level using either a treadmill or bicycle ergometer.

The first step is to calculate conversion factors to correct ventilation and gas exchange measurements to BTPS and STPD (this STPD factor is for conversion from BTPS), respectively:

1.

$$\text{BTPS factor} = \frac{P_B - P_{H_2O}}{P_B - 47} \times \frac{273 - 37}{273 + T}$$

$$= \frac{721}{703} \times \frac{310}{297}$$

$$= 1.07$$

2.

$$\text{STPD factor} = \frac{P_B - 47}{760} \times \frac{273}{273 + 37}$$

$$= \frac{703}{760} \times 0.881$$

$$= 0.815$$

Next, parameters of ventilation may be calculcated:

3.

$$\dot{V}_E \text{ (BTPS)} = \frac{V_{exhaled} \times 60}{\text{Collection time in seconds}} \times \text{BTPS factor}$$

$$= \frac{20.0 \text{ L} \times 60}{60} \times 1.07$$

$$= 21.4 \text{ L (BTPS)}$$

4.

$$V_T \text{ (BTPS)} = \frac{\dot{V}_E \text{ (BTPS)}}{f}$$

$$= \frac{21.4}{25}$$

$$= 0.856 \text{ L (BTPS)}$$

5.

$$V_D \text{ (BTPS)} = V_T \text{ (BTPS)} \times \left[1 - \frac{F_{E_{CO_2}} \times (P_B - 47)}{P_{a_{CO_2}}} \right] - V_{D_{mech}}$$

$$= 0.856 \times \left[1 - \frac{0.03 \times 703}{35} \right] - 0.018$$

$$= 0.856 \times [1 - 0.603] - 0.018$$

$$= (0.856 \times 0.397) - 0.018$$

$$= 0.340 - 0.018$$

$$= 0.322 \text{ L}$$

6.

$$\dot{V}_A \text{ (BTPS)} = \dot{V}_E \text{ (BTPS)} - [f \times V_D \text{ (BTPS)}]$$

$$= 21.4 - [25 \times 0.322]$$

$$= 21.4 - 8.05$$

$$= 13.4 \text{ L}$$

7.

$$V_D/V_T = \frac{0.322}{0.856}$$

$$= 0.38 \text{ (or 38\%)}$$

Next, gas exchange parameters are computed:

8.

$$\dot{V}_E \text{ (STPD)} = \dot{V}_E \text{ (BTPS)} \times \text{STPD factor}$$

$$= 21.4 \times 0.815$$

$$= 17.4 \text{ L}$$

9.

$$\dot{V}_{O_2} \text{ (STPD)} = \left[\left(\frac{1 - F_{E_{O_2}} - F_{E_{CO_2}}}{1 - F_{I_{O_2}}} \times F_{I_{O_2}} \right) - F_{E_{O_2}} \right] \times \dot{V}_E \text{ (STPD)}$$

$$= \left[\left(\frac{1 - 0.17 - 0.03}{1 - 0.2093} \times 0.2093 \right) - 0.17 \right] \times 17.4$$

$$= \left[\left(\frac{0.80}{0.79} \times 0.2093 \right) - 0.17 \right] \times 17.4$$

$$= [(1.01 \times 0.2093) - 0.17] \times 17.4$$

$$= [0.212 - 0.17] \times 17.4$$

$$= 0.042 \times 17.4$$

$$\dot{V}_{O_2} \text{ (STPD)} = 0.731 \text{ L}$$

10.

$$\dot{V}_{CO_2} \text{ (STPD)} = (F_{E_{CO_2}} - 0.003) \times \dot{V}_E \text{ (STPD)}$$

$$= (0.03 - 0.0003) \times 17.4$$

$$= 0.297 \times 17.4$$

$$= 0.517 \text{ L}$$

11.

$$R = \frac{\dot{V}_{CO_2} \text{ (STPD)}}{\dot{V}_{O_2} \text{ (STPD)}}$$

$$= \frac{0.517}{0.731}$$

$$= 0.71$$

12.

$$\dot{V}_E/\dot{V}_{O_2} = \frac{\dot{V}_E \text{ (BTPS)}}{\dot{V}_{O_2} \text{ (STPD)}}$$

$$= \frac{21.4}{0.731}$$

$$= 29.3 \text{L/L } \dot{V}_{O_2}$$

13.

$$\dot{V}_{O_2}/\text{HR} = \frac{\dot{V}_{O_2} \text{ (STPD)}}{\text{HR}} \times 1000$$

$$= \frac{0.731\text{L}}{100 \text{ beats}} \times 1000$$

$$= 7.31 \text{ mL } O_2/\text{beat}$$

The calculation of energy expenditure at any particular work load is described by the term METS, for multiples of the resting $\dot{V}_{O_2}$. The MET level for any work load can be calculated by one of two methods. In each method:

14.

$$\text{METS} = \frac{\dot{V}_{O_2} \text{ (STPD) exercise}}{\dot{V}_{O_2} \text{ (STPD) rest}}$$

but the means of estimating $\dot{V}_{O_2}$ (STPD) at rest differs. $\dot{V}_{O_2}$ (STPD) at rest can be measured or it may be estimated as 0.0035 L/min/kg (3.5 mL/kg). Using the second method in this example:

$$\text{METS} = \frac{0.731\text{L/min}}{0.0035\text{L/min/kg} \times 55 \text{ kg}}$$

$$= 3.80$$

If the subject's measured $\dot{V}o_2$ at rest had been 0.225 L/min (STPD) then:

$$\text{METS} = \frac{0.731\text{L/min}}{0.225\text{L/min}}$$

$$= 3.25$$

CALCULATION OF THE MEAN AND STANDARD DEVIATION

The mean ($\bar{X}$) and standard deviation (SD) are computed to determine the variability of a series of values. The SD is affected by every value in the series, especially extreme values. If the values are normally distributed, that is, each value has an equal chance of appearing, the standard deviation may be used to relate any subsequent value to the population of values already obtained. In the laboratory setting, this concept often is applied to determine the variability of blood gas electrodes or spirometers. By performing multiple measurements of the same quantity (i.e., the "control"), the mean may be determined and precision expressed by the SD of the measurements. Assuming that all of the values sampled are normally distributed, 68.3% of the values will be within ± 1 SD of the mean, 95.5% will be within ± 2 SD, and 99.7% within ± 3 SD. Once the mean and SD have been determined for a series of measurements, subsequent values may be checked to see if they are "in control." Values between ± 2 and ± 3 SD from the mean should occur only 5% of the time, and values more than ± 3 SD from the mean should occur less than 1% of the time.

The mean ($\bar{X}$) is calculated:

$$\bar{X} = \frac{\Sigma(X)}{N}$$

where:

Σ = a symbol meaning "the sum of"

X = individual data values

N = number of items sampled

The SD is calculated:

$$\text{SD} = \sqrt{\frac{\Sigma(X^2)}{N}}$$

where:

X^2 = deviations from the mean $(X - \bar{X})$ squared

N = number of items sampled

If the SD is computed from a sample of 30 items or less, $N - 1$ is substituted for N.

Example calculation of the mean and SD for a series of Pco_2 values:

Sample No.	Pco_2 (mm Hg)	Deviation from mean (X)	Deviation squared (X^2)
1	39	-0.9	0.81
2	40	0.1	0.01
3	43	3.1	9.61
4	42	2.1	4.41
5	39	-0.9	0.81
6	38	-1.9	3.61
7	40	0.1	0.01
8	41	1.1	1.21
9	38	-1.9	3.61
10	39	-0.9	0.81
Total	399		24.90
Mean	39.9		2.49

$$SD = \sqrt{\frac{24.9}{(10 - 1)}}$$

$$= \sqrt{2.77}$$

$$= 1.66$$

The range of Pco_2 values (in this example) within 2 SDs of the mean is $39.9 \pm (2 \times 1.66)$, or from 36.6 to 43.2 mm Hg

---

ANSWERS TO SELF-ASSESSMENT QUESTIONS

Chapter 1

1. c
2. c
3. 1.50 L (BTPS)
4. a
5. b
6. c
7. RV 2.6 L (BTPS)
   TLC 6.0 L (BTPS)
   RV/TLC% 43%
8. d
9. b
10. c
11. a
12. d

Chapter 2

1. a
2. c
3. $\dot{V}E$ 5.91 L/min (BTPS)
   V_T 493 mL (BTPS)

4. V_D/V_T 25%
5. $\dot{V}_A$ 4.61 L/min (BTPS)
6. c
7. b
8. d
9. b
10. a

Chapter 3

1. b
2. c
3. a
4. a
5. b
6. c
7. a
8. a
9. b
10. b
11. c
12. b

Chapter 4

1. d
2. b
3. c
4. d
5. a
6. d
7. a
8. b
9. c
10. a

Chapter 5

1. c
2. a
3. b
4. c
5. b

6. c
7. a
8. d
9. a
10. c

Chapter 6

1. b
2. b
3. c
4. d
5. c
6. c
7. a
8. c
9. b
10. c

Chapter 7

1. c
2. a
3. c
4. d
5. d
6. a
7. b
8. a
9. a
10. d
11. a
12. c

Chapter 8

1. c
2. c
3. c
4. d
5. a
6. b
7. b

9. a
10. c
11. b
12. b
13. a
14. b
15. c

Chapter 9

1. a
2. b
3. a
4. a
5. c
6. d
7. a
8. c
9. b
10. b
11. b
12. d
13. a
14. b
15. d
16. a
17. b
18. a

Chapter 10

1. c
2. d

3. d
4. d
5. b
6. b
7. b
8. b
9. b
10. a

Chapter 11

1. a
2. a
3. d
4. c
5. c
6. c
7. c
8. b
9. d
10. c
11. b
12. a
13. d
14. d
15. c

INDEX